MOTOR AREAS
OF THE
CEREBRAL CORTEX

Ciba Foundation Symposium 132

MOTOR AREAS
OF THE
CEREBRAL CORTEX

A Wiley – Interscience Publication

1987

JOHN WILEY & SONS

Chichester · New York · Brisbane · Toronto · Singapore

© Ciba Foundation 1987

Published in 1987 by John Wiley & Sons Ltd, Baffins Lane, Chichester, Sussex PO19 1UD, UK.

Ciba Foundation Symposium 132
x + 323 pages, 66 figures, 2 tables

Library of Congress Cataloging in Publication Data

Motor areas of the cerebral cortex. — (Ciba Foundation
    symposium; 132)
    "A Wiley–Interscience publication."
    Papers presented at a symposium held at the Ciba
Foundation, London, 24–26 Feb. 1987.
    Includes indexes.
    1. Motor cortex—Congresses. I. Ciba Foundation.
II. Series.
QP383.M68   1987   599'.01'852   87-19001
ISBN 0 471 91098 8

British Library Cataloguing in Publication Data

Motor areas of the cerebral cortex. — (Ciba Foundation
    symposium; 132)
    1. Cerebral cortex
    I. Ciba Foundation. II. Series.
    612'825   QP383
ISBN 0 471 91098 8

Typeset by Inforum Ltd, Portsmouth
Printed and bound in Great Britain by the Bath Press Ltd, Bath, Avon.

Contents

Participants

D.M. Armstrong   Department of Physiology, University of Bristol Medical School, University Walk, Bristol BS8 1TD, UK

D.B. Calne   Division of Neurology, University of British Columbia, Health Sciences Centre Hospital, 2211 Wesbrook Mall, Vancouver, British Columbia, Canada V6T 1W5

P.D. Cheney   Department of Physiology, University of Kansas Medical Center, Kansas City, Kansas 66103, USA

L. Deecke   Neurologische Universitätsklinik, Allgemeines Krankenhaus der Stadt Wien, Lazarettgasse 14, 1097 Vienna, Austria

E.E. Fetz   Department of Physiology & Biophysics, SJ-40, University of Washington School of Medicine, Seattle, Washington 98195, USA

H.-J. Freund   Neurologische Klinik, University of Dusseldorf, Moorenstrasse 5, 4000 Düsseldorf 1, Federal Republic of Germany

A.P. Georgopoulos   The Philip Bard Laboratories of Neurophysiology, Department of Neuroscience, Johns Hopkins University School of Medicine, 725 N Wolfe Street, Baltimore, Maryland 21205, USA

P.S. Goldman-Rakic   Section of Neuroanatomy, Yale University School of Medicine, C303 SHM, PO Box 3333, New Haven, Connecticut 06510-8001, USA

E.G. Jones   Department of Anatomy & Neurobiology, University of California, California College of Medicine, Irvine, California 92717, USA

J. Kalaska   Centre de Recherche en Sciences Neurologiques, Faculté de Médecine, Université de Montréal, Case Postale 6128, Succersale A, Montréal, Québec, Canada H3C 3J7

H.G.J.M. Kuypers   Department of Anatomy, University of Cambridge, Downing Street, Cambridge CB2 3DY, UK

R. Lemon   Department of Anatomy, University of Cambridge, Downing Street, Cambridge CB2 3DY, UK

C.D. Marsden   Department of Neurology, Institute of Psychiatry, De Crespigny Park, Denmark Hill, London SE5 8AF, UK

D.N. Pandya   Edith Nourse Rogers Memorial Veterans Hospital, 200 Springs Road, Bedford, Massachusetts 01730, USA

R.E. Passingham   Department of Experimental Psychology, University of Oxford, South Parks Road, Oxford OX1 3UD, UK

C.G. Phillips   Aubrey House, Horton-cum-Studley, Oxford OX9 1BU, UK

R. Porter (*Chairman*)   The John Curtin School of Medical Research, The Australian National University, GPO Box 334, Canberra City, ACT 2601, Australia

G. Rizzolatti   Istituto di Fisiologia Umana, University of Parma, Via A. Gramsci 14, 43100 Parma, Italy

P.E. Roland   Department of Clinical Neurophysiology, Karolinska Hospital, Box 60 500, S-10401 Stockholm 60, Sweden

Y. Shinoda   Department of Physiology, School of Medicine, Tokyo Medical & Dental University, 1-5-45 Yushima, Bunkyoku, Tokyo 113, Japan

P.L. Strick   Department of Physiology & Neurosurgery, Veterans Administration Medical Center, Research Service (151), 800 Irving Avenue, Syracuse, New York 13201, USA

J. Tanji   Department of Neurophysiology, Brain Research Institute, Tohoku University School of Medicine, Seiryo-machi 1-1, Sendai 980, Japan

W.T. Thach   Department of Anatomy & Neurobiology, Washington University, School of Medicine, Medical Center, Box 8108, 660 South Euclid Avenue, St Louis, Missouri 63110, USA

M. Wiesendanger   Institute of Physiology, University of Fribourg, Rue du Musée 5, CH-1700 Fribourg, Switzerland

Wu Chien-Ping   Shanghai Brain Research Institute, Chinese Academy of Sciences, 319 Yo-yang Road, Shanghai, People's Republic of China

Xi Ming-Chu (*Ciba Foundation Bursar*)   Shanghai Brain Research Institute, Chinese Academy of Sciences, 319 Yo-yang Road, Shanghai, People's Republic of China

Introduction

The John Curtin School of Medical Research, The Australian National University, GPO Box 334, Canberra City, ACT 2601, Australia

1987 Motor areas of the cerebral cortex. Wiley, Chichester (Ciba Foundation Symposium 132) p 1–3

The many new techniques introduced into clinical neurological practice in recent years have reawakened interest in the motor areas of the human cerebral cortex. The physiological role of these areas in influencing skilled voluntary movement has been studied anew, and the disorders produced when these regions of the cortex are damaged or diseased have been re-evaluated. Computer-aided tomography, for example, has allowed the sites of disordered structure in the brains of patients who suffer from movement disorders to be much more accurately delineated. Studies of regional cerebral blood flow and measurements of regional metabolic function using such methods as positron emission tomography (PET scanning) have enabled the brain locations associated with aspects of motor function to be examined in new ways in human subjects. And the resurrection of electrical and magnetic methods for stimulating the outflow pathways from the cerebral cortex in humans has been useful in clinical diagnosis and prognosis.

The detailed information that physiologists have traditionally sought about the connectivity of these outflow pathways in primates must also be re-evaluated. Some of the new methods demonstrate quite satisfactorily the regional structures associated with clinical disorders or involved in the physiological control of movement. But electrical methods must still be used for examining temporal characteristics, as opposed to spatial characteristics, because the time resolution of many of the computer-aided methods does not yet provide a satisfactory understanding of temporal order in sequences of events in the cerebral cortex.

These developments make it timely for us to review the present state of knowledge of the organization and function of the motor areas of the cerebral cortex. It is particularly important to do so at this stage because our understanding of regional associations with movement performance and its disorders has recently improved. This has occurred at the same time as the expansion of basic knowledge about the details of cell-to-cell connectivity and the intrinsic organization of both the internal structure of minute zones of cerebral cortex and the extrinsic connectivity with those zones. The exact definition of the

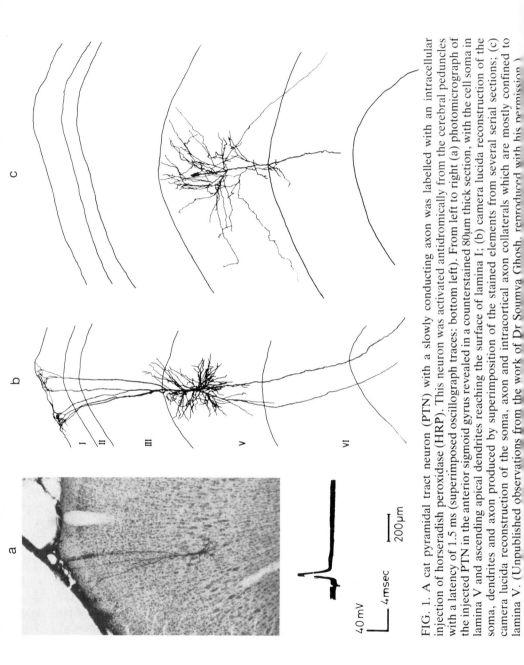

FIG. 1. A cat pyramidal tract neuron (PTN) with a slowly conducting axon was labelled with an intracellular injection of horseradish peroxidase (HRP). This neuron was activated antidromically from the cerebral peduncles with a latency of 1.5 ms (superimposed oscillograph traces: bottom left). From left to right (a) photomicrograph of the injected PTN in the anterior sigmoid gyrus revealed in a counterstained 80μm thick section, with the cell soma in lamina V and ascending apical dendrites reaching the surface of lamina I; (b) camera lucida reconstruction of the soma, dendrites and axon produced by superimposition of the stained elements from several serial sections; (c) camera lucida reconstruction of the soma, axon and intracortical axon collaterals which are mostly confined to lamina V. (Unpublished observations from the work of Dr Soumya Ghosh, reproduced with his permission.)

structures that make up the neuronal elements within a minute region of cerebral cortex has been aided enormously by the combination of refined anatomical and electrophysiological methods.

My colleague Dr Soumya Ghosh has described the morphology of pyramidal neurons in area 4 of the cerebral cortex in cat and monkey. He has made intracellular recordings, using horseradish peroxidase (HRP)-filled electrodes, to examine the electrophysiological responses of these neurons to stimuli delivered at a number of regions in the cerebral cortex, cerebral peduncles, spinal cord and thalamus. The structure of the dendritic trees of pyramidal cells in different laminae, their arborization within the cerebral cortex, and the extent of the collateral distribution of the axon collaterals can be revealed by such methods, which have been used extensively by Deschenes et al (1979) in Canada (Fig. 1).

These methods have been very useful in assisting our understanding of the minute organization of cellular elements in the cerebral cortex. When we add the emerging knowledge about the pharmacology of synaptic transmission between cells in the cortex and from projection fibres which enter a region of cortex, it is not too difficult to discern how the development of fundamental knowledge about the cerebral cortex and its structure has influenced clinical thinking about the management of patients, for example those with cerebral ischaemia after vascular accidents. Not long ago the understanding of the pharmacology of synaptic action within the cerebral cortex would have been considered much too esoteric for clinical neurologists to consider. Yet today the vocabulary of clinicians includes such names as N-methyl-D-aspartic acid (NMDA) receptors. Indeed, the management of stroke patients by treatment with antagonists of such substances is now undergoing clinical trials.

Motor areas of the cerebral cortex are multiple. As all human behaviour achieves its expression through movement the whole brain may be regarded as the organ of motor performance. Motor areas of the cerebral cortex may be determined to be relatively closely coupled to movement if weak electrical stimuli applied to those areas result in muscle contractions. But profound and sometimes disabling motor deficits may accompany lesions or damage in regions of the cerebral cortex which do not yield movements when they are so stimulated. The functional roles of frontal or parietal or midline areas of cerebral cortex have been re-examined recently in a variety of situations and in a number of animal species. I hope that the discussions during this meeting will allow the motor functions of these regions to be considered as well as those of the perirolandic cerebral cortex.

As I pointed out at the Ciba Foundation symposium on *Functions of the Basal Ganglia* (Porter 1984), it is not possible to consider the functions of certain deep structures of the brain without considering the dynamic interactions which continuously link those deep structures to the cerebral cortex. Conversely, it is not possible to discuss the motor areas of the cerebral cortex independently of the context which gives them their motor significance. We have to consider the targets of the outputs from the motor areas of cerebral cortex. Most easily interpreted may be the corticospinal projections which more or less directly influence motor neurons in the spinal cord.

Corticocortical connections link the cerebral motor areas in highly specific ways. Corticopontine projections make it essential to include the loops through the cerebellum in any consideration of motor functions of the cerebral cortex. In addition we will eventually have to try to understand how cortical interactions with the basal ganglia operate to produce the right amount of movement in natural function but too much or too little in disease. We will also have to examine whether and how the cortex regulates its own inputs via corticothalamic connections acting on projections to the cortex arriving through thalamic nuclei.

It would be too much to ask that we address all these matters in the present symposium; but it is appropriate that we have all of them in mind as we approach the discussion of a few aspects that can be examined with the unique expertise that is assembled here. The motor areas of the cerebral cortex have been among the longest-studied of any parts of the mammalian central nervous system. In the past the complaint has been made that the observations assembled by anatomists and physiologists studying monkeys or other mammals have been inconsistent with clinical neurological experience. That does not seem to be the case in 1987. It will be important for areas of agreement and areas of dissension to be clarified in meetings such as this. Experimental observations can then be directed to the future acquisition of the basic information that is still needed for understanding mechanisms of movement performance, the learning of skills, and the disorders of voluntary movement that accompany brain disease.

Many of us first became interested in motor physiology through experiments conducted by Charles Phillips. We are very fortunate in having him here to give us a historical background to the anatomical studies which other people will be discussing later in the symposium. He will also take us back to the early use of electrical stimulation of the brain to define motor areas of the cerebral cortex.

References

Deschenes M, Labelle A, Landry P 1979 Morphological characterization of slow and fast pyramidal tract cells in the cat. Brain Res 178:251–274
Porter R 1984 In: Functions of the basal ganglia. Pitman, London (Ciba Found Symp 107) p 266

Epicortical electrical mapping of motor areas in primates

C.G. Phillips

Horton-cum-Studley, Oxford, OX9 1BU, UK

Abstract. The neocortical motor areas of monkeys were discovered by epicortical electrical stimulation. Ferrier in 1875 drew non-overlapping circles for face, limbs and tail. His 'centres' were postcentral as well as precentral. In the 1880s Horsley added an arm and face area on the medial surface (where Penfield's supplementary motor area is now ensconced). At the turn of the century the newborn science of cortical architectonics discovered striking differences between precentral and postcentral areas. Sherrington got no responses from the postcentral gyrus of apes. At mid-century, however, Woolsey reinstated the postcentral motor map (his Sm 1). The discrepancies between these classical maps could probably be explained by sensitivity to levels of anaesthesia and to arbitrarily chosen configurations of stimuli whose intracortical actions remained obscure. Some of the modes of action of epicortical stimulation have since been worked out. These are relevant to the results of electrical and magnetic stimulation of the human brain through scalp and skull.

Today's research is differentiating the functions of the precentral and postcentral areas (4, 6_{PM}, 6_{SMA}, 3a, 3b,1): at the microscopic level, by studies of sampled neurons whose discharges can be related to specific components of learnt motor performances, and whose connectivities can be traced by electroanatomical and microscopical labelling of their perikarya, axons and synapses; at the macroscopic level, by studies of Bereitschaftspotential and regional cerebral metabolism in motor performances in intact humans.

1987 Motor areas of the cerebral cortex. Wiley, Chichester (Ciba Foundation Symposium 132) p 5–20

The neocortical motor areas were discovered by electrical stimulation of the convexities of gyri. The very extensive surfaces buried in the walls of sulci were not at first explored. It became common to speak of 'excitable' and 'inexcitable' areas of the cerebral cortex. Such distinction, however, makes little sense in the light of today's knowledge of the radial, quasi-modular arrangement of neuronal perikarya, dendrites and axons that are to be found, though with considerable local variation, in all areas of the laminated neocortex. It has to be assumed that all these areas are electrically excitable. The only problem is to detect that excitation has taken place. From the motor areas the corticobulbar and corticospinal projections to the segmental interneurons and motor neurons are dense enough, and focused sharply enough, to evoke movements at a single distal joint; or they are less dense, and distributed more diffusely, to evoke—at higher threshold—simultaneous movements at more than one joint, proximal as well as distal. These responses were originally detected by inspection of the joints and palpation of the muscles that were thus thrown into action. Today they can be recorded intracellularly from the target neurons. The latter method has the advantage that excitatory synaptic potentials (EPSP) can be recorded in response to stimuli that are well below the lowest thresholds for muscular contraction, and that inhibitory (IPSP) as well as excitatory actions can be detected. In area 4, epicortical stimulation can be made weak enough to evoke EPSP and IPSP in intracortical interneurons without causing any discharge of corticofugal neurons, but enabling the radial and tangential propagation of excitation and inhibition to be measured (Ezure et al 1985, Ezure & Oshima 1985). Similar experiments in 'inexcitable' areas will prove their electrical excitability, even if the distribution of their corticofugal projections is so diffuse and widespread as to make it hard to discover their cortico-subcortical or cortico-cortical targets. But the scope of this brief historical sketch is limited to the motor areas, and the detections to be considered will be the firing of corticospinal neurons. The story will stop short of Asanuma & Sakata's invention of the powerful technique of intracortical microstimulation (1967).

Gross epicortical mapping of motor areas

Ferrier's pioneering experiments on anaesthetized monkeys, done in 1875 (Ferrier 1886), set the fashion for repetitive stimulation of the cortex with the inductorium (probable frequency 30–40 Hz). Ferrier preferred this 'faradization' to the galvanic stimulation used by Fritsch & Hitzig (1870), which 'causes only a sudden contraction in certain groups of muscles' at the make of the current, 'but fails to call forth the definite purposive combination of muscular contractions, which is the very essence of the reaction, and key to its interpretation.' Like Fritsch & Hitzig, Ferrier used bifocal ('bipolar') electrodes. He gauged the strength of stimulation by adjusting the inter-coil distance and applying the electrodes to his tongue. His 'motor' centres' he represented as circles on his maps, but with 'no exact line of demarcation from each other'; 'where they adjoin stimulation is apt to produce conjointly the effect peculiar to each.' The circles were distributed widely over the dorsolateral surface of the hemisphere, postcentral as well as precentral. The 'motor centres' for the fingers were on the postcentral gyrus. In one monkey Ferrier explored the medial surface of the hemisphere and found that 'irritation' of the fronto-parietal portion of the marginal convolution 'gave rise to movements of the head and limbs similar to those obtained by stimulation of the corresponding regions on the convex or external aspect.' This would have included what we now call the supplementary motor area (SMA).

Ferrier did not believe that all his 'centres' were 'truly motor, in the sense of being due to irritation of a part in direct connection with the motor strands of the crus cerebri and spinal cord. . . . for the stimulation of a sensory centre may give rise to reflex or associated movement.' Thus, stimulation of centre 14—'pricking of the opposite ear, head and eyes turn to the opposite side'—resembled a monkey's natural response to a loud whistle into its ear. Since a monkey deaf in consequence of bilateral lesion of centre 14 (whose failure to react to the explosion of a percussion cap was demonstrated at the International Medical Congress in 1881) was not paralysed at any stage of recovery from the operation, Ferrier included that centre 14 was not a 'truly motor' centre. But in those days, when staining of degenerating axons and myelin sheaths was still to come, loss of 'motor strands' could be detected only after massive fronto-parietal ablations, by gross scarring and loss of nerve fibres in the pyramidal and lateral corticospinal tracts. So the 'motor strands' issuing from a single 'truly motor centre' would have been invisible.

Horsley with his colleagues Beevor (Beevor & Horsley 1890) and Schäfer (Horsley & Schäfer 1888) got more detailed results in monkeys and in a single orang-utan, in regard to both the widespread distribution of excitable foci on the convexity and the foci on the medial surface of the hemisphere (now the SMA). Their finger responses also were postcentral.

At the turn of the century Grünbaum (later Leyton) and Sherrington started work on the 'excitable cortex' of chimpanzee, orang-utan and gorilla, work that was not fully published until 1917. Deliberately interesting themselves in near-threshold responses to unifocal ('unipolar') faradization with a stigmatic electrode, they found that the excitable foci were all precentral. 'Frequently the strength of faradism applied to post-centralis was carried far beyond the strength ordinarily permissible for reliable physiological observations, and still quite failed to evoke any detectable effect' (Leyton & Sherrington 1917). In 1905 the first major works on cortical architectonics were published quite independently by A.W. Campbell (1905), Sherrington's friend and neighbour at Liverpool, and by Brodmann (1905) in Germany. The differences between the thickness and lamination of precentral and postcentral gyri were very striking. Sherrington's maps were of unprecedented detail, richness and fineness of grain. Always alert to inhibitory as well as excitatory action, Sherrington noted (1906, p 288): 'A.S. Grünbaum and myself have seen that in the chimpanzee and gorilla any single manual digit can be moved isolatedly by stimulation of the cortex. We must not forget, however, that with even a *small* movement the field of inhibition may yet be wide, for I have on occasion noted inhibition of muscles of the shoulder, the shoulder previously being unrelaxed.'

Horsley (1909) accepted Sherrington's limitation of 'the so-called motor area of the brain' to the precentral gyrus. He had gained the impression that motor responsiveness to postcentral stimulation diminishes as one ascends the

primate scale. The thumb and finger movements he and Beevor had found in
monkeys (Beevor & Horsley 1890) had been 'restricted and feeble' or un-
obtainable, and in his stimulations in humans he had never been able to get
any motor responses from postcentral cortex.

In the 1950s interest settled on the existence of multiple motor areas, each
containing its own somatotopic map, and all contained within the wide
precentral and postcentral areas mapped by Ferrier and Horsley. Woolsey et
al (1953) and Woolsey (1958) using a 60 Hz alternating current, reinstated the
postcentral motor map. Woolsey called it Sm 1 (sensory > motor) in contrast
to the precentral map Ms 1 (motor > sensory). The postcentral map sur-
vived chronic ablation of the precentral gyrus, but thresholds were 'two or
three times those adequate to produce movement on stimulation of the
precentral gyrus.' Traces of a second motor map were found in the parietal
operculum where motor and sensory maps 'coincide somatotopically'
(Woolsey 1958). This would correspond to Penfield & Rasmussen's findings
in the superior bank of the Sylvian fissure in humans. A third somatotopic
map was 'the supplementary motor area of Penfield' (Woolsey et al 1952),
previously reported in humans by Penfield & Rasmussen (1950). Thresholds
for SMA were 'never as low as in the digital portion of the precentral area.'

Modes of action of epicortical stimulation

The chequered history of these maps from the 1870s to the 1950s might seem
rather puzzling to anyone without practical experience of this kind of work.
We have to assume that the underlying ('real') maps of the corticospinal
projection are relatively constant in a particular species of monkey. Their
boundaries may be more or less distinct and either spuriously sharpened or
further smudged by the experimental procedures. Many of the discrepancies
between the experimental maps drawn by different investigators could probably be ascribed to differences in the level of anaesthesia. It would nowadays
be mandatory to monitor as precisely as possible the level of anaesthesia at
the times of stimulation. A delicate and reliable monitor that can easily be
checked routinely is the threshold for a flick movement of contralateral
thumb and index in response to a single rectangular anodal epicortical pulse
of 5.0 ms duration applied to the lowest-threshold point within their large
cortical area.

Other differences might be found in the arbitrary choice of stimulus configurations by different workers: unifocal or bifocal ('bipolar') electrodes;
polarity, duration, amplitude, wave-form and repetition frequency of the
pulses; number of pulses in the trains. Obviously it is reasonable to choose
one's preferred electrodes and to adjust the dials of a modern stimulator until
a configuration is achieved that will elicit the largest repertory of well-
differentiated responses; but attached to this freedom of choice is the obli-

gation to describe quantitatively the configurations that have been used.

Disparities between experimental maps could be due to favourable or unfavourable effects of the foregoing factors on the distances from the point of stigmatic epicortical contact across which excitation could be propagated transcortically—physically, trans-synaptically or both. Suppose this 'point' to be uniquely capable of eliciting a highly circumscribed response at threshold, for example of a single finger. We cannot assume that the responding corticospinal neurons are all confined within an area as small as the 'point' of epicortical contact. That point might be merely the centre of an area containing enough corticospinal neurons to discharge any spinal motor neurons. (An area of smaller radius could be adequate to evoke EPSP and IPSP in some spinal motor neurons, but these effects could not have been detected in classical mapping experiments.) The classical maps were all drawn by repetitive stimulation, often continued for several seconds, at the chosen points. Spatial and temporal summation—transcortical and subcortical—are evidently necessary for muscular response. The preferential accessibility of hand, foot and face (Liddell & Phillips 1950) is due to the relatively dense connections that link their large cortical territories with their segmental motor neurons.

Transcortical spread can be estimated rather accurately by using a roving epicortical electrode and recording the responses of single corticospinal neurons whose location in the cortex is known (Phillips & Porter 1977). For *direct* excitation by physical spread of current, brief (0.2 ms) anodal pulses are required. A pulse too weak to elicit any movement (2.0 mA) will excite corticospinal neurons lying as far distant horizontally as 10 mm from the stigmatic contact, as well as corticospinal neurons in the depth of the central sulcus, about 8 mm below the convexity of the gyrus. The threshold for corticospinal neurons nearest to (that is, immediately underlying) the contact is 0.3 mA. These minimal responses do not spread transcortically in response to repetitive stimulation. For epicortical cathodal stimulation the lowest thresholds are higher. Excitation of corticospinal neurons is *indirect* (trans-synaptic), and engages an enlarging population of these neurons in response to each successive pulse of a repetitive train. The transcortical extent of this trans-synaptic propagation of excitation has yet to be measured. Experiments with bifocal ('bipolar') electrodes reveal their actions to be complex, and not at all confined to the interpolar region as has sometimes been claimed (Phillips & Porter 1962). For gross epicortical mapping they have nothing to recommend them.

With such a wide spread of corticospinal neurons directly excited by punctate anodal epicortical stimulation there cannot fail to be overlapping of adjacent areas projecting from area 4 to the spinal cord. Such overlap has been demonstrated between the colonies of corticospinal neurons that project monosynaptic excitation to single spinal motor neurons (Landgren et al 1962).

Epicortical mapping has by no means outlived its usefulness, for example in helping to decide whether the motor effects of stimulating SMA are complicated by transcortical spread to area 4 (Wiesendanger et al 1973), or in locating cortical areas in ablation experiments. Whenever possible, estimates of the extent of spread, based on the thresholds of excitation of identified neurons at different distances from the epicortical stigmatic electrode in the relevant sulci and gyri, would surely be worth making to improve the accuracy of the mapping. For discharging minimal, well-circumscribed corticofugal volleys from the convexities of gyri, or from any cytoarchitectonic area of a lissencephalic brain, punctate stimulation with brief surface-anodal pulses of 0.3 mA is convenient and atraumatic.

Very recently it has been found possible to send a brief burst of volleys at high frequency down the human corticospinal tract by applying a strong anodal or magnetic pulse to the scalp overlying the cortical arm area in healthy volunteers (Day et al 1987), to record the passage of the volleys down the spinal cord in patients undergoing spinal surgery (Boyd et al 1986), and to detect the monosynaptic actions of the corticomotoneuronal volleys on the motor neurons of intrinsic muscles of the contralateral hand by gross electromyographic and single motor unit recording. The first and last of these procedures are non-invasive and are enabling the clinical neurologist for the first time in history to examine directly the state of the corticomotoneuronal pathway in patients with cerebrovascular injury, mutliple sclerosis and other illnesses.

The different actions of the anodal and magnetic pulses are of the greatest neurophysiological as well as clinical importance. Kernell & Wu Chien-ping's analysis (1967a,b) of the actions of strong epicortical anodal pulses in baboons is directly relevant to the actions of strong anodal pulses delivered through scalp and skull to the underlying arm area in humans. It has long been known that a strong epicortical pulse evokes a sequence of volleys in the corticospinal tract (Patton & Amassian 1954, 1960). The first volley ('D wave') is due to direct excitation of corticospinal neurons, the later volleys ('I waves') to indirect (synaptic) excitation. Kernell & Wu Chien-ping (1967a) proved that the I waves are due to repetitive firing of the same fast corticospinal neurons that had contributed to the D wave (Fig. 1). To generate such synchronized repetitive firing the brief pulse must have started some self-sustaining excitatory mechanism whose action outlasts the flow of stimulating current. Patton & Amassian's hypothesis was that the I waves are due to a 'periodic bombardment of Betz cells through chains of neurons with fixed temporal characteristics.'

Another hypothesis can however be proposed. Suppose that the epicortical anodal pulse excites, *simultaneously*, a large synchronous corticospinal volley (D wave) and a large synchronous thalamocortical volley at some point in the subcortical white matter which, after conduction time plus one synaptic

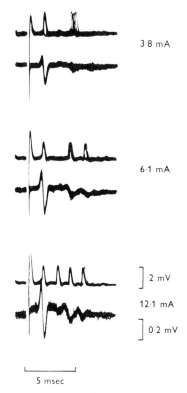

FIG. 1. *Lower trace of each pair:* Records of D and I waves from lateral corticospinal tract at upper cervical level in response to 0.2 ms anodal epicortical pulses delivered to contralateral arm area of baboon's area 4. Current strengths noted at right of each pair. *Upper trace of each pair:* records from a fast corticospinal axon to show relation of its repetitive impulse-discharge to the sequence of D and I waves recorded simultaneously at each current strength. All records formed by superimposition of about 10 sweeps. (From Kernell & Wu Chien-ping 1967a.)

delay, starts a monosynaptic EPSP *simultaneously* in a large population of corticospinal neurons. The impulse-generating pacemaker of a corticospinal neuron has the property of responding repetitively to a depolarizing current at a frequency related to its intensity. The upper limit of frequency (about 1000 impulses s^{-1}) is set by the refractory period (Fig. 2). It is assumed that an EPSP of a particular wave-form and amplitude will always elicit an identical stereotyped pattern of corticospinal impulses, certified by more or less exact superimposition of their action potentials in many superimposed traces.

The bottom pair of records in Fig. 1 show the fully developed responses to a very strong pulse (12.1 mA). The lower trace shows the D wave followed by three I waves, recorded from the surface of the lateral corticospinal tract. The upper trace shows the four impulses recorded simultaneously from a fast

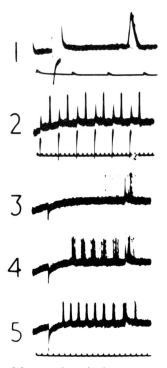

FIG. 2.   Discharges of fast corticospinal axon recorded from C_{4-5} junction of cat's spinal cord in response to contralateral anodal epicortical stimulation of area 4. Each trace formed by superimposition of 20–30 sweeps. Time scales: ms. 1: Brief epicortical pulse, 0.4 mA; 2: same pulses at 250 Hz; 3: long pulse, 0.165 mA; 4: long pulse, 0.22 mA; 5: long pulse, 0.295 mA; discharge of nine impulses, frequency falling from over 650 Hz to 500 Hz. (From Hern et al 1962.)

corticospinal axon. These impulses will be referred to as D, I_1, I_2 and I_3. Their frequency of firing is about 600 impulses s^{-1}.

In the top pair of records (stimulus 3.8 mA) the D impulse is followed by the I_2 impulse. The hypothesis proposes that the EPSP of corticospinal neurons rises relatively slowly, reaching the pacemaker's firing threshold at I_2 latency (though with enough jitter to suggest a near-threshold response). This EPSP would have fallen below the firing threshold before the neuron had recovered from the I_2 refractory period, hence the absence of an I_3 impulse. I_2 and I_3 waves are just visible (lower traces).

Stimulus 6.1 mA (middle records) fires the corticospinal neurons at I_2 and I_3 latencies. The hypothesis proposes that a larger population of thalamocortical axons is excited by the stronger pulse, generating a corticospinal neuron EPSP that rises steeply enough to fire I_2 at a fixed latency; and persisting at an intensity sufficient to fire an I_3 impulse after recovery from the I_2 refractory period (though with slight latency jitter and failure to fire in some trials). The lower records show that the I_2 and I_3 waves are now well developed.

Stimulus 12.1 mA (bottom records). The hypothesis proposes that a still larger population of thalamocortical axons has been excited, causing a still more steeply rising EPSP that reaches firing threshold at I_1 latency and persists at supraliminal level for long enough to fire I_2 and I_3. The I_1, I_2 and I_3 waves (lower traces) are all well developed.

The sequence of D and I waves in humans in response to anodal pulses resembles the sequence in the baboon and may turn out to have a similar mechanism. But the magnetic method evokes I waves only. This suggests that excitation is not occurring in the cortex but at some deeper locus in the brain (Day et al 1987).

Collateral experiments on monkeys will surely be needed to discover the subcortical locus or loci at which induced currents of sufficient intensity, flowing in appropriate orientations, are producing their motor effects. Similar problems arise in regard to the phosphenes aroused when the head is placed in a fluctuating magnetic field. There would be great gains to clinical and basic neuroscience if such effects could be targeted on any structure in the depths of the brain. But we cannot overlook the longer-term possibility of such methods falling into evil hands.

The areas today

In his eighth Silliman Lecture Sherrington (1906, p. 307) confessed his disappointment at the limited contribution of the excitation method to the understanding of cortical function.

> As to the meaning of this whole class of movements elicitable from the so-called 'motor' cortex, whether they represent a step towards psychical integration or on the other hand express the motor result of psychical integration, or are participant in both, is a question of the highest interest, but one which does not seem as yet to admit of satisfactory answer. . . . [They] furnish evidence confirmatory of points mentioned before in regard to lower reflex action. This is interesting, since they must be admitted to be movements of higher order than any of those others. Nevertheless they are to my thinking merely fractional movements. . . . The results before you must appear a meagre contribution towards the greater problems of the working of the brain; their very poverty may help to emphasize the necessity for resorting to new methods of experimental inquiry in order to advance in this field.

Sherrington's experiments had certainly furnished 'evidence confirmatory of points mentioned before in regard to lower reflex action' (e.g. coordination, reciprocal inhibition, etc); indeed, many of the responses evoked from the cortex could also be evoked as spinal reflexes—'the local reflex movements obtained from the bulbospinal animal and the reactions elicitable from the motor cortex of the narcotized animal fall into line as similar series'

(1906, p. 299). Ferrier's 'definite purposive combination of muscular contractions, which is the very essence of the reaction' (Ferrier 1886) would also
seem to 'fall into line' as a spinal mechanism that can be set going by either
peripheral or cortical stimulation.

It seems fair to say that the subsequent discovery of multiple somatotopic
areas by gross epicortical stimulation has not thrown much light on cortical
function. It does however tell us where to look. Is neuronal activity within
these areas related to 'the motor result of psychical integration' rather than
being 'a step towards psychical integration'? Taken together, the epicortical
and cytoarchitectonic maps challenge us to differentiate the functions of areas
4, 6 (premotor and SMA), 3a, 3b, 1, 5 and 7, all of which would have been
included within the 19th century motor maps. The much-needed 'new
methods of experimental inquiry' had to wait another 60 years for Evarts
(1966) to take up the challenge. His experiments and those of the people who
are now advancing them the world over are at the very heart of this symposium. Large samples of neurons can be harvested from the laminae of the
different areas of relatively few monkeys performing tasks learnt for reward.
The neurons can be sorted into different categories by the relation of their
discharges to specific components of the performance. The discharging
neurons can be visualized *post mortem* by microchemical imaging of their
perikarya, dendrites, axons and synapses. At the macroscopic level, studies of
the Bereitschaftspotential and of regional cerebral metabolism are revealing
the activity of the different areas in motor performance in intact humans.
'Motor' interests centre on the roles of area 6 (premotor and SMA) in the
preparatory stages of movement, especially in response to visual and auditory cues, and on the role of area 4—the Final Common Path leading out of
the forebrain and cerebellum—in its execution.

References

Asanuma H, Sakata H 1967. Functional organisation of a cortical efferent system
    examined with focal depth stimulation in cats. J Neurophysiol 30:35–54
Beevor CE, Horsley V 1890 A record of the results obtained by electrical excitation of
    the so-called motor cortex and internal capsule in an Orang-Outan (*Simia satyrus*).
    Philos Trans R Soc Lond B Biol Sci 181:129–158
Boyd SG, Rothwell JC, Cowan JMA et al 1986 A method of monitoring function in
    corticospinal pathways during scoliosis surgery with a note on motor conduction
    velocities. J Neurol Neurosurg Psychiatry 49:251–257
Brodmann K 1905 Beiträge zur histologischen Lokalisation der Grosshirnrind. J
    Psychol Neurol Lpz 4:176–226
Campbell AW 1905 Histological studies on the localisation of cerebral function.
    Cambridge University Press, Cambridge
Day BL, Thompson PD, Dick JPR, Nakashima K, Marsden CD 1987 Different sites
    of action of electrical and magnetic stimulation of the human brain. Neurosci Lett,
    in press
Evarts EV 1966 Representation of movements and muscles by pyramidal tract neurons

of the precentral motor cortex. In: Yahr MD, Purpura DP (eds) Neurophysiological basis of normal and abnormal motor activities. Raven Press, New York, p 215–253

Ezure, K, Oshima T 1985 Lateral spread of neuronal activity within the motor cortex investigated with intracellular responses to distant epicortical stimulation. Jpn J Physiol 35:223–249

Ezure K, Oguri M, Oshima T 1985 Vertical spread of neuronal activity within the cat motor cortex investigated with epicortical stimulation and intracellular recording. Jpn J Physiol 35:193–221

Ferrier D 1886 The functions of the brain, 2nd edn. Smith Elder, London, 323 p

Fritsch G, Hitzig E 1870 Über die elektrische Erregbarkeit des Grosshirns. Arch Anatomie Physiol Wiss Med Lpz 37:300–332

Hern JEC, Phillips CG, Porter R 1962 Electrical thresholds of unimpaled corticospinal cells in the cat. QJ Exp Physiol 47:134–140

Horsley V 1909 The Linacre Lecture on the function of the so-called motor area of the brain. Br Med J 2:125–132

Horsley V, Schäfer EA 1888 A record of experiments upon the functions of the cerebral cortex. Philos Trans R Soc Lond B Biol Sci 179:1–45

Kernell D, Wu Chien-ping 1967a Responses of the pyramidal tract to stimulation on the baboon's motor cortex. J Physiol (Lond) 191: 653–672

Kernell D, Wu Chien-ping 1967b Post-synaptic effects of cortical stimulation of forelimb motor neurones in the baboon. J Physiol (Lond) 191:673–690

Landgren S, Phillips CG, Porter R 1962 Cortical fields of origin of the monosynaptic pyramidal pathways to some alpha motoneurones of the baboon's hand and forearm. J Physiol (Lond) 161:112–125

Leyton ASF, Sherrington CS 1917 Observations on the excitable cortex of the chimpanzee, orang-utan and gorilla. Q J Exp Physiol 11:135–222

Liddell EGT, Phillips CG 1950 Thresholds of cortical representation. Brain 73: 125–140

Patton HD, Amassian VE 1954 Single- and multiple-unit analysis of cortical stage of pyramidal tract activation. J Neurophysiol 17:345–363

Patton HD, Amassian VE 1960 The pyramidal tract: its excitation and functions. In: Field J (ed) Handbook of physiology—neurophysiology. American Physiological Society, Washington, vol 2:837–861

Penfield W, Rasmussen AT 1950 Cerebral cortex of man. A clinical study of localisation of function. Macmillan, New York

Phillips CG, Porter R 1962 Unifocal and bifocal stimulation of the motor cortex. J Physiol (Lond) 162: 532–538

Phillips CG, Porter R 1977 Corticospinal neurones: their role in movement. Academic Press, London (Monogr Physiol Soc 34) p 158–161

Sherrington CS 1906 The integrative action of the nervous system. Constable & Co, London

Wiesendanger M, Séguin JJ, Künzle H 1973 The supplementary motor area—a control system for posture? In: RB Stein et al (eds) Control of posture and locomotion. Plenum, New York, p 331–346

Woolsey CN 1958 Organization of somatic sensory and motor areas of the cerebral cortex. In: Harlow HF, Woolsey CN (eds) Biological and biochemical bases of behavior. University of Wisconsin Press, Madison, p 63–81

Woolsey CN, Settlage PH, Meyer DR, Sencer W, Hamuy TP, Travis AM 1952 Patterns of localization in precentral and 'supplementary' motor areas and their relation to the concept of a premotor area. Res Publ Assoc Res Nerv Ment Dis 30:238–264

Woolsey CN, Travis AM, Barnard JW, Ostenso RS 1953 Motor representation in the postcentral gyrus after chronic ablation of precentral and supplementary motor areas. Fed Proc 12:160

DISCUSSION

Roland: When the cortex is electrically stimulated, multiple voltage-sensitive ion channels may open in a variety of neurons, some of which are inhibitory, others excitatory; then—by some miracle—an axon potential may travel down to the spinal cord. How can we extract any information about somatotopy from electrical stimulation if we excite inhibitory neurons or restrict the influences of stimulation to pyramidal cells? Can we get a clear idea of what somatotopy means in electrical stimulation experiments by looking at the properties of ion channels and the microphysiological properties of the neurons that are stimulated?

Phillips: Those fundamental biophysical questions can only be solved by intracellular recording from single identified cortical neurons. Oshima and his colleagues (Koike et al 1970, 1972) made beautiful records of intracellularly stimulated pyramidal tract neurons in the cat. At the level of a single neuron, identified by antidromic stimulation of the pyramidal or lateral corticospinal tract, it will be possible to see what happens to conductances and membrane potentials at different levels of activity.

The term punctate has often been used in connection with somatotopy. That is a sort of *double entendre* because not only is the stimulating electrode making a punctate epicortical contact but it is also assumed that the response was punctate. That is what I was trying to torpedo in my paper: it isn't a punctate response but a spreading response. It has to spread far enough from the point of contact to engage enough neurons with a common output before any output can be detected macroscopically.

At the microscopic level, Bob Porter and I (Phillips & Porter 1964) found that with stronger stimuli the monosynaptic corticomotoneuronal EPSPs and disynaptic IPSPs were followed by abundant polysynaptic actions on the spinal motor neurons, inhibitory as well as excitatory. Some showed only polysynaptic actions, some only inhibition, particularly in the motor neurons of the forearm. In the hand monosynaptic excitation is predominant.

Marsden: In experiments on anaesthetized animals we may miss one of the crucial features of the human motor map. With electrical or magnetic stimulation of the human motor cortex through the scalp you can choose which part of your anatomy will twitch by voluntarily contracting it. How does that work?

Phillips: In light general anaesthesia, and when there is no spontaneous movement, the baboon's spinal motor neurons are hyperpolarized by 10 mV or more with respect to their firing threshold. So even the largest corticomotoneuronal EPSPs, those for hand and foot (maximal amplitude about 3 mV), cannot reach the firing threshold. They can only do so when the corticomotoneuronal synapses are facilitated by a brief burst of corticospinal volleys at 500 Hz. Motor neurons of other muscle groups receive a less dense corticomotoneuronal projection and are thus relatively inaccessible to this mode of cortical stimulation. Now suppose that your motor apparatus resembles the baboon's. When you are relaxed, a burst of D and I volleys evoked electrically, or of I volleys evoked magnetically, will make your hand twitch but will fail to activate muscles of less accessible groups. If, however, you make a sustained voluntary contraction confined to one of these groups, you will close the 10 mV gap in the spinal motor neurons you are firing tonically, and narrow it in the motor neurons you are keeping poised, say, 1 or 2mV below their firing threshold. (Presumably the voluntary contraction would be sustained by one or more descending pathways in addition to the pyramidal tract.) Then, when an electrical or magnetic pulse evokes its characteristic burst, the resulting EPSPs, though too small to reach the firing threshold of any motor neurons in the relaxed condition, will now bring many of them to threshold simultaneously and elicit a twitch from the appropriate part of your anatomy.

Porter: Conscious animals can be trained to maintain a low level of contraction in particular muscles and one can then test the effect of the cortical stimulus. This is not unlike the human experiments. But what is being set at a new level? Is it the cerebral cortex or the state of activation of all the segmental machinery in the spinal cord? Clinical observations may provide some answers to that question.

Marsden: In so far as one can test this in human beings it seems to be a cortical focusing event rather than a spinal event. I would like to hear other people's views on where and how focusing occurs in the motor cortex.

Porter: Should we conclude that a particular output pathway is mapped by electrical stimulation methods and that because the inhibitory processes are not mapped one cannot find a deficit related to that output pathway by making a lesion, even though many other things may be influenced by that lesion?

Lemon: There has been more than a century of discussion on the different effects of electrical stimulation on the cerebral cortex. Has too much of that discussion been about the effects of electrical stimulation on the brain and not enough about the real function of the areas that are being stimulated? The 'processes of movement' described by Hughlings Jackson cannot be imitated by electrical stimulation.

Phillips: I have always regarded the electrical map as a map of outputs. It is surely extremely valuable to use epicortical stimulation for finding where you are and deciding what you are going to ablate. It is not very interesting for function but it is for connectivity.

Fetz: Some of your records for higher stimulus intensities showed repetitive EPSPs, but those usually seemed to occur under conditions in which there was also repetitive firing of the corticomotoneuronal cells. How predominant do you think the disynaptic excitatory pathway is on these distal motor neurons?

Porter: In the anaesthetized monkey, the possibly oligosynaptic, disynaptic or polysynaptic excitatory events are not very obvious in motor neurons that innervate the small muscles of the hand, even with massive stimulation of the cerebral cortex. Like you, I would conclude that many of the successive waves in the complex EPSP can be accounted for by repetitive firing in corticomotoneuronal fibres. We haven't made such detailed studies of motor neurons innervating muscles that act more proximally.

Thach: Dr Lemon asked whether cortical electrophysiology could be tied to normal mechanisms of motor control. The amount of inhibition within the cortex may be relevant to normal motor neuron control. Is the cortex so wired as to excite the independent movement of one digit and inhibit (by 'lateral inhibition') the movement of adjacent digits? We have come to accept this as one of the cardinal functions of cerebral motor cortex, yet do we know the mechanism accounting for it?

Secondly, a property of motor cortex that is often regarded as pathological is its ability to sustain discharge and develop a seizure or epileptic pattern. In recent years there has been more interest in whether neurons can maintain a signal extended over time in the absence of any external triggering situations— the so-called set discharge. Could this epileptic discharge be a substrate, by a loop mechanism such as the reverberating loop of Lorente de Nó or by an iterative membrane discharge, for maintaining the signal across time?

Phillips: David Armstrong did some nice work on how inhibition is built up in pyramidal neurons. There is abundant evidence that it builds up and spreads transcortically. The problem is to measure how far it spreads.

Armstrong: It is a long time since I stimulated pyramidal tract axons and produced IPSPs in pyramidal tract neurons which were not themselves being antidromically invaded. Certainly the IPSPs were enormous and the latencies quite short (Armstrong 1965).

Shinoda: We stained single corticospinal axons arising from the 'forelimb area' of the motor cortex in the monkey, using the method of intra-axonal injection of horseradish peroxidase (HRP), and found that many of them have very strong projections to forelimb motor neuron pools. However, there are very few axon collaterals from those axons to the intermediate zone of the spinal cord. So I have an impression that there must be very few disynaptic or oligosynaptic excitatory connections to motor neurons at the spinal segmental level.

Porter: Would the results you get by filling corticospinal fibres with HRP allow you to say whether, at some other segmental level, there are collaterals that innervate cells of origin of propriospinal pathways?

Shinoda: At present we can stain axons for lengths of about 30 mm, which cover only one to three segments. Therefore, we do not know whether the same axons innervate propriospinal neurons in the upper cervical cord of the monkey. But our previous electrophysiological data showed that corticospinal axons projecting to forelimb motor neuron pools have multiple axon collaterals to C_3

and C_4 in the monkey spinal cord (Shinoda et al 1979). Those collaterals probably terminate on propriospinal neurons.

Calne: To what extent do the maps generated by stimulation correspond to the maps of deficits deriving from lesions in these regions? What are the differences and what are the similarities?

Kuypers: My experience is that there is a very strong correlation between the stimulation maps and the maps of the deficits after lesions in the various areas. For example, a relatively small lesion restricted to the hand area of the macaque's motor cortex (including the anterior bank of the central sulcus) abolishes the animal's capacity to execute individual finger movements for at least two to three years, while closing the hand as a whole remains possible.

Calne: Is that quite different from a lesion of, say, the pyramidal tract?

Kuypers: Yes, it is different because a pyramidotomy involves all corticospinal fibres, while a lesion of the precentral hand area involves only a portion of them. However, the pyramidotomy produces roughly the same effect on the motor capacity of the hand as the precentral lesion, i.e. it permanently abolishes the capacity to execute highly fractionated movements, such as individual finger movements (Lawrence & Kuypers 1968).

Calne: I thought that a lesion in the medullary pyramid, for example, would lead to a problem with selecting movements of the hand rather than causing the same extent of paralysis that would occur with a cortical lesion.

Kuypers: If you transect the pyramidal tract you deprive the animal of the capacity to execute highly fractionated movements, which capacity is in all likelihood dependent on the direct corticomotoneuronal fibres embedded in the pyramidal tract. However, ultimately you are not interfering with the animal's capacity to select the appropriate movements to try to reach a certain goal. The animal still knows exactly what it wants and it can achieve this because all its brainstem connections to the spinal cord are still intact.

Passingham: If you make a unilateral cortical lesion in the motor area, at first the animal will not use the contralateral hand. But if you then restrain the other hand the animal will now use the affected hand. So you get the same effect.

Goldman-Rakic: From the published work it seems that large areas of the motor cortex have to be removed to get these deficits. This fits with microstimulation work where you have to have a considerable amount of spread. We might think of it as somewhat analogous to the visual system, where we don't think that a single neuron or even several neurons are sufficient to put together a perception of a stimulus at a given point in space. Similarly, when we speak of motor control from motor cortex, are we really talking about a population of cells generating the signal for a given motor command rather than a single neuron?

Phillips: Edward Evarts (1967) pointed out that you can injure a pyramidal tract neuron with an extracellular microelectrode, causing it to discharge at high frequency during the few seconds between injury and death of the cell; and that such discharges fail to elicit any movements.

References

Armstrong DM 1965 Synaptic excitation and inhibition of Betz cells by antidromic pyramidal volleys. J Physiol (Lond) 178:37–38P

Evarts EV 1967 Representation of movements and muscles by pyramidal tract neurons of the precentral motor cortex. In: Yahr MD, Purpura DP (eds) Neurophysiological basis of normal and abnormal motor activities. Raven Press, New York, p 253

Koike H, Mano K, Okada Y, Oshima T 1970 Repetitive impulses generated in fast and slow pyramidal tract cells by intracellularly applied current steps. Exp Brain Res 11:263–281

Koike H, Mano K, Okada Y, Oshima T 1972 Activities of the sodium pump in cat pyramidal tract cells investigated with intracellular injection of sodium ions. Exp Brain Res 14:449–462

Lawrence DG, Kuypers HGJM 1968 The functional organization of the motor system in the monkey. I. The effects of bilateral pyramidal lesions. Brain 91:1–14

Phillips CG, Porter R 1964 The pyramidal projection to motoneurones of some muscle groups of the baboons's forelimb. In: Eccles JC, Schadé JP (eds) Physiology of spinal neurones. Elsevier, Amsterdam (Prog Brain Res vol 12) p 222–242

Shinoda Y, Zarzecki P, Asanuma H 1979 Spinal branching of pyramidal tract neurons in the monkey. Exp Brain Res 34:59–72

Ascending inputs to, and internal organization of, cortical motor areas

E.G. Jones

Department of Anatomy and Neurobiology, University of California, Irvine, CA 92717, USA

Abstract. Modern anatomical studies show that, contrary to the long-held dogma, there appears to be essentially no convergence of lemniscal, cerebellar, pallidal, or substantial nigral afferents in the thalamus. Each afferent stream defines its own thalamic territory and, through the projection of these thalamic territories to separate cortical territories, the independence of the projections of subcortical motor nuclei upon the cortex is preserved. Only the spinothalamic system appears to gain access to both sensory and motor cortex.

A further principle of organization in the sensorimotor thalamus is the presence of individual anatomically and physiologically defined channels, composed of separate afferent inputs and groups of neurons relaying to the cortex. In the somatic sensory relay nuclei the dissociation of cutaneous, deep slowly and rapidly adapting channels is clear-cut in the thalamus and at the input level of the cortex. In the motor system, inputs from each of the deep cerebellar nuclei appear to be dissociated from one another in the thalamus and these in turn from the vestibular and spinothalamic systems. Just as pallidal, nigral and cerebellar pathways are in position to control separate premotor and motor areas of the cortex, so separate channels leading through VLp appear to be in a position to control separate functional units in area 4.

Within the cortex itself the absence of corticocortical connections passing from areas 3a and 3b to area 4 appears to indicate that information flow out of these areas is back to areas 1 and 2 for further processing before transmission to area 4 with all the consequences that entails for sensory convergence. Presumably, this route is sufficiently rapid for sensory inputs to reach area 4 at short latency. Although many data are beginning to accrue on the intrinsic structure and connectivity of the sensorimotor cortex, we are still distant from a complete wiring diagram. Circuitry involving thalamic afferents is becoming known slowly and the nature of the cells that are present and their transmitter characteristics are becoming evident from morphological and immunocytochemical studies, along with information on the patterns of axonal ramification of specific cell types, especially of GABAergic cells and of excitatory corticocortical cells.

1987 Motor areas of the cerebral cortex. Wiley, Chichester (Ciba Foundation Symposium 132) p 21–39

Thalamic inputs to motor areas

Lemniscal, cerebellar and pallidal regions of the thalamus. Older studies using

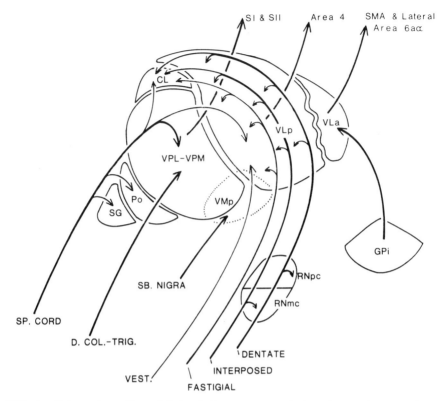

FIG. 1. Schematic outline of thalamic input–output relations imposed on a sagittal view of the monkey ventral nuclei and associated thalamic nuclei. This scheme emphasizes segregation of lemniscal, cerebellar and pallidal routes through to cerebral cortex. Cortical areas refer to those shown in Fig. 2. Substantia nigra relay (VMp) may include supplementary motor area (SMA) in its cortical target. Spinal cord and vestibular relays are also shown. Note projection of former to both sensory and motor cortex. (From Jones 1986.)

the Marchi method indicated that the brachium conjunctivum terminated in the ventral nuclei of monkeys at levels anterior to those of the medial lemniscus, and that the ansa lenticularis, arising from the globus pallidus, terminated anterior to the brachium conjunctivum. The idea of a tripartite functional organization of inputs to motor cortex, however, did not take hold and it became customary to assume that pallidal, substantial nigral and cerebellar inputs converged in the thalamic relay to motor cortex and that there was a substantial degree of overlap between the thalamic terminations of lemniscal, spinothalamic and cerebellar afferents. Direct vestibulothalamic connections were discounted until recently.

Studies conducted within the last five years have radically altered our view of the connectivity of the primate motor thalamus (Fig. 1). Separate lemnis-

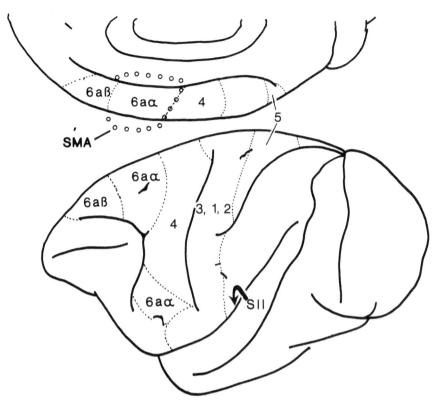

FIG. 2.   Schematic view of the positions of the fields of the premotor (6aβ, 6aα), motor (4), somatic sensory (3,1,2, SII) and anterior parietal (5) cortex in Old World monkeys (after Vogt & Vogt 1919). The medial part of area 6aα is probably coextensive with the supplementary motor area (SMA).

cal, cerebellar, pallidal and nigral relays seem to exist in the thalamus and project on independent sensory, motor and premotor cortical fields. The spinothalamic and vestibulothalamic afferents have also been better clarified.

The ventral thalamic nuclei in monkeys. The ventral nuclear complex of the thalamus in Old World monkeys has been re-evaluated on the basis of afferent connections (Jones 1986). Four main groups exist: ventral anterior (VA), ventral lateral anterior (VLa), ventral lateral posterior (VLp), and ventral posterior (VP). A ventral medial (VM) nucleus may be a continuation of VA.

Afferent connectivity. Recent anatomical studies in monkeys reveal that the VLa nucleus is the thalamic target of the internal segment of the globus pallidus (DeVito & Anderson 1982). The VLp nucleus is the target of all

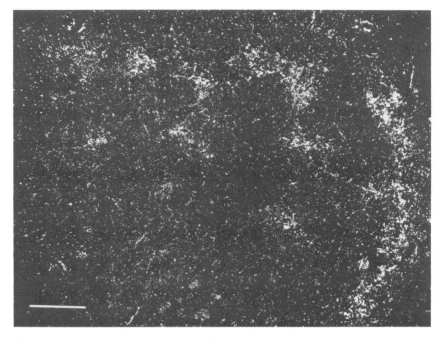

FIG. 3. · Autoradiographic, oblique frontal section showing lattice-like arrangement of interpositothalamic terminations in VLp nucleus. Gaps are filled, with little overlap by terminations of dentate and fastigial fibres. (From Asanuma et al 1983b.) Bar 300 μm.

three contralateral deep cerebellar nuclei and of the ipsilateral fastigial nucleus (Asanuma et al 1983a, b). The medial lemniscus, including its trigeminal component, ends in the ventral posterior (VPL and VPM) nuclei (Jones et al 1982). There is little evidence in my material, much of it involving double-labelling strategies, that indicates significant overlap in the terminations of cerebellar and pallidal fibres or of cerebellar and lemniscal fibres (Fig. 2), although the latter has been suggested. Spinothalamic fibres, however, terminate throughout the VPL nucleus and extend into the ventral part of the VLp nucleus to end among the cerebellar terminations (Asanuma et al 1983b).

Nigrothalamic terminations appear to lie medial to those of cerebello-thalamic, pallidothalamic and lemniscal fibres (Carpenter et al 1976) in the principal ventral medial nucleus (VMp) but may extend into VA. Vestibulo-thalamic fibres (Lange et al 1979, Asanuma et al 1983b), terminate in the ventral part of the VLp nucleus. None of the afferent pathways mentioned here has been found to terminate in the ventral posterior inferior (VPI) nucleus.

At present it appears that pallidal, cerebellar and lemniscal thalamic territories have separate access to selected fields of the cerebral cortex. The only convergence in the thalamus appears to be in the VLp nucleus in which afferents from the three deep cerebellar nuclei, the spinothalamic tract and the vestibular nuclei terminate. Even these inputs, however, appear to be segregated, since they contact separate clusters of cells in VLp (Asanuma et al 1983b).

Representation in the ventral posterior nuclei (VPL and VPM) and ventral lateral posterior (VLp) nucleus

VPL and VPM. There are clearly at least two parts to the VPL nucleus: a large central core region in which neurons are all activated by light tactile stimuli, including stimuli that activate slowly or rapidly adapting mechanoreceptors, receptors around hairs or receptors in glabrous skin; and a thin shell region, anterior, dorsal and to some extent posterior to the core, in which neurons are activated only by deep pressure, movement of joints or stimulation of Group 1 muscle afferents (Friedman & Jones 1981, Maendly et al 1981). This region is part of the VPL, not an overlap or transition zone with VLp (Friedman & Jones 1981, Jones et al 1982). There are hints that all parts of the contralateral half of the body are represented in both the shell and core regions but evidence is incomplete.

VLp nucleus. Recently it has become evident that the deep cerebellar nuclei both collectively and individually project in a topographically organized manner on the contralateral VLp nucleus (Asanuma et al 1983a,b, Fig. 1). Assuming that there is likely to be a body representation in the deep cerebellar nuclei, although evidence for this is sketchy, such a representation would therefore be projected onto the VLp nucleus. The nature of the map has been variously interpreted (Asamuma et al 1983a, Schell & Strick 1984); it is not clear whether it is single or multiple.

Selective labelling of the various inputs to VLp reveals a finer organization in VLp (Asanuma et al 1983b). Each deep cerebellar nucleus projects as a series of disjunctive focal groupings of axon terminations within the VLp nucleus (Fig. 3). The dentate foci are rod-like and anteroposteriorly elongated, like lemniscal terminations in VPL (Jones et al 1982). The foci formed by interpositial and fastigial fibres are more lattice-like, and those from the vestibular nuclei and spinal cord are focal but widely dispersed. Double-labelling experiments show that rods or foci from two different cerebellar nuclei or from other sources do not overlap to any significant extent at the light microscope level (Fig. 3). There is some physiological evidence in the cat, however, that some individual cells receive convergent input from two or more sources.

The data suggest that the great afferent systems are segregated from one another in the thalamus and that individual groups of axons terminate in relation to separate groupings of cells within those nuclei. In the somatosensory nuclei this is manifested as a functional segregation of neuronal types responding to different types of peripheral receptors (Jones et al 1982). In the VLp there is a segregation according to fibre origin but what this means in terms of function is not yet evident.

Thalamocortical connectivity

Maps of the motor areas. In the motor cortex, partial mapping of the sensory responses of movement-related neurons has suggested a dual body representation in the old cytoarchitectonic field, area 4 (Tanji & Wise 1981). These two representations, however, seem to exclude area 6aα of Vogt & Vogt (1919), which Brodmann had included in area 4 (Fig. 2). The part of area 6a α lying below area 4 of Vogt & Vogt and a part of area 4 lying in the posterior bank of the arcuate nucleus have, on anatomical grounds, been divided into two further putative motor representations (Schell & Strick 1984), but the areas have not been clearly defined. The medial part of area 6aα of Vogt & Vogt (1919) includes the supplementary motor area medially, with a coherent bilateral motor representation, and an area on the lateral surface that is far less responsive to microstimulation than the other motor areas, but which may be movement-related. Area 6aβ of Vogt & Vogt, in front of it, is virtually unexplored territory.

Afferent inputs to sensory and motor cortical maps. Individual thalamic nuclei (and thus the individual afferent systems discussed above) gain selective access to individual cortical territories, and separate constellations of thalamic cells may separately innervate different maps or parts of maps within the larger cortical territories.

There appears to be a complete segregation of afferent inputs to area 4 and to the first somatic sensory area (SI). All recent evidence is against any overlap or collateralization in the projections of VP to SI or of VLp to area 4 (Friedman & Jones 1981, Jones 1983).

The anterior border of area 4 is a source of much confusion but there appears to be a fairly distinct separation of the thalamic inputs from VLp and from VLa in a region that includes areas 4 and 6aα of Vogt & Vogt (1919). The evidence is not complete, and the existing evidence is subject to varying interpretations (Asanuma et al 1983b, Schell & Strick 1984). My own position is that VLp and the cerebellum provide input to area 4, and VLa and the globus pallidus provide the input to the supplementary motor area and lateral parts of area 6, area 4 being defined as area 4 and area 6 as area 6aα of Vogt & Vogt (1919). Schell & Strick's interpretation is the same except that they treat the part of area 4 in the arcuate sulcus as a prearcuate motor area separate from area 4. In their hands, as in ours, this region receives fibres from part of VLp and, therefore, from the cerebellum. The basic finding is that there is a cerebellar cortical motor territory and a pallidal cortical motor territory, both of which may be further divided. There is, thus, a segregation of lemniscal, cerebellar and pallidal routes not only through the thalamus but also at the cortex. Only the spinothalamic route appears to be unsegregated because, by ending in both VPL and VLp, it appears to gain access to both sensory and motor cortex.

The cortical targets of the thalamic relay for the substantia nigra have not been thoroughly worked out in the primate. It is likely that SI, area 4 and the greater part of area 6 are free of thalamic inputs from the VMp (and/or VA nucleus). The VMp nucleus projects rather diffusely to cortex along the medial surface of the hemisphere, so it is possible that it exerts some influence over the supplementary motor area.

Within the systems projecting on area 4 there may be independent relay channels formed by separate sets of thalamic cells projecting on individual subrepresentations in those areas. In the VLp nucleus, the evidence for a subnuclear organization comparable to that in VPL (Jones et al 1982) is not extensive. Neurons in ventral parts of the nucleus have cutaneous receptive fields (Lemon & Van der Burg 1979) and project to posterior parts of area 4, which contains neurons with cutaneous receptive fields (Tanji & Wise 1981). Dorsal parts have neurons with less easily detectable receptive fields project-ing to anterior parts of area 4, which contains neurons with deep receptive fields. There may also be an anteroposterior fractionation of the VLp, with anterior and posterior regions further segregated in respect to their cortical projections (Schell & Strick 1984). By analogy with the VPL projection to SI, one might expect to find that the rods or other foci of cells contacted in VLp by differential inputs would project to separate 'columns' in the motor cortex (Jones et al 1982, Asanuma et al 1983b). There may therefore be components of area 4 that are selectively influenced by dentate, interpositus, fastigial, spinal or vestibular inputs. This possibility has not yet been explored.

Neurons in the primate motor cortex can respond to natural peripheral stimulation or to electrical stimulation of peripheral nerves at remarkably short latencies. The routes taken by these short-latency afferent inputs are still controversial. Section of the dorsal columns of the spinal cord in monkeys leads to the disappearance of the peripheral receptive fields of motor cortex neurons, though this does not seem to affect their discharges in relation to the performance of movements (Brinkman et al 1978). The involvement of the dorsal columns, coupled with the short latency of response in the motor cortex and the presence of neurons with somatic sensory receptive fields in the VLp nucleus, led to the view that the medial lemniscal system would project directly to motor cortex (Asanuma et al 1980). However, from the previous discussion, the possibility of the medial lemniscus gaining synaptic

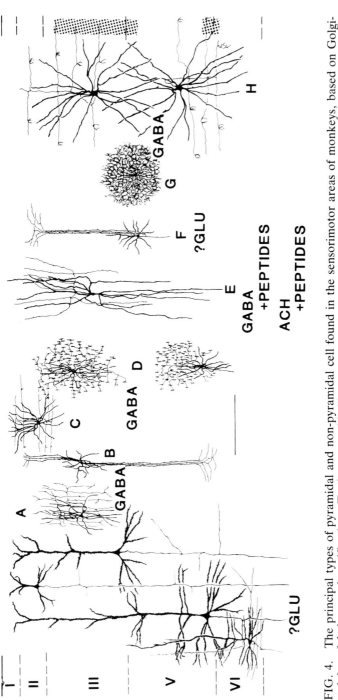

FIG. 4. The principal types of pyramidal and non-pyramidal cell found in the sensorimotor areas of monkeys, based on Golgi-staining of their axonal ramifications. To these are added known or putative transmitter agents associated with each type. A, typical arcade cell; B, double bouquet cell; C, small basket cell of layer II; D, chandelier cells; E, peptidergic cell; F, spiny cell of layer IV; G, neuroglia form or spiderweb cell; H, basket cells. GABA, γ-aminobutyric acid; GLU, glutamic acid. Bars to right indicate layers of thalamic terminations in motor cortex. (After Jones 1975.)

access to thalamocortical neurons projecting to area 4 is quite remote. The spinothalamic fibres relaying in VLp would seem an obvious choice for a direct somatic sensory route to area 4 but against this possibility are the observations on the essential role of the dorsal columns of the spinal cord (Brinkman et al 1978, Asanuma et al 1980). The deep cerebellar nuclei as sources of short latency input to motor cortex can be ruled out on several grounds (Asanuma et al 1983b).

We are left with the possibility of lemniscal inputs to motor cortex via corticocortical connections from areas 1 and 2, although Brinkman et al (1985) have recently reported that cooling of area 2 in conscious monkeys does not affect the short-latency discharges of motor cortex neurons to passively imposed peripheral stimuli.

Layers of thalamocortical terminations. Although it is now well-established that thalamic afferents terminate differentially among the fields of SI in the monkey (Jones & Burton 1976, Jones 1983), remarkably little work has been done at the same level of resolution on motor cortex. The major layer of termination of thalamic afferents in area 4 appears to be the rather wide layer III (Jones 1975) (Fig. 4). No subsidiary layers of thalamic terminations have yet been reported and the cells of termination and their properties are completely unknown. By analogy with the visual and somatic sensory areas, a variety of cortical cell types can probably receive direct (monosynaptic) connections from thalamocortical axons. In the visual cortex of the cat, cells of virtually every receptive field type receive at least some direct thalamic influences, and in rodent SI most morphological cell types receive some thalamic synapses (White 1986). In monkey SI, thalamic axons end on both GABAergic and non-GABAergic neurons (Hendry et al 1981). The GABAergic neurons include basket cells (DeFelipe et al 1986b) as well as other types, and the non-GABAergic recipient cells include small spiny non-pyramidal cells and large pyramidal cells that send their axons into the corpus callosum (Hendry & Jones 1983). By analogy with these findings and, again, with results from the mouse, it is possible that the large population of subcortically projecting pyramidal cells in the motor cortex (Jones 1986) may also be in a position to be influenced monosynaptically from the thalamus.

Corticocortical connections

Connectivity between the motor cortex and between the fields of SI is not diffuse or generalized but organized in specific patterns. In SI, areas 3a, 3b, 1 and 2 are interconnected in a complex manner but only areas 1 and 2 are interconnected with the motor cortex, area 4. The second somatic sensory area (SII) appears to project to area 4 but may not receive axons from area 4. SI also projects to area 5 of parietal cortex and to the supplementary motor area, both of which are interconnected and both of which project to area 4.

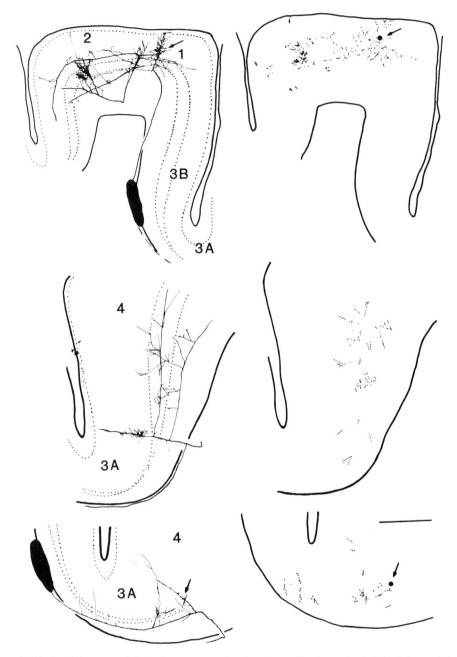

FIG. 5.   Upper: multiple, long-range, focal collateralization of a labelled layer III pyramidal cell in area 2 of SI in a monkey in which horseradish peroxidase was injected into the white matter beneath the cortex to involve corticocortical fibres passing forward to motor cortex (dotted line). Middle and lower: layer III pyramidal cells in area 3a and area 4 showing similar focal patterns of axon collateralization. Dots indicate axon terminals. (From DeFelipe et al 1986a.)

In all of these connections the somatotopy is preserved so that in any two areas only representations of the same body part tend to be connected.

The principal corticocortical input to the motor areas is from areas 1, 2 and the anterior part of area 5, to all three of which area 4 returns corticocortical fibres, as well as to area 3a. Yet area 4 receives no input from area 3a and appears to be totally unconnected with area 3b. The supplementary motor area receives inputs from areas 1, 2, 5 and 4 but not, apparently, from areas 3a and 3b. In virtually all motor and parietal fields, therefore, cutaneous and group I muscle afferents operating through these last two areas would only seem able to exert their effects on area 4 through areas 1 and 2. The major population of corticocortical cells in all the areas of the sensorimotor cortex are pyramidal cells of all sizes with somata in layers II and III (Figs. 4, 5). In general, the larger, deeper cells have the longest axons (see Jones 1986). Some corticocortical cells have been reported in other layers, particularly layer VI. The cells in layers II and III form patchy concentrations of somata and a single injection of tracer at one point in any of the sensorimotor fields leads to retrograde labelling of multiple patches of corticocortical cells in the same field and in the other connected fields. A single patch of corticocortical cells will also project to multiple foci in the same and adjacent fields, as indicated by anterograde labelling.

Corticocortical axons arising from single pyramidal neurons in any one of the fields of SI, including those identified as projecting forwards to area 4, have collateral branches that can terminate in focal concentrations in all the other fields of SI, and in area 5 as well (Fig. 5) (DeFelipe et al 1986a). Many such axons also have multiple focal concentrations of terminals in the field in which their parent cell soma lies (Fig. 5). Similar axon arborizations are seen on the ends of corticocortical axons in area 4. The axons of most of the corticocortical cells have major long horizontal collaterals arising in layers III and V of the parent area. These can then extend for distances of 1–1.5 mm or more, giving off focused terminal ramifications at wide intervals.

These multiple intra-areal and interareal focused connections, many formed by branches of the same corticocortical axon, might serve to interconnect comparable representations of the same body part in several functional areas. But they might also serve to promote convergence of influences from cells with different classes of inputs in the motor cortex—for example, a convergence of dentate, interpositus and fastigial influences along lines similar to those proposed by Iwamura et al (1983) in the SI cortex.

Corticocortical fibres joining the fields of SI to one another and to areas 4 and 5 have their major concentrations of terminals in layers I through IV (through III in motor cortex), though some may be seen in other layers as well. The terminal pattern suggests that the corticocortical fibres form terminals primarily on apical and basal dendrites of layer III pyramidal cells, as these dendrites ascend through layers I–III and descend into layer IV respectively. Sloper & Powell (1979) have shown electron microscopically that corticocortical fibres in the monkey SI probably terminate on pyramidal and non-pyramidal cells, but the proportions of different types of these cells that are contacted has not been determined.

Intrinsic connectivity of the sensorimotor cortex. Corticocortical and subcortically projecting cells of the sensorimotor areas are all pyramidal and their axons characteristically give rise to intracortical collaterals before they leave the parent cortical area. The collaterals of corticocortical cells may form an essential component of the intrinsic circuitry of a cortical area. Collaterals of subcortically projecting axons would presumably be similarly involved in the intrinsic circuitry and they have been the subject of much work in the cat visual cortex. Other intrinsic cortical circuits are formed by the several varieties of non-pyramidal neurons, all with intrinsic axons. In the sensorimotor regions there are eight well-defined varieties when classified according to their axonal distributions (Jones 1975, Fig. 4). The potential role of several of these in the intracortical elaboration of afferent messages has been the subject of several recent reviews. The transmitter characteristics of the intrinsic neurons in the primate sensorimotor areas are also beginning to be determined and a substantial majority, perhaps all the non-spiny types, are GABAergic (Houser et al 1983). Two morphological types, the basket and chandelier cells (Fig. 4), are confirmed as GABAergic (Houser et al 1983, DeFelipe et al 1986a,b) and the narrow, stringy bipolar or bitufted type of cell is not only GABAergic but also contains one or more of the known cortical neuropeptides—cholecystokinin, somatostatin, neuropeptide Y and substance P (Hendry et al 1984).

The selective uptake and retrograde transport of ^{3}H-GABA, which many feel is indicative of the GABAergic nature of the consequently labelled neurons, indicates a strong, bidirectional connection through the thickness of the SI and area 4 cortex. Mini-injections of ^{3}H-GABA made in layers II and IIIA retrogradely label neuronal somata primarily in layer IV; similar injections in layer VI and the deep part of layer V retrogradely label somata selectively in layers II and IIIA (DeFelipe & Jones 1985); injections in the middle layers do not label somata either above or below them (DeFelipe & Jones 1985). Thus, selective retrograde cell labelling invariably occurs superficial or deep to an appropriately placed injection of ^{3}H-GABA, but not lateral to it to any extent. If it can be accepted that the high affinity uptake and retrograde transport of a transmitter indicates its use by the affected cells, then one form at least of GABA-mediated inhibition may occur vertically within narrow columnar domains of cortex, and not to any extent on either side of functional columns. Long-range intracortical effects might be mediated by the collaterals of output neurons, which would be expected to be excitatory, although the (GABAergic) basket cells form long-range inhibitory connections as well (DeFelipe et al 1986b). It is assumed that there will also be GABA-mediated inhibition within local parts of a column, and intracolumn'ar excitatory effects, possibly mediated by the small spiny cells with vertical axons that are major recipients of thalamic inputs in most cortical areas.

Contralateral connections

The overall distribution of callosal fibres. Fibres traversing the corpus callosum have been known for some time to terminate in only certain parts of SI and SII of monkeys and there has been a lot of recent work on the relationships of the callosal fibre terminations to the architectonic subfields of SI and to the parts of the body representations in both SI and SII.

The callosal connectivity of the motor and premotor cortex also displays a variety of connectional patterns in relation to the different fields and, in some of the fields, parts of the motor representation are not connected across the midline. The reports on this subject are limited (see Jones 1986). The following overall scheme appears likely: area 4 sends to and receives fibres from its contralateral counterpart; within area 4, particularly in its posterior part where neurons with cutaneous receptive fields are found, parts of the representation, seemingly those devoted to the hands and feet, are not connected; these unconnected regions are relatively much smaller than the unconnected regions in SI; the supplementary motor area appears to be interconnected with its counterpart of the opposite side and to receive fibres from the contralateral area 4. In lateral parts of the premotor cortex there appear to be a number of callosally connected regions that become labelled after injections of tracer in the contralateral precentral region. Whether these are separate premotor body representations or merely parts of a single representation in which other parts are unconnected is not clear. Schell & Strick (1984) consider that they are separate representations, and this forms their basis for identifying different fields within the motor cortex.

Acknowledgements

Personal work reported in the text was supported by Grant Numbers NS10526, NS21377 and NS22317 from the National Institutes of Health, United States Public Health Service.

References

Asanuma C, Thach WT, Jones EG 1983a Anatomical evidence for segregated focal groupings of efferent cells and their terminal ramifications in the cerebellothalamic pathway of the monkey. Brain Res Rev 5:267–297
Asanuma C, Thach WT, Jones EG 1983b Distribution of cerebellar terminations and

their relation to other afferent terminations in the thalamic ventral lateral region of the monkey. Brain Res Rev 5:237–265

Asanuma H, Larsen K, Yumiya H 1980 Peripheral input pathways to the monkey motor cortex. Exp Brain Res 38:349–355

Brinkman J, Bush BM, Porter R 1978 Deficient influences of peripheral stimuli on precentral neurones in monkeys with dorsal column lesions. J Physiol (Lond) 276:27–48

Brinkman J, Colebach JG, Porter R, York DM 1985 Responses of precentral cells during cooling of post-central cortex in conscious monkeys. J Physiol (Lond) 368: 611–625

Carpenter MB, Nakano K, Kim R 1976 Nigrothalamic projections in the monkey demonstrated by autoradiographic techniques. J Comp Neurol 165:401–415

DeFelipe J, Jones EG 1985 Vertical organization of γ-aminobutyric acid-accumulating intrinsic neuronal systems in monkey cerebral cortex. J Neurosci 5:3246–3260

DeFelipe J, Conley M, Jones EG 1986a Multiple, long-range focal collateralization of axons arising from single neurons in monkey sensory-motor cortex. J Neurosci 6: 3749–3766

DeFelipe J, Hendry SHC, Jones EG 1986b A correlative electron microscopic study of basket cells and large GABAergic neurons in monkey sensory-motor cortex. Neuroscience 17:991–1009

DeVito JL, Anderson ME 1982 An autoradiographic study of efferent connections of the globus pallidus in Macaca mulatta. Exp Brain Res 46:107–117

Friedman DP, Jones EG 1981 Thalamic input to areas 3a and 2 in monkeys. J Neurophysiol 45:59–85

Hendry SHC, Jones EG 1983 Thalamic inputs to identified commissural neurons in the monkey somatic sensory cortex. J Neurocytol 12:299–316

Hendry SHC, Houser CR, Jones EG, Vaughn JE 1981 Synaptic relations of GABA-ergic intrinsic neurons in monkey somatic sensory cortex. Neurosci Abstr 7:833

Hendry SHC, Jones EG, DeFelipe J, Schmechel D, Brandon C, Emson PC 1984 Neuropeptide containing neurons of the cerebral cortex are also GABAergic. Proc Natl Acad Sci USA 81:6526–6530

Houser C, Hendry SHC, Jones EG, Vaughn JE 1983 Synaptic organization of im-munocytochemically identified GABAergic neurons in monkey sensory-motor cortex. J Neurocytol 12:617–638

Iwamura Y, Tanaka M, Sakamoto M, Hikosaka O 1983 Converging patterns of finger representation and complex response properties of neurons in area 1 of the first somatosensory cortex in the conscious monkey. Exp Brain Res 51:327–337

Jones EG 1975 Varieties and distribution of non-pyramidal cells in the somatic sensory cortex of the squirrel monkey. J Comp Neurol 160:205–267

Jones EG 1983 Lack of collateral thalamocortical projections to fields of the first somatic sensory cortex in monkeys. Exp Brain Res 52:375–384

Jones EG 1986 Connectivity of the primate sensory-motor cortex. In: Jones EG, Peters A (eds) Cerebral cortex. Plenum, New York, vol 5:113–183

Jones EG, Burton H 1976 Areal differences in the laminar distribution of thalamic afferents in cortical fields of the insular, parietal and temporal regions of primates. J Comp Neurol 168:197–247

Jones EG, Friedman DP, Hendry SHC 1982 Thalamic basis of place- and modality-specific columns in monkey somatosensory cortex: a correlative anatomical and physiological study. J Neurophysiol 48:545–568

Lange W, Büttner-Ennever JA, Büttner U 1979 Vestibular projections to the monkey thalamus: an autoradiographic study. Brain Res 177:3–18

Lemon RN, van der Burg J 1979 Short-latency peripheral inputs to thalamic neurones projecting to the motor cortex in the monkey. Exp Brain Res 36:445–462

Maendly R, Rüegg DG, Wiesendanger M, Wiesendanger R, Lagowska J, Hess B 1981 Thalamic relay for group I muscle afferents of forelimb nerves in the monkey. J Neurophysiol 46:901–917

Schell GR, Strick PL 1984 The origin of thalamic inputs to the arcuate premotor and supplementary motor areas. J Neurosci 4:539–560

Sloper JJ, Powell TPS 1979 An experimental electron microscopic study of afferent connections to the primate motor and somatic sensory cortices. Philos Trans R Soc Lond 285:199–226

Tanji J, Wise SP 1981 Submodality distribution in sensorimotor cortex of the unanesthetized monkey. J Neurophysiol 45:467–481

Vogt C, Vogt O 1919 Allgemeinere Ergebnisse unserer Hirnforschung. J Psychol Neurol Lpz 25:277–462

White EL 1986 Termination of thalamic afferents in the cerebral cortex. In: Jones EG, Peters A (eds) Cerebral cortex, vol 5. Plenum, New York

DISCUSSION

Cheney: Are pyramidal tract cells among the targets of the postcentral neurons that send collaterals to motor cortex?

Jones: We don't know yet where they terminate. Most of those terminals are up in layer III, where the dendrites of many pyramidal tract neurons reside. From our electron microscope studies and those of Tom Powell and his group, and by analogy with visual cortex where similar work has been done, we know that the terminations should include a combination of smooth dendrite neurons (probably GABA inhibitory neurons) and spiny neurons, which could include pyramidal tract neurons.

Rizzolatti: I am not very happy with your 'imperialistic' area 4, which I think includes at least three areas. From a physiological point of view the best map of the agranular frontal cortex is that of von Bonin & Bailey (1947). According to them the inferior part of the agranular cortex is constituted by areas FA, FBA and FCBm. To postulate a single large area 4 may lead one to conclude that there is only one major thalamic input to it. This is wrong. We injected wheatgerm agglutinin–horseradish peroxidase (WGA–HRP) into area FBA and found that the main thalamic projection to this area is from VLo (unpublished work). So in the area 4–6 complex there is a pallidal stripe between two cortical zones, FA and FCBm, that are essentially under cerebellar control.

Jones: I don't want to be called imperialistic. The area I showed to be the cerebellar terminal projection *has* been called area 4 by some but my main point is that there is a large cerebellar territory. Our work with retrograde labelling shows that this territory is totally cerebellar, with no part receiving from the thalamic target of the globus pallidus; nor does the cerebellar thalamic nucleus project to other territories in the cortex.

Porter: But you haven't excluded a spinothalamic input, have you?

Jones: No. Other projection zones and other representations are probably buried in this cerebellar territory. Some of these may be based simply on the differentiation of deep and cutaneous inputs, as shown for the postcentral gyrus. In addition one can talk about a dentate region, an interposed region, a fastigial region, and probably spinothalamic regions as well. However, this has not yet been shown at a sufficient level of resolution.

Rizzolatti: Have you also studied that part of the cortex which lies between the real area 4 (FA) and the postarcuate gyrus, or are you drawing inferences on the thalamic organization of this region from data obtained injecting tracers in the cortices near the arcuate and the central sulcus?

Jones: Peter Strick has shown that injections near the arcuate sulcus label part of what I regard as the cerebellar territory of the thalamus.

Rizzolatti: Our findings there agree with his, but area FBA receives mostly from the basal ganglia.

Deecke: Is this area devoted to tongue and face movements?

Jones: At one level of resolution it could be a face area, but only Woolsey's map is equated with the projection of a medial part of a topographically organized thalamic nucleus, which goes back to Walker. It is not necessarily concerned with facial movements.

Shinoda: How do you reconcile your single body map in the ventrolateral nucleus of the thalamus with Peter Strick's double body map representation in the motor cortex?

Jones: I am not committed to a single map. In the postcentral gyrus one can show a single map based on surface evoked potential recordings, which can then be further fractionated into at least two and probably four maps, depending on how much one believes the rather limited results reported from areas 2 and 3a. A similar kind of concept can prevail in this area as well. This is a single map in the broadest sense but I think it can be fragmented much further.

Roland: The pallidal output is to some extent somatotopically organized, so have you any evidence for rod-like organization in a somatotopic fashion in the VLa? How far would a projection from a rod-like segment of the VLA extend into the 6aα area?

Jones: Some topography is implicit in the earlier retrograde degeneration work by Tom Powell and Max Cowan. DeVito & Anderson (1982) used autoradiography and the distribution of label in the thalamus varied in different experiments, suggesting that there may be some differential topography. That is also similar to a broad map which might be further fractionated, one part going to the supplementary motor area and another into the rest of the 6aα area. But I want to stress that so far nobody has done those experiments thoroughly.

Georgopoulos: What is the relative distribution of GABA inhibitory neurons at different layers?

Jones: We have looked at both numbers and laminar distributions in 10 areas. In all areas the numbers in the supragranular layers are always higher than in the infragranular layers. In addition, in areas with well-defined zones of thalamic termination, such as certain of the subsidiary layers of layer IV in visual cortex, there are increased numbers of GABA neurons. In the motor cortex 100% of the neurons in layer I are GABAergic, there is a high peak in layer II, and then there is a gradual fall down to the deep layers. This may well reflect the large number of thalamic afferents to motor cortex that extend through layer III and maybe into the upper part of layer V.

Georgopoulos: What is the distance between the multiple terminations you showed from areas 1 and 2?

Jones: We regularly traced collaterals of over 6 mm in length. Gaps of about 800 μm are common.

Xi: You showed that there are no anatomical connections between area 4 and area 3a, which is one of the main receiving areas of group 1 muscle afferents in the monkey. We know that in the cat there are connections between area 4 and area 3a. How do neurons in area 4 in the monkey use the muscle afferents as feedback signals to adjust output when the animal performs movements? Do you think that in the monkey there is a direct projection from thalamus relaying peripheral muscle afferents to the motor cortical area?

Jones: I am fairly convinced that in the monkey area 3a is not furnishing a direct connection to area 4. Certainly we have not been able to demonstrate a connection in these single-cell preparations. One possibility is that a direct input from the thalamus conveys group I muscle afferents to area 4. I don't like this idea because our work indicates that the anterior part of the ventral posterior nucleus in which those afferents terminate projects solely to area 3a. Something may come up through the spinothalamic tract, but I don't like this idea either. My last resort is that something is projecting back from area 3a into areas 1 and 2, and these are known to project to area 4. I believe that some of these corticocortical axons are large enough for the latency to be quite short.

Marsden: Is the thalamic nucleus in humans that some stereotactic surgeons call VIM (and lesion to relieve tremor) equivalent to your anterior VP?

Jones: They are probably recording in the anterior part of VP, but this is not the equivalent of VIM in humans. The equivalent of VIM is the cerebellar territory. Recently, Tasker's group in Canada has reported new stereotactic results that seem to confirm this.

Marsden: So the VIM projects directly to motor cortex?

Jones: Yes.

Marsden: Does VIM receive a proprioceptive input anatomically?

Jones: By analogy with the monkey any proprioceptive input can only be through the cerebellum itself or through the spinothalamic tract, not through the medial lemniscus. That is not via directly projecting group I muscle afferents.

Porter: That will remain a problem for some time between those who have recorded electrophysiological responses in the thalamus and motor cortex and those who have done the anatomy of projections from muscle afferents.

Jones: You just can't do the anatomy on the human.

Kuypers: When you talk about the motor cortex do you mean area 4?

Jones: Not necessarily.

Kuypers: If I interpret your drawings properly then I must conclude that corticospinal fibres which descend from your VLo area show a very different termination in the spinal cord than the fibres from, e.g., the hand area which would form part of the cerebellar area. I wonder what is the meaning of a VLo projection to the rostral part of the corticospinal area, which, according to Woolsey (1958), carries representation of axial and girdle movements?

Jones: One has to use some of the older nomenclature but I would be quite happy to throw out the old names and talk about the pallidal region and the cerebellar region. But then, as you rightly say, there are other ways of dividing this up in terms of output.

Lemon: We made recordings some years ago from the border zone between Olszewski's VPL and the tissue just rostral to it. A microelectrode penetration in this border zone would encounter clusters of cells which projected to the postcentral gyrus and had typical 'lemniscal' properties. In the same penetration, less than 250 μm from these cell clusters we found other cells which projected to the precentral gyrus and also had 'lemniscal'-type responses at very short latency (4–8 ms) (Lemon & Van der Burg 1979). The thalamic boundaries are therefore not as precise as is sometimes suggested, so some of the cells in area 4 may get a fast input from the periphery, via either a spinothalamic or a lemniscal route. Bob Porter's experiments with sections of the dorsal columns seemed to abolish most of the fast sensory responses in area 4 cells in the monkey (Brinkman et al 1978).

Jones: The boundaries between thalamic nuclei in atlases are always straight lines but in reality there is always a lot of interdigitation. I agree entirely that you can jump within a space of 100 μm to postcentrally and precentrally projecting cells.

The second part of your question is more difficult to answer. Obviously if cells are side by side the dendrites could well be intermingling and there could easily be some cross-talk. Hirai and I have recently tried to look at that intracellularly in the cat. We have not been able to demonstrate any activation from lemniscus, or from dorsal horn stimulation, of cells projecting to the equivalent of the precentral gyrus, though the terminations of those studied are anatomically very close together.

References

Brinkman J, Bush BMJ, Porter R 1978 Deficient influences of peripheral stimuli on precentral neurones in monkeys with dorsal column lesions. J Physiol (Lond) 276:27–48

DeVito JL, Anderson ME 1982 An autoradiographic study of efferent connections of the globus pallidus in Macaca mulatta. Exp Brain Res 46:107–117

Lemon RN, Van der Burg J 1979 Short-latency peripheral inputs to thalamic neurones projecting to the motor cortex in the monkey. Exp Brain Res 36:445–462

von Bonin G, Bailey P 1947 The neocortex of Macaca mulatta. University of Illinois Press, Urbana, Illinois

Woolsey CN 1958 Organization of somatic sensory and motor areas of the cerebral cortex. In: Harlow HF, Woolsey CN (eds) Biological and biochemical bases of behavior. University of Wisconsin Press, Madison, p 63–81

Input and output organization of the supplementary motor area

M. Wiesendanger, H. Hummelsheim[1], M. Bianchetti[2], D.F. Chen, B. Hyland, V. Maier and R. Wiesendanger

Institut de Physiologie, Université de Fribourg, CH-1700 Fribourg, Switzerland

Abstract. Recent work on the supplementary motor area (SMA) in *Macaca fascicularis* led to the conclusion that this area is involved mainly in the preparation of self-paced movements. Results are presented indicating that the posterior portion of the SMA is also directly involved in movement execution and that it receives various sensory inputs. The main results are as follows: (1) The SMA has direct access to the spinal cord by way of corticospinal neurons, but the density of these neurons is lower than in the primary motor cortex (MI). (2) Intracortical microstimulation effects can be elicited in the SMA. Facilitatory effects on ongoing EMG activity can even be produced by single micropulses (8/s). The shortest latencies are compatible with an oligosynaptic or monosynaptic transmission. (3) SMA neurons respond (as do MI neurons) to external perturbations. (4) Anatomical tracing studies revealed that basal ganglia outflow to the SMA via the thalamus is important; our results suggest that dentate outflow contributes as well. (5) Many cells of the SMA may covary with conditioned movements in the same way as MI neurons do. It is argued that it is difficult to compare the lead-time of MI and SMA neurons since 'early' discharges may be coupled with anticipatory postural events.

1987 Motor areas of the cerebral cortex. Wiley, Chichester (Ciba Foundation Symposium 132) p 40–62

[1]*Present address:* Rehabilitationszentrum, University of Cologne, Cologne, FRG.
[2]*Present address:* Augenklinik, Kantonsspital Aarau, Aarau, Switzerland.

The supplementary motor area (SMA) was originally defined with the mapping technique of electrical stimulation of the cortical surface. The name was coined by Penfield who applied this technique during neurosurgery. Penfield & Welch (1951) also explored the monkey cortex, where the SMA was found to occupy a strip of mesial cortex approximately congruent with cytoarchitectonic area 6 on the mesial wall. The well-known simiusculus representation, derived from the work of Woolsey and coworkers (1952), conveys the notion of a secondary motor cortex with a complete body representation, exerting its control of the motor apparatus in parallel with and independently of the primary motor cortex (MI) of area 4. However, recent discoveries about the SMA have led to a remarkable change in views about this area, in that it is now believed to be hierarchically superior and crucially involved in movement initiation and in the programming of motor subroutines. Many of the relevant and fascinating results were obtained from studies of neurological deficits in patients with localized lesions, studies of regional cerebral blood flow and recordings of electrical macropotentials preceding the onset of voluntary movements (cf. recent reviews of Goldberg 1985 and Wiesendanger 1986). It was rarely possible in these human studies to identify precisely the areal involvement in cytoarchitectonic terms, and it is likely that the 'mesial, bilaterally organized premotor system' transgressed cytoarchitectonic boundaries, sometimes also including the medial prefrontal cortex and the limbic cortex.

The question then arises of whether the SMA is a 'supramotor' associational cortical field or whether it is part of the motor cortex as originally proposed.

One classical way to answer this type of question is to identify the principal inputs and outputs of the given structure. Thereby one can hope to gain insight into its functional 'specialization'. Since one of the goals of this symposium is to differentiate subfields of the motor cortex, some problems will be addressed in this paper that are related to the input–output organization of the SMA, as revealed by anatomical and electrophysiological techniques. Experimental results obtained in monkeys have led us to the conclusion that the SMA indeed shares many features with MI and that the SMA, at least in monkeys, can still be considered to be a subfield of the motor cortex. Our electroanatomical work revealed that the SMA is particularly (but not exclusively) related to trunk and shoulder muscles. We present preliminary results which tend to support the proposition (Wiesendanger 1986) that neurons within the SMA are involved in postural preparation for learnt movements.

Inputs to the SMA

The SMA as here defined, i.e. mesial area 6, is part of the agranular frontal cortex. The transition from area 4 into area 6 is gradual, with disappearance of the giant Betz cells and a thinning of the cortex. Rostrally, the SMA lies beside mesial area 8, which gradually acquires the features of the frontal granular cortex. We have explored the thalamic (Wiesendanger & Wiesendanger 1985a) and other connections with the SMA by injecting retrograde and anterograde tracers into various portions of area 6 (SMA). In agreement with a similar study by Schell & Strick (1984), we found heavy anterograde and retrograde labelling in that subdivision of the 'motor thalamus' known to receive a major contingent of pallidal afferents, i.e. the VLo nucleus. Some of our SMA injections, however, also labelled thalamic nuclei previously shown to receive cerebellar nuclear inputs. Thus, an injection centred in the rostral

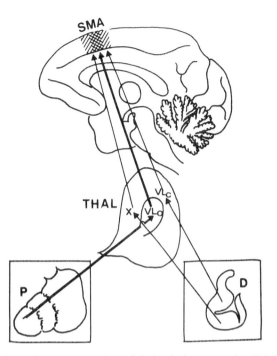

FIG. 1.   Schematic representation of thalamic inputs to the SMA (based on Wiesendanger & Wiesendanger 1985a, b). A major source is the oral part of the ventrolateral
nucleus (VLo) which in turn receives its afferents from the pallidum (P). In addition,
the SMA also receives thalamic afferents from the caudal portion of the ventrolateral
nucleus (VLc) and from area X. These two latter thalamic nuclei relay signals from the
cerebellar dentate nucleus (D) to the SMA.

SMA labelled a thalamic slab occupying some of both VLc and area X (this
labelled area was medial to the one labelled after postarcuate injections and
lateral to that labelled after mesial prefrontal cortex injections). These
observations led us to suggest that cerebellar information has access to the
SMA via the thalamus. This proposition was supported by the discovery that
a lectin-bound tracer substance (wheat germ agglutinin-horseradish peroxidase; WGA–HRP) injected into the SMA labelled portions of the contralateral dentate nucleus via trans-synaptic transport (this transport occurred
after a survival period of five days and was possibly favoured by the intimate
glomerular encapsulation of cerebellar afferent terminals and thalamocortical
neurons). From these observations (Wiesendanger & Wiesendanger 1985b)
we concluded that both basal ganglia outflow and cerebellar outflow are
routed to the SMA. There is a gradual shift from the central portion of the
SMA, dominated by signals from the basal ganglia, to the anterior and the
most posterior portions which are more influenced from the cerebellum. Fig.
1 serves to illustrate, in a simplified way, the major transthalamic re-entrance

loops to the SMA. This anatomical scheme invites two comments regarding function. One is that patients with lesions of the SMA have a characteristic, although transient, poverty of voluntary movements (somewhat akin to parkinsonian akinesia), probably finding its explanation in the powerful transthalamic pallidal inflow to the SMA. The other comment concerns the proposition of a rostro-caudal gradient of inputs that does not reflect a simple somatotopical layout. In monkeys, the anterior SMA furthermore appears to control eye movements (Schlag & Schlag-Rey 1987) and some types of vocalization (Kirzinger & Jürgens 1982). This is consistent with the differential thalamic input, the connections with the lateral frontal eye field (Wiesendanger & Wiesendanger 1984, Hummelsheim et al 1986a), and the relations with some other association areas (Jürgens 1984).

Do SMA neurons have sensory properties?

It is well known that MI neurons receive from mechanoreceptors a massive input that is likely to play an important role in active touch (Phillips 1986). It was found that SMA neurons are much less sensitive to peripheral perturbations or skin stimuli (Wise & Tanji 1981, Brinkman & Porter 1979). In our studies in the monkey, *Macaca fascicularis* (Wiesendanger et al 1985), we confirmed that, as a rule, cutaneous stimulation does not activate SMA neurons. However, systematic microelectrophysiological explorations in the caudal half of the SMA revealed clusters of neurons responding powerfully to passive elbow flexions and extensions (Fig. 2). Although the overall incidence of responsive neurons to that particular kinaesthetic stimulus was only 15% (the same as in the study of Wise & Tanji 1981), we feel that this low proportion in part reflects the intermingled and patchy somatotopy (see below). 'Good' penetrations (i.e. with clusters of cells with striking somatosensory responses) alternated with many penetrations without responding neurons. This positive finding suggests that in the appropriate somatotopical locations of the posterior SMA, somatosensory feedback signals may play an important role. The responsive SMA neurons were not antidromically excited by peduncle stimulation (with two exceptions) and may therefore represent a population without descending projections. When SMA neurons were tested manually with various manoeuvres of passive limbs, a trend towards rostro-caudal somatotopy emerged from the pooled results. In individual monkeys the striking feature was, however, the intermingling and overlap in the somatotopic representation. It is now clear from the work of Tanji and coworkers (e.g. Tanji & Kurata 1985, Kurata & Tanji 1985) that not only somatosensory but also auditory and visual signals are transmitted to the SMA. In their experiments, the sensory signals often evoked a response only if they served as a trigger for the conditioned movement. In this respect, SMA neurons appear to be similar to those of the premotor cortex (Kurata & Tanji 1986).

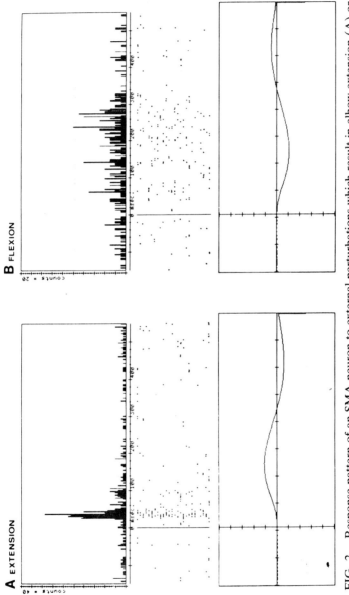

FIG. 2.   Response pattern of an SMA neuron to external perturbations which result in elbow extension (A) or flexion (B). Upper panels are peristimulus time histograms with dot rasters below. Lower panels show the handle displacements produced by a brief (80 ms) load pulse applied to the handle. Peak-to-peak excursion was 15°. Note that the response for elbow extension occurs at about 20 ms when the displacement is minimal. (Unpublished record from experiments on awake, passive monkeys; Wiesendanger et al 1985.)

Addressing the spinal cord and other outputs of the SMA

It is now firmly established that the SMA projects directly to the spinal cord, as corticospinal cells have been identified both anatomically and microelectrophysiologically (Murrary & Coulter 1981, Macpherson et al 1982a, b). The density is, however, clearly inferior to that of the limb representations of area 4. The average cell size is relatively small and the conduction velocity is accordingly low. That the SMA is part of the 'excitable cortex' was also demonstrated by intracortical microstimulation. Positive evidence (with currents lower than 30 μA) was found in the posterior half of the SMA. The microexcitable regions were small and 'patchy'. Threshold intensities were, on average, higher than in area 4. As with sensory responses, intracortical microstimulation effects revealed a fine-grained somatotopical relationship with a weak trend towards rostro-caudal organization (Hummelsheim et al 1986b). The efferent microzones of the SMA appear to be more intermingled, with nearby foci addressing relatively distant muscle groups. The corticospinal neurons of the SMA may also have many collaterals embracing distant segments of the spinal cord.

Repetitive surface stimulation complicates the interpretation because some of the effects were found to be relayed via the precentral cortex (Penfield & Welch 1951, Wiesendanger et al 1973). This may also be the case with prolonged intracortical microstimulation (Macpherson et al 1982a, Mitz & Wise 1987). Furthermore, motor effects may also be mediated indirectly via brainstem centres. To circumvent this difficulty we have used the method of single-pulse triggered averaging of ongoing EMG activity, introduced by Cheney & Fetz (1985). This method allows one to detect short-latency modulations in the EMG after single-pulse stimulation in area 4. Micropulses (30 μA) were applied at rates of 8/s in the SMA and, for comparison, in area 4 at sites where train intracortical microstimulation was effective. It became clear that post-pulse modulations were rarely seen when the SMA was stimulated. Nevertheless at positive sites ($n = 20$) the modulations occurred at surprisingly short latencies (6.2–12 ms for trunk and arm muscles) in the same range as those obtained by stimulation of MI. This is electrophysiological evidence for a sparse but fairly direct (oligosynaptic or even monosynaptic) projection to spinal motor neurons from the SMA. Whether corticospinal fibres originating in the SMA terminate in the ventral horn has not been settled by anatomical methods (Brinkman 1982, Cheema et al 1983).

To what extent does the SMA contribute to the transcerebellar corticocortical loop via the pontine nuclei and the thalamus, or to the trans-striatal loop via the pallidum and the thalamus? Anterograde tracers revealed a patchy projection in the most medial portion of the ipsilateral pontine nuclei, with occasional patches also contralaterally in the same area. The projection was situated more medially and was less powerful than the projection from area 4 (Dhanarajan et al 1977, Wiesendanger & Wiesendanger 1985b). The SMA projection to the corpus striatum is heavy. Our results confirm those of Künzle (1978) showing labelled segments near the caudate nucleus and the putamen, near where these nuclei are separated by the capsular fibres. It has been suggested that the putamen is mainly a component of a 'motor loop' traversing the basal ganglia and that the caudate nucleus is a component of 'complex' loops (DeLong et al 1983). It is interesting to note that the projection from the SMA appears to be straddling both loops. This perhaps reflects the dual nature of an SMA with 'motor' functions caudally and more complex functions rostrally.

Motor commands, sensory cues and preparatory set

In the past eight years recordings from single units in secondary motor areas have revealed a wide variety of activity patterns related to some aspects of learnt movements. Typically, MI neurons discharge with a sharp peak of about 80–100 ms before movement onset. Similar discharge patterns were also observed in SMA neurons and in premotor cortex neurons. However, the major interest in these latter regions was focused on those neurons which discharged in association with movement preparation, i.e. 'while the monkey waits' (cf. Evarts et al 1984 for review, and Tanji, this volume). Covariations with sensory cues providing advance information about the required forthcoming movement, or changes of activity with 'set', have been seen to precede the focal movement by several hundred milliseconds. The results are of particular interest in view of the proposed role of the human SMA in the programming and initiating of movements, and they seem compatible with the modern view that the SMA is 'upstream' from MI. In the context of this paper, the question may be asked whether the above results, obtained in the monkey, necessarily reflect the transmission of instruction signals from the SMA to MI, the alternative being that the SMA acts in parallel with MI. As might be expected, such a general and perhaps also somewhat naive question cannot be answered in a simple way. Although the discovery of cellular activity related to advance information or set provides strong arguments in favour of the 'supramotor' hypothesis, one has to remember that similar set-related neurons were also seen in MI (e.g. Tanji & Evarts 1976). Here we wish to offer an additional explanation for 'early' lead times of neuronal discharges in the SMA. It has been suggested (Wiesendanger 1986) that early activity preceding movements may be related to anticipatory postural preparation or to muscle tensing when the animal expects a signal to move. We have collected preliminary but potentially revealing results from a monkey trained to perform rapid arm movements, holding and moving a handle in either flexion or extension direction in response to visual cues (choice reaction task). Electromyographic activity was recorded in the prime movers

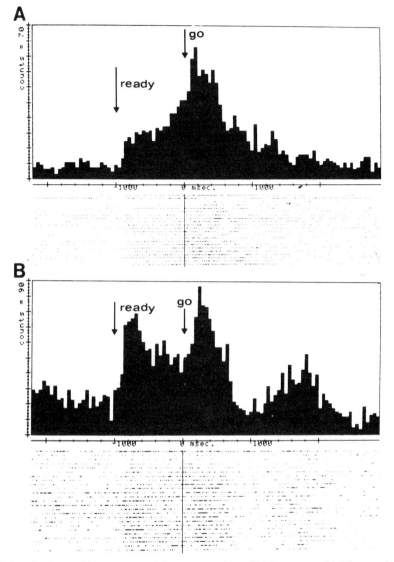

FIG. 3.   Perievent histograms and dot rasters of two SMA neurons (A,B) recorded in a monkey during the performance of a highly trained choice-reaction time task. A yellow light signal tells the monkey to be *ready* for the forthcoming trial, the signal to *go* (green for elbow flexion and red for elbow extension) occurs at time 0. Note increase in activity shortly after the ready signal occurs and a peak of activity after the go signal. No advance information about the required movement direction is provided with the ready signal. In A, there is a gradual build-up of activity during the preparatory phase (ready–go interval), whereas in B there is a more phasic response to the ready signal. Only one movement direction is shown in the histograms of neurons A and B; the preparatory activity was very similar for both movements. (Unpublished data from experiments of Chen, Hyland, Maier and Wiesendanger.)

(biceps and triceps) as well as in a number of shoulder, forearm and trunk muscles. About 150 neurons have so far been recorded in the SMA and in the MI arm area. Handle position, rectified and filtered EMG and neuronal spike data were digitized on-line (sampling interval 5 ms). The computer also controlled the timing of the experimental protocol and recorded the following events: (1) onset of a light inviting the monkey to prepare for the following trial, (2) onset of the 'go' signal telling the monkey to flex or to extend, (3) onset of movement, (4) target reaching and (5) reinforcement. Position, EMG and neuronal activity were then plotted off-line, separately for the two movement directions and aligned to any of the above events. We report here on a subset of SMA neurons that displayed activity changes after the ready signal and before the go signal (Fig. 3).

Thus far, we have recorded 69 SMA and, for comparison, 57 MI neurons which showed some relation with the behavioural paradigm. Among these neurons, we found 27 SMA neurons (39%) and an equal proportion of 22 MI neurons (39%) which changed their activity between the ready signal and the go signal. (No advance information about the direction of the next movement was given by the ready signal.) Typically, the activity change was expressed as a slow tonic build-up (seven SMA neurons and four MI neurons) or as a tonic increase followed by a peak or trough of activity around the time of move-ment onset (20 SMA neurons and 18 MI neurons). Such early neuronal changes (up to about 900 ms before movement onset) may indeed reflect programming of subsequent activity in MI neurons controlling prime movers. However, in contrast to Mauritz & Wise (1986), who found no anticipatory EMG activity in their behavioural paradigm, we observed early EMG changes in some muscles in the preparatory (waiting) period. An example of such 'preparatory' EMG activity in the pectoralis is shown in Fig. 4. Similar changes were also seen in wrist flexors and extensors and even in the prime movers. This striking result suggests that SMA neurons with early pre-movement activity changes may be engaged in direct control of postural and ancillary muscles during an evolving synergy. Of course, these observations in no way invalidate the interpretation that SMA neurons also transmit in-structions or signals about set to MI neurons (as one might also anticipate from the anatomical data).

The arguments about the hierarchically superior position of the SMA often concern the timing of activity changes in the SMA compared to MI, in relation to a focal movement. However, movement onset may be defined either by the first deviation of a kinematic variable or by EMG onset, or even by still earlier pre-movement EMG silence (Conrad et al 1983). For most natural arm movements the synergies, as revealed by multi-EMG rcordings, show a relatively complex pattern and timing of the various muscles. For example, in our task the activation of some shoulder muscles preceded that of the biceps and triceps muscles by about 100 ms. Thus, the lead time of neural

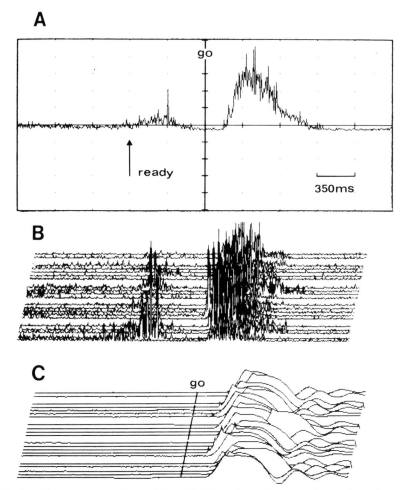

FIG. 4.   Electromyographic activity (EMG) and position signals obtained from the
same monkey performing a choice-reaction task. A: average of rectified EMG activity
recorded with surface electrodes from the biceps muscle (22 trials of flexion movements only). B: EMG activity of successive single trials. C: angular position signal
provided by the potentiometer of the handle. Choice-reaction time was about 200 ms.
Note anticipatory EMG activity (without movement of the handle) occurring during
the preparatory period (i.e. between ready and go signals). All traces are aligned to
the go signal. (Unpublished data from experiments of Chen, Hyland, Maier and
Wiesendanger.)

activity in these muscles would be different. Perhaps it will be possible in the
future to establish the principal relation by means of intracortical microstimulation at the recording sites. Furthermore, statements about the lead
time become difficult if, as in the present experiments, muscular activity
changes even before the start signal, i.e. during the preparation time.

Conclusions

Considerable interest in the function of the SMA has been produced by observations on the human brain that suggest this area is a supramotor rather than a supplementary motor area (e.g. Orgogozo & Larsen 1979). However, it is not so clear whether the SMA, as originally defined by electrical surface stimulation and cytoarchitectonics, accounts for all the invoked complex ('higher') functions. Moreover, with the phylogenetic expansion of the frontal lobe, including the medial frontal cortex, in the human brain, it is difficult to establish homologies with the subhuman primate brain. This paper has considered the input–output organization of the SMA in the macaque. Many anatomical and physiological properties of the SMA are, in essence, similar to those of MI. In our opinion, it is therefore justified to include the SMA as a subfield of the motor cortex. Nevertheless, there are notable differences in the organizational details of the SMA and MI. These differences include the thalamic inputs, the corticocortical connections, the descending connections with subcortical targets (especially with the corpus striatum, the red nucleus, and the pontine nuclei), and the density of corticospinal connections. We have shown that neurons in the SMA, similarly to MI neurons, display a transient modulation just before and during movements. We have also shown that, in a considerable proportion of SMA neurons, there is a slow build-up of activity long before movement onset, i.e. during the preparatory period. We argued that this early change in cellular activity may reflect not only motor set but also the control of anticipatory postural changes or tensing when the start signal is expected.

However, similar early discharges during movement preparation have also been found in neurons of the prefrontal and premotor cortex (e.g. Kubota et al 1974, Fuster et al 1982, Mauritz & Wise 1986), and even in MI (Kubota & Funahashi 1982, Tanji & Evarts 1976, Lecas et al 1983). The difference is probably mainly in the number of such 'preparatory neurons', with a decreasing gradient from the prefrontal cortex to the primary motor cortex (Kubota 1985). Even within the SMA it seems that there is also a rostro-caudal gradient, with the caudal portion being more akin to MI and the rostral portion more like the prefrontal cortex. It may well be that, in the human brain, the rostral division of the SMA with its complex function expands more than the caudal division.

Acknowledgements

The work in our laboratory was supported by the Swiss National Science Foundation (Grant No. 3.522–0.83) and the Thomas Stanley Johnson Foundation. We are grateful to Mrs S. Rossier for typing the manuscript. Brian Hyland was supported by the New Zealand MRC and Neurological Foundation. D.F. Chen was an IBRO fellow, and H. Hummelsheim was a DFG fellow. We also thank R. Jensen for computer programming.

References

Brinkman C 1982 Supplementary motor area (SMA) and premotor area (PMC) of the monkey brain: distribution of degeneration in the spinal cord after unilateral lesions. Neurosci Lett Suppl 8:S36

Brinkman C, Porter R 1979 Supplementary motor area in the monkey. Activity of neurons during performance of a learned motor task. J Neurophysiol 42:681–709

Cheema S, Rustioni A, Whitsel BL 1983 Corticospinal projections from precentral and supplementary cortices in macaques as revealed by anterograde transport of horseradish peroxidase. Neurosci Lett Suppl 14:S62

Cheney PD, Fetz EE 1985 Comparable patterns of muscle facilitation evoked by individual corticomotoneuronal (CM) cells and by single intracortical microstimuli in primates: evidence for functional groups of CM cells. J Neurophysiol 53:786–804

Conrad B, Benecke R, Goehmann M 1983 Premovement silent period in fast movement initiation. Exp Brain Res 51:310–313

DeLong MR, Georgopoulos AP, Crutcher MD 1983 Cortico-basal ganglia relations and coding of motor performance. Exp Brain Res Suppl 7:30–40

Dhanarajan P, Rüegg DG, Wiesendanger M 1977 An anatomical investigation of the corticopontine projection in the primate (*Saimiri sciureus*). The projection from motor and somatosensory areas. Neuroscience 2:913–922

Evarts EV, Shinoda Y, Wise SP (eds) 1984 Neurophysiological approaches to higher brain functions. Wiley, New York, 198 p

Fuster JM, Bauer RH, Jervey JP 1982 Cellular discharge in the dorsolateral prefrontal cortex of the monkey in cognitive tasks. Exp Neurol 77:679–694

Goldberg G 1985 Supplementary motor area structure and function: reviews and hypotheses. Behav Brain Sci 8:567–616

Hummelsheim H, Pause M, Hefter H, Mauritz KH 1986a Afferent and efferent connections of the supplementary motor area (SMA) with other cortical motor centres. Neurosci Lett Suppl 26:S490

Hummelsheim H, Wiesendanger M, Bianchetti M, Wiesendanger R, Macpherson J 1986b Further investigations of the efferent linkage of the supplementary motor area (SMA) with the spinal cord in the monkey. Exp Brain Res 65:75–82

Jürgens U 1984 The efferent and afferent connections of the supplementary motor area. Brain Res 300:63–81

Kirzinger A, Jürgens U 1982 Cortical lesion effects and vocalization in the squirrel monkey. Brain Res 233:299–315

Kubota K 1985 Prefrontal and premotor contributions to the voluntary movement in learned tasks. Exp Brain Res 58:A8

Kubota K, Funahashi S 1982 Direction-specific activities of dorsolateral, prefrontal and motor cortex pyramidal tract neurons during visual tracking. J Neurophysiol 47:362–376

Kubota K, Iwamoto T, Suzuki H 1974 Visuokinetic activities of primate prefrontal neurons during delayed-response performance. J Neurophysiol 37:1197–1212

Künzle H 1978 An autoradiographic analysis of the efferent connections from premotor and adjacent prefrontal regions (areas 6 and 9) in *Macaca fascicularis*. Brain Behav Evol 15:185–234

Kurata K, Tanji J 1985 Contrasting neuronal activity in supplementary and precentral motor cortex of monkeys: II. Responses to movement triggering vs. nontriggering sensory signals. J Neurophysiol 53:142–152

Kurata K, Tanji J 1986 Premotor cortex neurons in macaques: activity before distal and proximal forelimb movements. J Neurosci 6:403–411

Lecas JC, Requin J, Vitton N 1983 Anticipatory neuronal activity in the monkey precentral cortex during reaction time foreperiod: preliminary results. Exp Brain Res Suppl 7:120–127

Macpherson JM, Marangoz C, Miles TS, Wiesendanger M 1982a Microstimulation of the supplementary motor area (SMA) in the awake monkey. Exp Brain Res 45:410–417

Macpherson J, Wiesendanger M, Marangoz C, Miles TS 1982b Corticospinal neurones of the supplementary motor area of monkeys. A single unit study. Exp Brain Res 48:81–88

Mauritz KH, Wise SP 1986 Premotor cortex of the rhesus monkey: neuronal activity in anticipation of predictable environmental events. Exp Brain Res 61:229–244

Mitz AR, Wise SP 1987 The somatotopic organization of the supplementary motor area: intracortical microstimulation mapping. J Neurosci 7:1010–1021

Murray EA, Coulter JD 1981 Organization of corticospinal neurons in the monkey. J Comp Neurol 195:339–365

Orgogozo JM, Larsen B 1979 Activation of the supplementary motor area during voluntary movements in man suggests it works as a supramotor area. Science (Wash DC) 206:847–850

Penfield W, Welch K 1951 The supplementary motor area of the cerebral cortex. Arch Neurol Psychiatry 66:289–317

Phillips CG 1986 In: Movements of the Hand. The Sherrington Lectures XVII. Liverpool University Press, Liverpool, p 125–126

Schell GR, Strick P 1984 The origin of thalamic inputs to the arcuate premotor and supplementary motor areas. J Neurosci 4:539–560

Schlag J, Schlag-Rey M 1987 Evidence for a supplementary eye field. J Neurophysiol 57:179–200

Tanji J 1987 Neuronal activity in the primate non-primary cortex is different from that in the primary motor cortex. This volume, p 142–150

Tanji J, Evarts EV 1976 Anticipatory activity of motor cortex neurons in relation to direction of an intended movement. J Neurophysiol 39:1062–1068

Tanji J, Kurata K 1985 Contrasting neuronal activity in supplementary and precentral motor cortex of monkeys. I. Responses to instructions determining motor responses to forthcoming signals of different modalities. J Neurophysiol 53:129–141

Wiesendanger M 1986 Recent developments in studies of the supplementary motor area of primates. Rev Physiol Pharmacol Biochem 103:1–59

Wiesendanger M, Wiesendanger R 1984 The supplementary motor area in the light of recent investigations. Exp Brain Res Suppl 9:382–392

Wiesendanger M, Séguin JJ, Künzle H 1973 The supplementary motor area—a control system for posture? In: Stein RB et al (eds) Control of posture and locomotion. Plenum, New York, p 331–346

Wiesendanger M, Hummelsheim H, Bianchetti M 1985 Sensory input to the motor fields of the agranular frontal cortex: A comparison of the precentral, supplementary motor, and premotor cortex. Behav Brain Res 18:89–94

Wiesendanger R, Wiesendanger M 1985a The thalamic connections with medial area 6 (supplementary motor cortex) in the monkey (*Macaca fascicularis*). Exp Brain Res 59:91–104

Wiesendanger R, Wiesendanger M 1985b Cerebello-thalamic linkage in the monkey as revealed by transcellular labeling with the lectin wheat germ agglutinin conjugated to the marker horseradish peroxidase. Exp Brain Res 59:105–117

Wise SP, Tanji J 1981 Neuronal responses in sensorimotor cortex to ramp displacements and maintained positions imposed on hindlimb of the unanesthetized monkey. J Neurophysiol 45:482–500

Woolsey CN, Settlage PH, Meyer DR, Spencer W, Hamuy TP, Travis AM 1952 Patterns of localisation in precentral and 'supplementary' motor areas and their relation to the concept of a premotor area. Res Publ Assoc Res Nerv Ment Dis 30:238–264

DISCUSSION

Freund: What is known about the effect of sensory inputs, other than proprioceptive inputs, on the activity of SMA cells?

Wiesendanger: We never saw responses to pure cutaneous stimuli; all somatosensory responses were obtained with passive movements of the limbs or of the trunk, suggesting that the SMA is indeed dealing mostly with proprioceptive input. Although we did not study visual or auditory stimuli systematically, we never saw responses to such stimuli in the passive monkey. But we know from Jun Tanji's study (Tanji & Kurata 1982) that visual and auditory signals may readily activate SMA cells if these signals have a definite meaning for the monkey's performance.

Tanji: I agree. If you give the monkey a meaningless visual or auditory stimulus the neurons do not respond, but if the stimulus triggers a movement or is an instruction for forthcoming movement, the neuron reacts.

Deecke: The idea that SMA is upstream of MI is very acceptable. Although macropotentials cannot really prove this, there is evidence that the readiness potential preceding finger movement starts earlier at the midline than it does at the lateral precentral region. However, the instruction to initiate movement may be conveyed from SMA to MI not only directly but also via the cerebellum or basal ganglia and back to the motor cortex.

Wiesendanger: In my opinion it is difficult to classify cortical areas in terms of their hierarchical position. Although the 'upstream' or 'supramotor' hypothesis has been in the foreground in recent discussions about the SMA, I wanted to emphasize the bulk of evidence suggesting that the primary motor cortex and the SMA also operate much in *parallel*.

Kuypers: Cheema et al (1983) injected WGA–HRP into the macaque's supplementary motor cortex and obtained anterograde labelling of fibres to the spinal intermediate zone but not to the motor neuronal cell groups.

In the context of the present discussion, it is perhaps worth remembering that the cortex is a sandwich. One slice characteristically contains the neurons of the descending projections while the other contains only neurons which establish corticocortical connections. Projections from the supplementary motor cortex to the precentral motor cortex come mainly out of the top slice (Muakkassa & Strick 1979), while the projections to the spinal cord come out of the bottom slice.

Jones: I don't like the idea of the cortex as a sandwich but the layers are certainly inextricably linked. It would be difficult to divorce superficial layer activity from deep layer activity.

Cheney: It is pleasing to see that others are beginning to use single-pulse microstimulation in the presence of background EMG activity to analyse the organization of descending input to motor neuron pools. Single-pulse microstimulation has several advantages over using high frequency trains of microstimuli to evoke movements, including (1) the ability to accurately measure the latency of output effects, (2) detection of inhibitory as well as excitatory effects, and (3) quantification of the magnitude of effects. This approach should continue to prove useful in examining linkages between various brain areas and motor neuron pools.

Jones: In looking at connectivity as a mechanism for activity and behaviour we tend to focus on single channels but there are numerous levels of connectivity within the thalamus and cortex. There is a basic relay channel for information flow, and in terms of the SMA this is still composed primarily of the outflow from the pallidum. On top of that there is a series of what we might call diffuse or non-specific connections running through thalamus and all of these seem to be associated with the cortical arousal system in its wider sense. We should not think of any cortical area as being unifunctional, nor should we think of the layers as unifunctional: the layers are interrelated. Any cortical area has multiple inputs and these may terminate in a whole variety of different layers. The visual system, for example, has a multiplicity of different cell types even within one thalamic nucleus, and these can activate different layers and different constellations of neurons within the visual cortex. Some of these may not even talk to one another. The channels they form may project separately right out to the paravisual areas. Although it is good to focus on a single level, which is about all we can resolve in most of our techniques, multiple levels of analysis may be involved.

Wiesendanger: The SMA is a relatively small area and it doesn't make sense that the whole of the huge output from the basal ganglia is concentrated there alone. In fact there is good, mainly anatomical, evidence that almost the entire frontal cortex receives ascending inputs from the basal ganglia. Alexander et al (1986) recently reviewed these data, which so far have revealed five relatively independent trans-striatal loops that feed back to the frontal lobe, including the prefrontal association cortex, the frontal eye field and cingulate areas as well as SMA. Some of these 'complex' trans-striatal loops, which involve association cortex, are systems that in the human brain develop relatively more than the system making up the 'motor loop'.

Roland: Are there two separate functional areas, a rostral part in front of SMA and a more caudal part, the SMA proper, with limb-regulating functions? Jürgens (1984) showed that the rostral part, which may belong to area 6 or area 8, also receives afferents from area 7. If so, it is certainly organized quite differently from the SMA. Melamed & Larsen (1979) found increases in front of the SMA proper. Other laboratories have also found that oculomotor responses are located in front of the SMA, or at least in the rostral part of SMA. In experiments in which there were several oculomotor responses per minute but no other motor activity we found that the rostral part of SMA was activated whereas SMA itself was not (Roland 1982, Roland et al 1981). Furthermore, I am told by the neuroanatomists that it is very difficult to make a sharp distinction between dysgranular and agranular frontal areas. So should we regard the rostral part as functionally and anatomically different from the caudal area?

Wiesendanger: This becomes a matter of definition. If we accept the criteria of surface stimulation, lesions and cytoarchitectonics (mesial area 6), then the portion of the SMA which is anterior to Peter Strick's SMA 'arm area', but within mesial area 6, indeed appears to have different connections and functions from the posterior arm area of SMA.

Strick: The question of whether separate 'rostral' and 'caudal' subdivisions exist within the SMA is a difficult one to answer. Even defining the anatomical borders of the SMA is not easy. Our approach to the general problem of functional borders has been to define and focus our studies on the *arm area* of each cortical region. This ensures that we don't fall into the trap of comparing the connections and functional properties of the arm area of one cortical area with the face area of another.

Using this approach there are a number of general conclusions that can be made about the topographic organization of the SMA. The arm area of the SMA lies in area 6 on the medial wall of the hemisphere (Woolsey et al 1952). It is located at levels largely caudal to the posterior extent of the arcuate sulcus. This region of the SMA projects directly to the arm area of primary motor cortex and to cervical segments of the spinal cord (e.g. compare Muakkassa & Strick 1979 with Martino & Strick 1987). Furthermore, forelimb movements can be evoked by intracortical stimulation of this region (e.g. Macpherson et al 1982). The representations of the face and hindlimb in the SMA lie rostral and caudal to the arm representation. However, the exact extent of these representations and their borders with adjacent cortical areas have not been easy to determine.

Calne: In these elegant comparisons between the motor cortex and SMA can one use drugs (such as 1-methyl-4-phenyl-1,2,3,6-tetrahydropyridine, MPTP) which knock out the striatal system to separate the kinds of responses that you are obtaining?

Wiesendanger: The idea of using drugs that modify basal ganglia output for studying possible functional changes in the SMA is intriguing. One might predict that MI and SMA neurons would behave differently under a drug such as MPTP. Although there has been a large amount of work, mostly biochemical, on MPTP-treated monkeys, there is to my knowledge no published work on activity patterns of MI and SMA neurons related to disordered behaviour.

Goldman-Rakic: I am confused about whether you think SMA is upstream or not. You seemed to be raising a very interesting possibility, that SMA may issue motor commands independently of the motor cortex.

Wiesendanger: We were asked to be provocative, and I therefore stressed the 'parallel hypothesis'. But I also mentioned that our own results do not allow us to reject the 'upstream' hypothesis.

Porter: This raises an important issue about whether sequential events in the central nervous system drive movement or whether many parallel events in different parts of the brain are operating simultaneously to drive movement.

Goldman-Rakic: Anatomically we might be over-emphasizing the parallel nature of the systems. There may be some convergence in these pathways, although I would not deny that the parallelism is still there. For example, prefrontal cortex projects to both caudate and putamen and both of these project to globus pallidus, but we don't know what happens in between. Furthermore, we now know for several thalamic nuclei that a given nucleus can project to multiple cortical targets, thus introducing some divergence into the thalamocortical projections (Kievit & Kuypers 1977, Goldman-Rakic & Porrino 1985). It therefore remains to be seen whether corticostriatal systems are strictly parallel or whether some more complicated processing is going on.

Thach: One question is whether SMA has a hierarchical role in triggering activity of motor cortex in addition to having its own independent output. To answer this question one must look for timing differences between SMA and motor cortex in relation to the onset of movement, and inactivate SMA to see if motor cortex activity is delayed or abolished. I believe Dr Tanji may have done this.

Tanji: I have cooled the area, but not in a paradigm suitable for detecting the timing of the discharge.

Passingham: Another way is to remove SMA completely on both sides. If it is important in triggering behaviour you might expect to see akinesia, for example, but in our experiments we never see it. A week after surgery the monkeys look completely normal.

Porter: The immediate effect of cooling of the cortex may be quite different to the effect of lesions in animals.

Marsden: In relation to parallel distribution of multiple corticocortical circuits through the basal ganglia, what note should one take of Percheron et al's (1984) observation that the large dendritic fields of globus pallidus neurons may embrace the axons of many striopallidal neurons? Doesn't this suggest convergence of striatal output onto pallidal cells?

Porter: That relates to the dendritic fields of cells in all the territories we are discussing. It also relates to the way the output of any one of those cells is distributed. That output goes to a territory in a particular target position but, by means of collaterals, the output from even a single cortical cell can also go to other regions of the cerebral cortex. That other projection greatly increases the problem you are talking about. Very few people other than Dr Shinoda have looked for contacts between incoming fibres and the receiving cells in any particular territory. It is not just a matter of the explosion of the zone occupied by the dendritic tree: it is also a question of the distribution of the input fibres that come within that territory.

Jones: There is, surprisingly, topography within a system in which the fine level of resolution seems to break down. One could always argue for the specificity of connections at different levels of the dendritic tree. At the moment that is how we explain some of these effects but I am not sure how specific some of them really are.

Porter: But large numbers of inputs may be needed for activation to be effective in forwarding transmission from an input system to an output cell.

Jones: That is true for some areas but in others, such as the ventral posterior nucleus, a single EPSP sets cells discharging furiously.

Porter: But you don't know whether that EPSP arises from one fibre.

Marsden: I would like to explore the parallel hypothesis that Mario Wiesendanger introduced, that SMA not only addresses the motor cortex but also is itself a direct motor output zone, receiving its major input from the basal ganglia. What is the relative power of the corticomotoneuronal connections from SMA to different muscles, i.e. proximal versus distal? What proportion of SMA corticomotoneuronal axons have bilateral versus unilateral distributions? In other words, if SMA is a motor output zone, what part of the motor system could it control?

Wiesendanger: In terms of its direct control on the spinal cord, the SMA is certainly weaker than the precentral area. The intracortical microstimulation experiments may emphasize the more direct connections and in those experiments we gained the impression that the SMA controls mainly, but not exclusively, trunk and proximal muscles. The fairly wide distribution of motor effects may mean that the corticospinal neurons originating in the SMA are necessary for linking fractions of movements into a synergy.

*Deecke:*Goldberg (1985), relying on Sanides (1970), pointed out that SMA and MI come from different telencephalic 'bubbles' in ontogeny and also in phylogeny. What implications does this have for their function?

Wiesendanger: Assuming that the SMA acquires hierarchically superior properties in motor control, as seems to be the case for the human brain, the hypothesis of Sanides (1964) that the SMA is phylogenetically old turns out to be a paradox.

Deecke: Its phylogenetic age may reflect the fact that it is more closely related to limbic aspects of brain function.

Kuypers: The two functions of the SMA may be subserved by two different populations of neurons in this area, one of which may be subserved by the

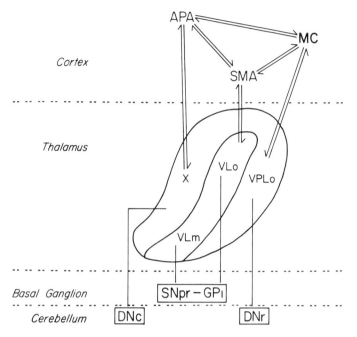

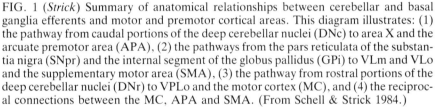

FIG. 1 (*Strick*) Summary of anatomical relationships between cerebellar and basal ganglia efferents and motor and premotor cortical areas. This diagram illustrates: (1) the pathway from caudal portions of the deep cerebellar nuclei (DNc) to area X and the arcuate premotor area (APA), (2) the pathways from the pars reticulata of the substantia nigra (SNpr) and the internal segment of the globus pallidus (GPi) to VLm and VLo and the supplementary motor area (SMA), (3) the pathway from rostral portions of the deep cerebellar nuclei (DNr) to VPLo and the motor cortex (MC), and (4) the reciprocal connections between the MC, APA and SMA. (From Schell & Strick 1984.)

neurons located mainly in the upper slice of the sandwich, the other by those in the lower slice.

Strick: Not so long ago we believed that there was a single nucleus in the thalamus, the ventrolateral nucleus (VL), which received a convergent input from the cerebellum and the basal ganglia. All of VL was thought to project to a single cortical area, the primary motor cortex. According to this view, the output of the motor cortex was determined in part by the integration of cerebellar and basal ganglia inputs which took place in VL. Recent findings have led to some important changes in these anatomical concepts. It is now clear that the ventrolateral thalamus contains a number of subdivisions. Each subdivision receives input from a distinct subcortical region and projects to a different *motor* area in the frontal lobe. I would like to summarize some of our recent results on this topic. Many of these findings have been more completely presented and discussed in Schell & Strick (1984) and Strick (1985).

At present, it has been possible to define three systems which connect the basal ganglia and cerebellum with motor areas in the cerebral cortex (Fig. 1). At the cortical level these systems include the primary motor cortex (MC) and the two 'premotor' areas in the frontal lobe which project most densely to it, i.e. the supplementary motor area (SMA) on the medial wall of the hemisphere and the arcuate premotor area (APA) in the caudal bank of the arcuate sulcus (e.g. Muakkassa & Strick 1979, Schell & Strick 1984, Strick 1985, Primrose & Strick 1985). Each cortical area is the site of termination of a distinct subcortical pathway. One system originates in the internal segment of the globus pallidus (GPi) and projects to a region of the ventrolateral thalamus (VLo) which innervates the SMA. A second system originates in rostral portions of all three deep cerebellar nuclei (DNr) and projects to a region of the ventrolateral thalamus (VPLo) which innervates the MC. The third system originates in caudal portions of all three deep cerebellar nuclei (DNc) and projects to a region of the ventrolateral thalamus (area X) which innervates the APA.

Another important source of input to each system originates from the parietal lobe. Our analysis of this input (Galyon & Strick 1985) indicates that separate regions of areas 5 and 7 project to each cortical motor area. Furthermore, although some parietal lobe regions project to both the primary motor cortex and a premotor area, no region in the parietal lobe has substantial projections to both premotor areas. Thus, each cortical motor area is a nodal point for inputs from distinct subcortical and parietal lobe regions.

Fig. 1 emphasizes that the three systems are largely parallel and independent at subcortical levels. The possibility for interactions occurs largely at the cortical level where dense interconnections exist between the cortical motor areas. When we examined the pattern of intracortical connections between the primary motor cortex and the two premotor areas (Primrose & Strick 1985) we found that projections to and from the primary motor cortex originate from neurons located in both infragranular and supragranular layers. This pattern of intracortical connections does not define a clear direction of information flow for these motor areas. In fact, recent observations on the origin of corticospinal projections suggest that, for some aspects of their function, the SMA and APA may operate at the same hierarchical level as the primary motor cortex (Martino & Strick 1987). We found that the regions of the SMA and APA which project to the arm area in the precentral gyrus also have direct projections to cervical segments of the spinal cord (Fig. 2). Thus, the premotor areas can influence the control of movement at the spinal level. Furthermore, the independence and parallel organization which characterizes the input organization of these systems is also present in their output organization.

Our concepts regarding the anatomical organization of the central systems involved in the control of movement are thus undergoing significant revision. Descending systems which have direct access to spinal cord mechanisms originate not only from the primary motor cortex but also from premotor areas in the frontal lobe. The spinal projections from the SMA and APA may provide

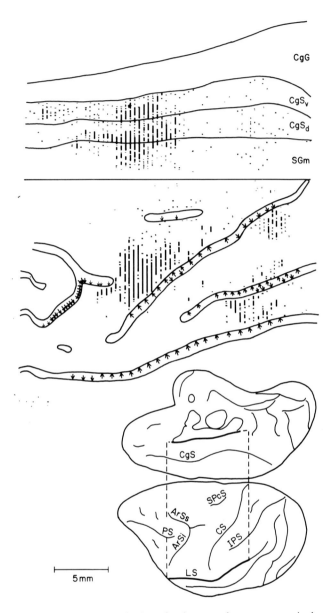

FIG. 2 (*Strick*) Origin of corticospinal projections to the upper cervical segments of macaque spinal cord. A lateral view of the left hemisphere (top) is displayed in this figure. The location of this cortical area is indicated by the dashed lines on the cortical diagram at the bottom. The medial wall is reflected upwards and the cingulate sulcus (CgS) is opened to display its dorsal (CgSd) and ventral banks (CgSv). Labelled neurons on the surface of the cortex are indicated by interrupted lines. Labelled neurons in sulci are indicated by arrows. Note the large number of arrows pointing to labelled neurons in the caudal bank of the arcuate sulcus (ArSi). ArSs, superior limb of the arcuate sulcus; CgG, cingulate gyrus; CgS, cingulate sulcus; CS, central sulcus; IPS, intraparietal sulcus; LS, lateral sulcus; PS, principal sulcus; SGm, medial superior frontal gyrus; SPcS, superior precentral sulcus. (From Martino & Strick 1987.)

important routes for the basal ganglia, cerebellum and parietal lobe to exert their influence on motor output. Furthermore, these routes may be independent of those from the primary motor cortex. Certainly, the primary motor cortex can no longer be viewed as the 'upper motor neuron' or sole 'final common pathway' for the central control of movement.

References

Alexander GE, DeLong MR, Strick PL 1986 Parallel organization of functionally segregated circuits linking basal ganglia and cortex. Annu Rev Neurosci 9:357–381

Cheema SS, Whitsel BL, Rustioni A 1983 Cortico-spinal projections from the pericentral and supplementary cortices in macaques as revealed by anterograde transport of horse-radish peroxidase. Neurosci Lett vol 40 S14:S62

Galyon DD, Strick PL 1985 Multiple and differential projections from the parietal lobes to the premotor areas of the primate. Soc Neurosci Abstr 11:1274

Goldberg G 1985 Supplementary motor area structure and function: review and hypotheses. Behav Brain Sci 8:567–615

Goldman-Rakic PS, Porrino LJ 1985 The primate mediodorsal (MD) nucleus and its projections to the frontal lobe. J Comp Neurol 242:535–560

Jürgens U 1984 The efferent and afferent connections of the supplementary motor area. Brain Res 300:63–81

Kievit J, Kuypers HGJM 1977 Organization of the thalamo-cortical connexions to the frontal lobe in the rhesus monkey. Exp Brain Res 29:299–322

Macpherson JM, Marangoz C, Miles TS, Wiesendanger M 1982 Microstimulation of the supplementary motor area (SMA) in the awake monkey. Exp Brain Res 45:410–416

Martino AM, Strick PL 1987 Corticospinal projections originate from the arcuate premotor area. Brain Res 404:307–312

Melamed E, Larsen B 1979 Cortical activation pattern during saccadic eye movements in human: localization by focal cerebral blood flow increases. Ann Neurol 5:79–88

Muakkassa KF, Strick PL 1979 Frontal lobe inputs to primate motor cortex: evidence for four somatotopically organized 'premotor' areas. Brain Res 177:176–182

Percheron G, Yelnik J, Francois C 1984 A Golgi analysis of the primate globus pallidum. III Spatial organisation of the striopallidal complex. J Comp Neurol 227:214–227

Primrose DC, Strick PL 1985 The organization of interconnections between the premotor areas in the primate frontal lobe and arm area of primary motor cortex. Soc Neurosci Abstr 11:1274

Roland PE 1982 Cortical regulation of selective attention in man. A regional cerebral blood flow study. J Neurophysiol 48:1059–1078

Roland PE, Skinhoj E, Lassen NA 1981 Focal activations of the human cerebral cortex during auditory discrimination. J Neurophysiol 45:374–386

Sanides F 1964 The cyto-myeloarchitecture of the human frontal lobe and its relation to phylogenetic differentiation of the cerebral cortex. J Hirnforschung 6:269–282

Sanides F 1970 Functional architecture of motor and sensory cortices in primates in the light of a new concept of neocortex evolution. In: Noback C, Montagna W (eds) The primate brain. Appleton-Century-Crofts, New York (Adv Primatol vol 2)

Schell GR, Strick PL 1984 The origin of thalamic inputs to the arcuate premotor and supplementary motor areas. J Neurosci 4:539–560

Strick PL 1985 How do the basal ganglia and cerebellum gain access to the cortical motor areas? Behav Brain Res 18:107–123

Tanji J, Kurata K 1982 Comparison of movement-related activity in two cortical motor
    areas of primates. J Neurophysiol 48:633–653
Woolsey CN, Settlage PH, Meyer DR, Sencer W, Hamuy TP, Travis AM 1952 Patterns
    of localization in the precentral and "supplementary" motor areas and their relation
    to the concept of a premotor area. Res Publ Assoc Res Nerv Ment Dis 30:238–264

Some aspects of the organization of the output of the motor cortex

H.G.J.M. Kuypers

Department of Anatomy, University of Cambridge, Downing Street, Cambridge, CB2 3DY, UK

Abstract. The precentral motor cortex in the macaque is defined here as that portion of the precentral motor-sensory areas which projects to the intermediate zone and motor neuronal cell groups in the spinal cord and their bulbar counterparts, i.e. the lateral reticular formation and motor nuclei of the lower brainstem. In this respect the precentral motor cortical areas differ from postcentral areas such that the descending projections from the latter are focused on the spinal dorsal horn and the spinal V complex. Differences in the distribution of the corticospinal fibres in different species are mentioned and differences in findings obtained by means of different tracing techniques are discussed. The projections from the precentral motor cortex to various brain-stem cell groups are also discussed and the areas of origin of these projections are delineated. The presence of branching neurons distributing collaterals to several of these areas is considered.

1987 Motor areas of the cerebral cortex. Wiley, Chichester (Ciba Foundation Symposium 132) p 63–82

The neuronal networks of the brain create behaviour by ordering the execution of different movements and movement complexes which allow the organism to achieve certain goals. The descending connections from the motor cortex constitute one of the channels through which the messages that ultimately will be translated into movements and movement complexes are transmitted to the effector organs, i.e. the assembly of motor neurons and muscles. The general organization of these descending connections in cat and monkey are the subject of this paper.

The motor cortex in the macaque will be defined as the precentral corticospinal area which projects to the spinal intermediate zone, containing the bulk of the interneurons, and to spinal motor neuronal cell groups (Kuypers 1964). This corticospinal area comprises area 4 and probably also the caudal portion of area 6 (Catsman-Berrevoets & Kuypers 1976). This corticospinal area corresponds roughly to the precentral motor cortex of Woolsey and his collaborators (Woolsey 1958). This precentral corticospinal area is distinct from the supplementary motor cortex which projects only to the spinal intermediate zone and not to the motor neuronal cell groups. In the macaque, the entire precentral corticospinal area projects to the spinal intermediate zone, but only the caudal parts of this cortical area also project to motor neuronal cell groups (Kuypers 1960). In the chimpanzee (and probably also in the human) a slightly different arrangement may exist because in the lower third of the precentral gyrus the corticobulbar fibres from the rostral bank of the central sulcus are distributed exclusively to bulbar motor neuronal cell groups, while the fibres from the convexity of the precentral gyrus also project to interneurons (cf. Kuypers 1964).

In cat and monkey the corticospinal fibres from the different parts of the precentral corticospinal area are distributed to different parts of the spinal cord and to different parts of the spinal grey matter. The present paper deals mainly with this distribution pattern. In order to clarify the structure of this distribution pattern, it is useful first to sketch briefly the terminal distribution of the descending brainstem pathways in the spinal grey matter, because these pathways recognize certain subdivisions of the intermediate zone which are also recognized by the corticospinal fibres.

At least three groups of descending brainstem pathways to the spinal cord can now be distinguished. Two of these groups, i.e. the ventromedial and the lateral groups, terminate mainly in the intermediate zone. They appear to form each other's counterparts, in that they terminate in opposite parts of this zone. The third group of descending brainstem pathways distributes fibres to all subdivisions of the spinal grey matter, i.e. the dorsal horn, intermediate zone and motor neuronal cell groups. The ventromedial group of brainstem pathways descends through ventral and medial parts of the medullary cross-section. This group is composed of the fibres descending from the interstitial nucleus of Cajal, the mesencephalic and pontine medial reticular formation, the superior colliculus, the dorsal part of the magnocellular medullary reticular formation and the vestibular nuclei (Nyberg-Hansen 1966, Basbaum et al 1978, Holstege & Kuypers 1982). These pathways, some of which terminate bilaterally, have largely overlapping termination areas in the ventromedial parts of the intermediate zone, i.e. in lamina VIII and the adjoining medial parts of lamina VII (Fig. 1). Several of these pathways tend to be of the diffuse type, with many of their fibres distributing collaterals to both the cervical and the lumbar cord (Wilson & Peterson 1981). These pathways also distribute some fibres to the motor neuronal cell groups, especially those innervating axial and proximal muscles (Shapovalov 1972). The cell groups which give rise to these various pathways all distribute fibres to the pontine and medullary medial reticular formation, but avoid the lateral reticular formation (Kuypers 1964).

The lateral group of brainstem pathways descend laterally through the brainstem into the spinal dorsolateral funiculus. The most outstanding component pathways are the rubrobulbar and rubrospinal tracts which originate from the contralateral red nucleus and the dorsally adjoining mesencephalic reticular formation (Holstege & Kuypers 1982, Holstage 1987). The fibres of these tracts are distributed to the lateral reticular formation of the brainstem, the lateral part of the facial nucleus (innervating muscles around the eye and the mouth) and the arca of the dorsal column nuclei (cf. Fig. 5 in Kuypers 1964, Holstege 1987). In the spinal cord the rubrospinal fibres terminate in the dorsal and lateral parts of the intermediate zone (i.e. lateral parts of lamina V, lamina VI and dorsal parts of lamina VII) (Nyberg-Hansen 1966, Holstege & Kuypers 1982) (Fig. 1). Some rubrospinal fibres are also distributed to motor neuronal cell groups innervating distal extremity muscles (Shapovalov 1972, Holstege 1987). The laterally descending crossed pontospinal tract also distributes fibres to dorsal and lateral parts of the intermediate zone, but in addition provides a limited projection to the most superficial layers of the dorsal horn (Holstege & Kuypers 1982). The rubrospinal tract in monkey and cat represents a relatively focused system in that most of its fibres are distributed to one of the two enlargements, while relatively few fibres give off collaterals to both (Huisman et al 1982). The crossed pontospinal tract, on the other hand, is much more diffuse (Huisman et al 1982).

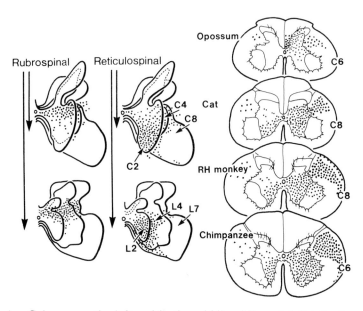

FIG. 1.   Columns on the left and in the middle: differential distribution of rubrospinal and reticulospinal fibres in intermediate zone. (Redrawn from Giovanelli-Barilari & Kuypers 1969.) Column on right: distributions of corticospinal fibres in spinal cord of opossum, cat, rhesus monkey and chimpanzee (updated). (Adapted from Kuypers 1981.)

The differential termination of the two groups of brainstem pathways in the spinal grey matter (Fig. 1) suggests that they subserve different functions. This is supported by several functional findings. Our lesion studies in cat and monkey (Kuypers 1964, Lawrence & Kuypers 1968) suggested that the ventromedial group of brainstem pathways is mainly concerned with steering postural and orienting movements of head or body and with synergistic movements of body and limbs, while the rubrospinal tract is mainly concerned with steering movements of the extremities, especially their distal parts. These conclusions are supported by several other findings (Alstermark et al 1981), especially those from chronic recordings in red nuclei in conscious monkeys (Kohlerman et al 1982).

The functional differences between these two groups of brainstem pathways, in regard to the steering of movements, probably reflects the different ways in which the recipient neurons in the two different parts of the intermediate zone (Fig. 1) are related to the motor neurons. This would imply that the fibre connections from the cortex to these two different parts of the intermediate zone would, like the two groups of brainstem pathways, show differences in function.

Anterograde degeneration findings showed that in the macaque monkey the corticospinal fibres from the pericentral cortical areas are distributed to the dorsal horn mainly contralaterally, to the dorsal and lateral parts of the intermediate zone mainly contralaterally, to the ventromedial parts of the intermediate zone bilaterally and to the motor neuronal cell groups of distal extremity muscles mainly contralaterally (Kuypers & Brinkman 1970) (Fig. 2). These anterograde degeneration findings are confirmed by recent anterograde transport findings with wheat germ agglutinin–horseradish peroxidase (WGA–HRP) (Cheema et al 1984). These findings also showed that the postcentral corticospinal fibres to the dorsal horn are distributed not only to lamina IV but also to laminae I, II and III (Cheema et al 1984).

The anterograde degeneration findings following various precentral lesions (Kuypers & Brinkman 1970) showed that in the macaque fibres from different parts of the precentral corticospinal area are distributed to different parts of the spinal cord and to different parts of the spinal grey matter (Fig. 2).

Small lesions in approximately the 'hand area' of the motor cortex (Woolsey 1958), extending 2–5 mm along the central sulcus and involving the anterior bank of the central sulcus as well as the immediately adjoining portion of the convexity of the precentral gyrus, produced fibre degeneration in the contralateral spinal grey matter from C_2 to T_4. This fibre degeneration involved the dorsal and lateral parts of the intermediate zone (i.e. lamina V, lamina VI, and the dorsal and lateral parts of the lamina VII), and the dorsal parts of the lateral motor neuronal cell groups in C_7, C_8 and T_1 (Fig. 2). Similar small lesions in approximately the 'foot area' on the convexity of the hemisphere and on its medial aspect (Woolsey 1958) produced fibre degen-

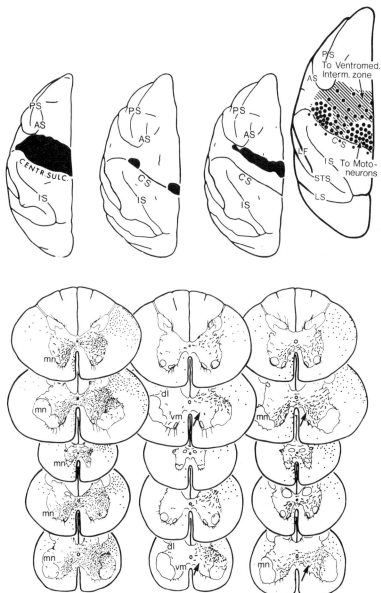

FIG. 2. Distributions of corticospinal fibre degeneration in ventromedial (vm) and dorsal-lateral (dl) parts of intermediate zone and motorneuronal (mn) cell groups in macaque after precentral lesions. Note: distributions to dorsal-lateral intermediate zone and motorneuronal cell groups after lesions of hand and foot areas and to ventromedial part of intermediate zone after rostral lesion. Upper right: diagram of precentral origin of projections to ventromedial intermediate zone and motorneuronal cell groups. (Adapted from Kuypers 1981).

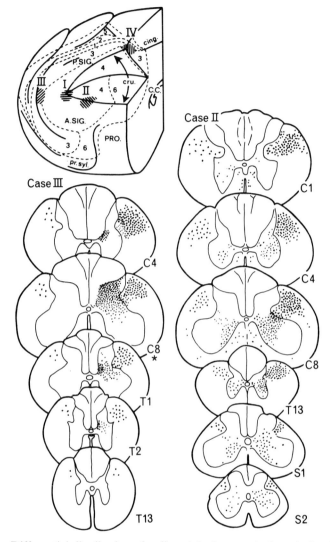

FIG. 3. Differential distribution of radioactivity in cat spinal cord after injections of small quantities of tritiated leucine in different parts of sensory motor cortex. Note presence of radioactivity in ventromedial intermediate zone in case II and absence in case III. Cruciate sulcus (cru.) is opened; A. Sig., anterior sigmoid gyrus; C.C., corpus callosum; pr. sylv., presylvian sulcus; P. Sig., posterior sigmoid gyrus; PRO, gyrus proreus. (Redrawn from Armand et al 1985.)

eration contralaterally in the dorsal and lateral parts of the intermediate zone of T_{10} to S_1, combined with degeneration in the dorsal parts of the motor neuronal cell groups in L_5, L_6, L_7 and S_1 (Fig. 2). Thus, the distribution of the degeneration in the intermediate zone in the cervical and the lumbosacral segments largely coincided with the distribution of the rubrospinal fibres in these areas.

When the lesion in the hand area was moved 5 mm medially along the central sulcus, the same distribution of degeneration was found in the cervical and upper thoracic segments as in the previous cases, except that the degeneration in the intermediate zone extended more ventrally and also involved its ventromedial part, i.e. the medial parts of lamina VII and lamina VIII, on both sides. This ventral extension of the distribution of the degeneration in the intermediate zone resembled the terminal distribution of the ventromedial group of brainstem pathways (Fig. 1) and was even more pronounced after a very narrow lesion extending 1 cm along the central sulcus at the level of the superior precentral dimple. In this case, the degeneration involved the ventromedial parts of the intermediate zone on both sides, throughout the length of the spinal cord, although it was most pronounced at the cervical levels. Further, virtually no degeneration was present in the cervical motor neuronal cell groups but some was present in the lumbosacral motor neuronal cell groups. A similar distribution pattern, but without any fibre degeneration in the motor neuronal cell groups, was observed throughout the spinal cord after mediolateral lesions involving the rostral parts of the precentral corticospinal area (Fig. 2) and in the caudal half of the spinal cord after a lesion on the medial surface of the hemisphere 1–1.5 cm rostral to the level of the central sulcus.

In the animals with a bilateral distribution of the degeneration in the ventromedial parts of the intermediate zone, some of the fibres in the dorsolateral part of the contralateral intermediate zone may have been fibres of passage. However, fibre termination in this area could not be excluded. Therefore, on the basis of the above findings, it could only be stated that the rostral parts of the precentral corticospinal area, together with a portion of the cortex along the central sulcus at the level of the superior precentral dimple, are characterized by a bilateral distribution of corticospinal fibres to the ventromedial parts of the intermediate zone, combined with a minimum or an absence of direct corticomotoneuronal projections. This distribution contrasts sharply with that obtained from the hand and foot representation areas along the central sulcus. These areas were found to represent the main sources of the direct corticomotoneuronal connections, and were found to project almost exclusively to the dorsal and lateral parts of the contralateral intermediate zone (Fig. 2).

A comparison of the above findings with those regarding the descending brainstem pathways (Fig. 1) suggested that the projections from the hand and foot representation areas to the intermediate zone, like those from the red nucleus, presumably deal mainly with steering movements of the extremities, in particular their distal parts. The additional direct corticomotoneuronal connections from these areas (Fig. 2) can be expected to provide the capacity to execute highly fractionated movements of the distal extremities (Lawrence & Kuypers 1968). The projections from the anterior portion of the precentral corticospinal area (and from the small intermediate area in the posterior part of the precentral gyrus) to the ventromedial parts of the intermediate zone (Fig. 2) probably subserve a function similar to that of the ventromedial brainstem pathways (Fig. 1). Thus, these projections probably contribute to the steering of movements of the body axis, of postural and orienting movements of head and body, and of synergistic limb–body movements. These projections could also be expected to contribute to guiding the direction of progression. Such an organization is in keeping with findings after lesions of different parts of the precentral corticospinal area and has much in common with the findings of Woolsey and his collaborators (Woolsey 1958).

In keeping with this general design, we found that the rostral part of the precentral corticospinal area, together with the rostral parts of area 6, represents the main source of the cortical projections to the upper medullary medial reticular formation (Kuypers & Lawrence 1967, Catsman-Berrevoets & Kuypers 1976) which contributes fibres to the ventromedial groups of brainstem pathways. According to anterograde degeneration (Kuypers & Lawrence 1967) and anterograde amino acid transport findings (Hartman-von Monakow et al 1979), the caudal part of the precentral corticospinal area, which includes the hand and foot representation areas, represents the main source of the somatotopically organized corticorubral projections to the ipsilateral magnocellular red nucleus which projects to the dorsolateral parts of the spinal intermediate zone. This conclusion is supported by some retrograde horseradish peroxidase transport findings (Catsman-Berrovoets et al 1979), but is slightly at variance with others. These projections from the rostral and caudal parts of the precentral corticospinal area to the upper medullary reticular formation and the magnocellular red nucleus are closely related to the cortical projections from these areas to the spinal cord, in that some of the cortical fibres to the magnocellular red nucleus and some of the fibres to the medial medullary reticular formation represent collaterals of the corticospinal fibres from the different parts of the precentral corticospinal area (Humphrey & Rietz 1976). As to the projections to the upper medullary reticular formation, the existence of such collaterals has been demonstrated recently by K. Keizer, H.G.J.M. Kuypers and R. van der Vlies (unpublished observations), using the retrograde fluorescent double labelling technique. (In this same study, we also found that many of the corticospinal neurons in the area of the supplementary motor cortex distribute collaterals to the upper medullary medial reticular formation.)

Recent anterograde WGA–HRP transport findings (Cheema et al 1984) and anterograde labelled amino acid transport findings (Armand et al 1985) showed that the corticospinal fibres in the cat are distributed to the spinal grey matter in roughly the same pattern as in the macaque, except that in cat no cortical fibres are distributed to the motor neuronal cell groups (Fig. 1). Several retrograde HRP transport findings (e.g. Armand & Kuypers 1980) demonstrated that the corticospinal motor cortex in cat, i.e. area 4 and the adjoining lateral part of area 6 (Keizer & Kuypers 1984), comprises two different types of cortical zones, i.e. a specific zone and a common zone. The specific zone consists of two areas, one in the medial and one in the lateral part of the motor cortex, corresponding approximately to the hand and foot representation areas (Nieoullon & Rispal-Padel 1976). These two areas distribute fibres only contralaterally and project to the cervical and the lumbosacral enlargements, respectively (e.g. Armand & Kuypers 1980). The common zone, on the other hand, occupies the medial part of the motor cortex next to area 6 and extends caudally into the region between the two specific areas. This common zone projects bilaterally to both enlargements (Armand & Kuypers 1980) and tends to carry the representations of axial movements, neck and body movements and proximal forelimb movements (Nieoullon & Rispal-Padel 1976). Anterograde labelled leucine transport findings (Armand et al 1985) indicated that at least part of this common zone and of the specific zone behave in much the same way as the corresponding parts of the monkey's motor cortex. The common zone (Fig. 3) projects bilaterally to the ventromedial parts of the intermediate zone throughout the spinal cord. The two areas of the specific zone, on the other hand, distribute fibres contralaterally to the dorsal and lateral parts of the intermediate zone (Fig. 3) of the cervical and the lumbosacral enlargements, respectively (Armand et al 1985). These findings, combined with those of Nieoullon & Rispal-Padel (1976), demonstrate that the spatial organization of the motor cortex in cat is very similar to that in the monkey (Woolsey 1958); the areas carrying the representation of axial and proximal movements, in cat and monkey, characteristically project bilaterally to the ventromedial parts of the intermediate zone and those carrying the hand and foot representations project contralaterally to the dorsal and lateral parts of the intermediate zone. However, these cortical areas in the cat do not project to the motor neuronal cell groups. Interestingly enough, in the cat these cell groups do receive such fibres from the red nucleus (Shapovalov 1972, Holstege 1987).

Anterograde degeneration findings (Kuypers 1964) showed that, in the cat, the caudal parts of the pericruciate motor cortex project to the magnocellular red nucleus. On the other hand, the area comprising the rostral and medial parts of the motor cortex, including area 6, represents the main source of the corticobulbar projections to the upper medullary medial reticular formation (Kuypers 1958). These findings are in keeping with the anterograde labelled leucine transport findings (Armand et al 1985). Electrophysiological findings have shown that some of these cortical fibres to the rubrospinal portion of the red nucleus represent collaterals of corticospinal fibres. Moreover, retrograde fluorescent double labelling (Keizer & Kuypers 1984) showed that some of

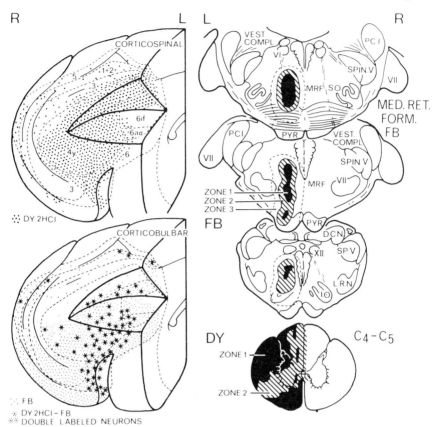

FIG. 4.   Distribution of double-labelled neurons in medial part of cat sensory motor cortex after injections of Fast Blue in lower brainstem medial reticular formation and ipsilateral injections of diamidino yellow dihydrochloride (DY.2HC1) in $C_4 - C_5$. (Adapted from Keizer & Kuypers 1984.)

the fibres from the medial parts of the motor cortex (i.e. the common zone) to the medullary medial reticular formation also represent collaterals of corticospinal fibres (Fig. 4).

    These various findings point to the existence of a common basic design in the organization of the efferent connections from cortex and brainstem in cat and monkey (Fig. 5). This basic design in the efferent connections pertains not only to the anatomy of the fibre connections but also to their functional contributions to the steering of movements. Further insight into the design hinges on further clarification of the differences in the interneuronal-motor neuronal relationships between the interneurons in the different parts of the intermediate zone. Perhaps the different sets of interneurons in the different parts of the intermediate zone possess the same characteristics as some of the

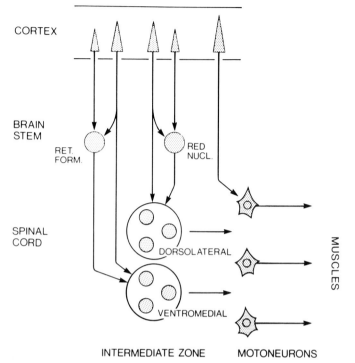

FIG. 5. Diagram illustrating cortical connections to brainstem cell groups, spinal intermediate zone and motor neuronal cell groups.

descending pathways which terminate on them, in that the interneurons in the ventromedial parts of the intermediate zone represent a diffuse system, while those in the dorsal and lateral parts represent a focused system. In other words, the individual interneurons in the former area may maintain widespread connections with a variety of motor neurons in a large portion of the spinal cord, while those in the latter area may maintain connections with a limited set of motor neurons in a rather restricted part of the spinal cord. However, it should be kept in mind that the data on the connections of the spinal motor neurons obtained by electrophysiological and retrograde transneuronal tracing techniques may not immediately reveal these types of differences in the connections of the various groups of interneurons.

Acknowledgements

The author wishes to thank Miss Susan Insole for her help with the illustrations and Miss Anne Wright for typing the manuscript.

References

Alstermark B, Lundberg A, Norsell U, Sybirska E 1981 Integration in descending motor pathways controlling the forelimb in the cat. Differential behavioural defects after spinal cord lesions interrupting defined pathways from higher centers to motoneurons. Exp Brain Res 42:299–318

Armand J, Kuypers HGJM 1980 Cells of origin of crossed and uncrossed corticospinal fibers in cat. A quantitative horseradish peroxidase study. Exp Brain Res 40:23–34

Armand J, Holstege G, Kuypers HGJM 1985 Differential corticospinal projections in the cat. An autoradiographic tracing study. Brain Res 343:351–355

Basbaum AI, Clanton CH, Fields HL 1978 Three bulbospinal pathways from the rostral medulla of the cat: An autoradiographic study of pain modulating systems. J Comp Neurol 178:209–224

Catsman-Berrevoets CE, Kuypers HGJM 1976 Cells of origin of cortical projections to the dorsal column nuclei, spinal cord and bulbar medial reticular formation in the Rhesus monkey. Neurosci Lett 3:245–252

Catsman-Berrevoets CE, Kuypers HGJM, Lemon RN 1979 Cells of origin of the frontal projections to magnocellular and parvocellular red nucleus and superior colliculus in cynomolgus monkey. An HRP study. Neurosci Lett 12:41–46

Cheema SS, Rustioni A, Whitsel BL 1984 Light and electron microscopic evidence for a direct corticospinal projection to superficial laminae of the dorsal horn in cats and monkeys. J Comp Neurol 225:276–290

Giovanelli-Barilari M, Kuypers HGJM 1969 Propriospinal fibers interconnecting the spinal enlargements in the cat. Brain Res 14:321–330

Hartman-von Monakow K, Akert K, Kuenzle H 1979 Projections of precentral and premotor cortex to the red nucleus and other midbrain areas in Macaca fascicularis. Exp Brain Res 34:91–106

Holstege G 1987 Rubrobulbar and rubrospinal pathways in the cat. An HRP and autoradiographic study. Behav Brain Res Special Issue: Red Nucleus, in press

Holstege G, Kuypers HGJM 1982 The anatomy of brain stem pathways to the spinal cord in cat. A labeled amino acid tracing study. In: Kuypers HGJM, Martin GF (eds) Descending pathways to the spinal cord. Elsevier, Amsterdam (Prog Brain Res vol 57) p 145–175

Huisman AM, Kuypers HGJM, Verburgh CA 1982 Differences in collateralization of the descending spinal pathways from red nucleus and other brain stem cell groups in cat and monkey. In: Kuypers HGJM, Martin G F (eds) Descending pathways to the spinal cord. Elsevier, Amsterdam (Prog Brain Res vol 57) p 185–217

Humphrey DR, Rietz RR 1976 Cells of origin of corticorubral projections from the arm area of primate motor cortex and their synaptic actions in red nucleus. Brain Res 110:162–169

Keizer K, Kuypers HGJM 1984 Distribution of corticospinal neurons with collaterals to lower brain stem reticular formation in cat. Exp Brain Res 54:107–120

Kohlerman NJ, Gibson Ar, Houk JC 1982 Velocity signals related to hand movements recorded from red nucleus neurons in monkeys. Science 217:857–860

Kuypers HGJM 1958 An anatomical analysis of cortico-bulbar connexions to the pons and lower brain stem in the cat. J Anat 92:189–218

Kuypers HGJM 1960 Central cortical projections to motor and somato-sensory cell groups. An experimental study in the Rhesus monkey. Brain 83:161–184

Kuypers HGJM 1964 The descending pathways to the spinal cord, their anatomy and function. In: Eccles JC, Schadé JP (eds) Organization of the spinal cord. Elsevier, Amsterdam (Prog Brain Res vol 11) p 178–200

Kuypers HGJM 1981 Anatomy of the descending pathways. In: Brooks VB (ed) Motor control, pt 1. American Physiological Society, Bethesda, MD (Handb Physiol sect 1 The nervous sytem vol 2) p 597–666

Kuypers HGJM, Brinkman J 1970 Precentral projections to different parts of the spinal intermediate zone in the Rhesus monkey. Brain Res 24:29–48

Kuypers HGJM, Lawrence DG 1967 Cortical projections to the red nucleus and the brain stem in the Rhesus monkey. Brain Res 4:151–188

Lawrence DG, Kuypers HGJM 1968 The functional organization of the motor system in the monkey. II. The effects of lesions of the descending brain-stem pathways. Brain 91:15–36

Nieoullon A, Rispal-Padel L 1976 Somatotopic localization in cat motor cortex. Brain Res 105:405–422

Nyberg-Hansen R 1966 Functional organization of descending supraspinal fibre systems in the spinal cord. Anatomical observations and physiological correlations. Ergebn Anat Entwickl-Gesch 39:6–47

Shapovalov AI 1972 Extrapyramidal monosynaptic and disynaptic control of mammalian alpha-motoneurons. Brain Res 40:105–115

Wilson VJ, Peterson BW 1981 Vestibulospinal and reticulospinal systems. In: Brooks VB (ed) Motor control, pt 1. American Physiological Society, Bethesda, MD (Handb Physiol sect 1 The nervous system vol 2) p 667–702

Woolsey CN 1958 Organization of somatic sensory and motor areas of the cerebral cortex. In: Harlow HF, Woolsey CN (eds) Biological and biochemical bases of behavior. University of Wisconsin Press, Madison, p 63–81

DISCUSSION

Cheney: How do you reconcile your results with those obtained by Humphrey & Reitz (1976) with electrophysiological techniques showing that the corticorubral projection is largely independent of the corticospinal projection?

Kuypers: I did not mean to imply that all cortical fibres to the rubrospinal part of the red nucleus are collaterals of corticospinal fibres. In fact the findings of Humphrey and Reitz clearly indicate the existence of an extensive cortical projection to the rubrospinal neurons which is independent of the corticospinal projection. However, I do not feel that their experiments have decided the relative importance of the two types of corticorubral projection systems. A further point is that stimulation of the red nucleus by Humphrey & Reitz would not have allowed them to distinguish cortical neurons projecting to the rubrospinal part of the red nucleus from cortical neurons projecting to its parvocellular part. For this reason, the observation that only a low proportion of slowly conducting corticorubral fibres were related to the corticospinal fibres (collaterals) may not be entirely accurate.

Cheney: How many cells have collaterals to the red nucleus and how many bypass it?

Kuypers: We have not studied this. However, using the fluorescent double-labelling technique one could approximate the percentage of corticospinal neurons that are branching neurons distributing collaterals to the magnocellular (i.e. the rubrospinal) red nucleus. We have done such a study in regard to the branching corticospinal fibres distributing collaterals to the medullary medial reticular formation (Keizer & Kuypers 1984). Approximating the percentage of cortical neurons distributing collaterals to the rubrospinal part of the red nucleus requires sharply delineated injections limited to the rubrospinal part of the red nucleus, not involving the parvocellular nucleus. Such injections are not easy to obtain. In addition, the rubrospinal part of the red nucleus in monkey extends further forward than is generally assumed (Huisman et al 1982).

Freund: Could you comment further on the output from the frontal eye fields? Secondly, bilateral interaction can be accomplished via the connections between the two hemispheres and the connectivity at the brainstem level. As the pyramidal system is strongly organized unilaterally, what do you regard as the major systems for integrating bilateral movements?

Kuypers: Let me focus on the bilaterality. There seems to be a persistent pattern, in that the cortical projections to the brainstem reticular formation and to the ventromedial parts of the spinal intermediate zone are distributed bilaterally, and the recipient neurons in this spinal area distribute descending propriospinal fibres bilaterally throughout the spinal cord. The ascending components, however, tend to be distributed mainly contralaterally (Molenaar & Kuypers 1978). The bilateral corticobulbar and corticospinal projections in question are derived in the monkey mainly from areas located in the rostral parts of the corticospinal area. These parts, according to Woolsey (1958), carry predominantly the representation of axial and proximal body-limb movements. The fibres from the caudal parts of the motor cortex and in particular those from the hand and foot representation areas are distributed mainly contralaterally. The recipient spinal areas of this contralateral projection contain almost exclusively 'short' propriospinal neurons which are distributed mainly ipsilaterally (Molenaar & Kuypers 1978). Thus the bilateral integration of arm movements, for example, may occur at almost all levels. This bilaterality is probably exemplified by the fact that one half of the brain can steer visually-guided reaching movements of either arm, but can steer visually-guided hand and finger movements only contralaterally (Brinkman & Kuypers 1973). However, the way in which the interhemispheric callosal connections contribute to the bilateral integration of hand and finger movements is unclear to me.

Wu: Could there also be a direct linkage in the cat between corticospinal fibres and the motor neurons, especially their dendritic trees?

Kuypers: Recently, Cheema et al (1984) observed in the cat some cortical fibres anterogradely labelled by WGA-HRP in the dorsolateral part of the lateral motor neuronal cell group. These fibres were present at somewhat odd segments (i.e. C_4–C_6 and L_6). These fibres might establish direct corticomotoneuronal connections, but I think the bulk of the possible direct connections would be established only with the most distal parts of motor neuronal dendrites. For example, according to Cajal the dendrites of the hypoglossal (XII) neurons extend deep into the bulbar lateral reticular formation, where many cortical fibres from the lower third of the precentral gyrus (face area) terminate. Here some direct corticomotoneuronal connections might be established. Further, in the spinal cord the dendrites of the motor neurons of the intrinsic foot muscles extend from this motor nucleus in the low sacral ventral horn dorsomedially into the lateral parts of the intermediate zone, where many of the corticospinal fibres terminate. Here also, some cortical connections with distal motor neuronal dendrites might be established.

Shinoda: Earlier Peter Strick mentioned that there are two corticospinal systems involved in the control of arm movement. In one, corticospinal neurons specifically project to the upper cervical cord and terminate on propriospinal neurons. These neurons, in turn, project to forelimb motor neurons in the lower cervical cord. As far as I understand Dr Lundberg's work, most of the propriospinal neurons at the upper cervical segment of the spinal cord are innervated by axon collaterals of corticospinal axons which project to the lower cervical cord (Illert et al 1975). Our findings of multiple branches of single corticospinal axons agree with his observations (Shinoda et al 1976). That is, virtually all corticospinal axons have multiple branches at different spinal segments. In the 'forelimb area' of the motor cortex very few neurons specifically project to the upper cervical cord without further descending to the lower cord, and the majority of the neurons in that area project to the lower cervical cord with axon collaterals to C_3 and C_4 (Futami et al 1979, Shinoda et al 1986). Therefore, I doubt whether there is a corticospinal system for controlling arm movement in which corticospinal neurons specifically project to the upper cervical cord. Do your data fit in with Peter Strick's interpretation?

Kuypers: Many corticospinal fibres go to those parts of the spinal grey matter where the Göteborg propriospinal neurons are located. Because of technical difficulties, such neurons seem to have been investigated only at C_3 to C_5. However, I expect this population of neurons to extend further caudally into C_8, where many corticospinal fibres also terminate (Armand et al 1985). I am sure that these more caudally located neurons also receive corticospinal collaterals, e.g. the ones you were able to visualize. This is in keeping with the fact that the degeneration after even the smallest lesion of the hand area in the monkey spans almost the whole of the cervical cord (Kuypers & Brinkman 1970).

Strick: You implied that the disynaptic corticospinal pathway which is mediated by interneurons in upper segments of cervical cord is concerned more with the control of axial and proximal musculature than with the control of distal musculature. However, Alstermark & Sasaki (1985) demonstrate that this pathway evokes potent effects on distal as well as proximal motor neurons.

Kuypers: That does not seem to fit, I realize. However, Alstermark and his collaborators (1981) postulated from their movement data after different funicular lesions that the C_3 to C_4 propriospinal neurons can transmit to forelimb motor neurons the command for target-reaching but not for food-taking (with the hand). They also state that this food-taking probably depends on direct activation of neuronal networks within the forelimb segments by way of the corticospinal or rubrospinal tract, or both. This fits entirely with my present data and our earlier data (Kuypers 1964, Lawrence & Kuypers 1968a,b).

Strick: The physiological studies of Lundberg and colleagues (e.g. Alstermark & Sasaki 1985, Illert et al 1976, 1977, 1978) appear to indicate that the disynaptic corticospinal pathway which is mediated by interneurons in upper cervical segments is as potent as the disynaptic pathway mediated by interneurons in lower cervical segments.

Kuypers: I understand what you mean but I can only point to the movement defects and to the postulation of Alstermark and his collaborators that I have just referred to.

Marsden: Do the two populations of interneurons with their different direct cortical and indirect inputs differ in their distribution at the segmental level, say at C_8?

Kuypers: Yes, our available data suggest that they do. Lesion-degeneration findings in the lumbar cord suggested that the intermediate zone neurons projecting to distal motor neurons are located dorsolaterally and in the middle of the intermediate zone, while the neurons projecting to axial motor neurons are located ventromedially. In the middle of the intermediate zone there is a mixture of interneurons projecting to motor neurons of distal and proximal extremity muscles (cf Fig. 4 in Kuypers 1981). Moreover, the neurons in the dorsal and lateral parts of the low cervical intermediate zone, for example, maintain only relatively 'short' propriospinal connections almost exclusively ipsilaterally. Many of the neurons in the ventromedial parts of the intermediate zone, however, maintain long descending propriospinal connections, which are distributed bilaterally (Molenaar & Kuypers 1978). Finally, HRP injections in the dorsolateral parts of the motor neuronal cell groups (distal muscles) produced virtually no retrograde neuronal labelling in the ventromedial parts of the intermediate zone (lamina VIII), while such labelling occurred after HRP injections in the ventral part of the lateral motor neuronal cell groups (proximal muscles) (Molenaar 1978).

Lemon: Michael Illert, who did the original studies with Lundberg on the C_3–C_4 propriospinal pathway in the cat, has been collaborating with us in experiments on the corticomotoneuronal system in the monkey. We were struck by the observation that stimulation of the medullary pyramid produced only weak or no disynaptic EPSPs in distal motor neurons (Fritz et al 1985). There are large monosynaptic EPSPs from the pyramid but the disynaptic EPSPs in these motor neurons are very weak. However, in some cases their existence may be masked by the strong disynaptic IPSPs produced by pyramidal stimulation in these motor neurons.

Shinôda: Did you examine the pyramidal input to biceps motor neurons in the monkey? Were there disynaptic EPSPs in those motor neurons?

Lemon: Yes. In biceps motor neurons the disynaptic EPSPs are more pronounced and the monosynaptic effects are weak or absent. In motor neurons that had a strong monosynaptic input the disynaptic inputs were more difficult to detect.

Strick: Dr Kuypers, in your plots of corticospinal projections to the spinal cord terminations one aspect has always puzzled me. The input to the ventral medial zone is not symmetrical. It is more dense to the ipsilateral cord and lighter to the contralateral ventral medial zone. Have you any explanation for that?

Kuypers: I started out thinking that the input was unilateral and in fact primarily contralateral. However, I could not get round the point that in the majority of cases these corticospinal projections were bilateral. Frequently, there seems to be an intensity difference with an emphasis either ipsilaterally or contralaterally. A certain asymmetry may also occur in human material (Schoen 1964). Such asymmetry might be related to the fact that the ascending fibres from lamina VIII, which are distributed throughout the spinal cord and probably also to the lowest part of the brainstem, are distributed contralaterally (Molenaar & Kuypers 1978).

Strick: You and others have observed that small lesions in the distal forelimb representation of primary motor cortex produce degeneration which extends from C_3 to T_1. Thus, the anatomical evidence is very clear that a localized region of even distal motor cortex innervates a widespread region of the spinal cord and not just the cord segments containing distal motor neurons.

Kuypers: I completely agree with you. However, in our cases it also spanned the upper part of the thoracic cord (Kuypers & Brinkman 1970).

Strick: It spans the cervical cord, even for the most localized lesion of the precentral gyrus.

Porter: That doesn't necessarily imply that motor neurons at all those levels of the cervical cord are engaged by those collaterals. The influence on motor neurons may be limited to a few of those segments of the spinal cord and the branches of a single descending fibre could still engage the motor neurons for only one muscle. As Jenny & Inukai (1983) showed, the motor neurons for a forelimb muscle may occupy a column distributed through three or four segments.

Strick: It is also possible that there are interneurons in upper cervical segments which mediate a disynaptic pathway from the motor cortex to motor neurons in lower cervical segments.

Tanji: In recording from the small area just caudal to the arcuate sulcus I am always impressed with the amount of activity, especially in relation to distal movement. Have you observed anything comparable to that?

Kuypers: The only distribution we found with the anterograde degeneration technique after lesions *rostral* to the arcuate sulcus was an extensive projection to the deeper layers of the superior colliculus (Kuypers & Lawrence 1967). Of course, from the area immediately caudal to the arcuate sulcus there are strong projections to the precentral gyrus, including the rostral bank of the central sulcus (Pandya & Kuypers 1969, Pandya & Vignolo 1971, Muakkassa & Strick 1979).

Marsden: How would you superimpose the input from group Ia afferents onto that spinal interneuronal machinery?

Kuypers: That is a difficult question. Not enough data about the location of the Ia inhibitory interneurons are available yet for that pattern to be compared with the one I presented.

Shinoda: Lundberg and his colleagues clearly showed the existence of propriospinal neurons in C_3 and C_4 innervating forelimb motor neurons, but we don't know whether propriospinal neurons innervating hindlimb motor neurons exist in the pyramidal system and where they are located, if they exist. Do your anatomical observations provide any information about that?

Kuypers: I expect that the same arrangement exists in the lumbosacral cord as in the cervical cord, from our degeneration findings in the macaque (Kuypers & Brinkman 1970), which showed that after very small lesions in the hand area and in the foot area of the precentral gyrus the degeneration spanned the whole length of the cervical and lumbosacral cords, respectively.

Strick: The region where Professor Tanji sees distal limb movements falls within the arcuate premotor area which projects to the arm area of primary motor cortex and upper segments of the cervical spinal cord. That is different from the prearcuate region which has connections with the superior colliculus.

Kuypers: As I said earlier, I agree.

Thach: Is that part of the ventral medial or dorsal lateral system?

Kuypers: I don't know. I have only seen the fluorescent retrograde labelling of corticospinal neurons in the postarcuate area. We have not used injections in this area to determine the spinal distribution of these fibres by the anterograde transport technique. However, the bulk of the postarcuate neurons which project to the hand area of the motor cortex, according to Strick and Muakkassa, are located in the upper part of the cortex. The projecting neurons must be located in deeper parts.

Lemon: Microstimulation studies in area 4 of behaving monkeys that are developing a certain level of voluntary muscle activity show that this muscle activity is often strongly suppressed by microstimulation (Lemon et al 1987). This suppression has probably escaped notice in many studies where people were looking for overt movement or EMG activation, not for suppression of movement or of muscle activity. Corticospinal disynaptic inhibitory pathways might have very widespread effects within the cervical spinal cord. Some of the interneurons that we are seeing in the upper cervical segments may be inhibitory interneurons interposed in this pathway. Perhaps that ties in with the group Ia projection which is another important source of disynaptic inhibition (Jankowska et al 1976).

References

Alstermark B, Sasaki S 1985 Integration in descending motor pathways controlling the forelimb in the cat. 13. Corticospinal effects in shoulder, elbow, wrist and digit motoneurons. Exp Brain Res 59:353–364

Alstermark B, Lundberg A, Norsell U, Sybirska E 1981 Integration in descending motor pathways controlling the forelimb in the cat. Differential behavioural defects after spinal cord lesions interrupting defined pathways from higher centers to motoneurons. Exp Brain Res 42:299–318

Armand J, Holstege G, Kuypers HGJM 1985 Differential corticospinal projections in the cat. An autoradiographic tracing study. Brain Res 343:351–355

Brinkman J, Kuypers HGJM 1973 Cerebral control of contralateral and ipsilateral arm, hand and finger movements in the split-brain rhesus monkey. Brain 96:653–674

Cheema SS, Rustioni A, Whitsel BL 1984 Light and electron microscopic evidence for a direct corticospinal projection to superficial laminae of the dorsal horn in cats and monkeys. J Comp Neurol 225:276–290

Fritz N, Illert M, Kolb FP, Lemon RN, Muir RB, Van der Burg J, Wiedemann E 1985 The cortico-motoneuronal input to hand and forearm motoneurones in the anaesthetized monkey. J Physiol (Lond) 366:10p

Futami T, Shinoda Y, Yokota J 1979 Spinal axon collaterals of corticospinal neurons identified by intracellular injection of horseradish peroxidase. Brain Res 164:279–284

Huisman AM, Kuypers HGJM, Verburgh CA 1982 Differences in collateralization of the descending spinal pathways from red nucleus and other brain stem cell groups in cat and monkey. In: Kuypers HGJM, Martin GF (eds) Descending pathways to the spinal cord. Elsevier, Amsterdam (Prog Brain Res vol 57) p 185–217

Humphrey DR, Reitz RR 1976 Cells of origin of corticorubral projections from the arm area of primate motor cortex and their synaptic actions in the red nucleus. Brain Res 110:162–169

Illert M, Lundberg A, Padel Y, Tanaka R 1975 Convergence on propriospinal neurones which may mediate disynaptic corticospinal excitation to forelimb motoneurones in the cat. Brain Res 93:530–534

Illert M, Lundberg A, Tanaka R 1976 Integration in descending motor pathways controlling the forelimb in the cat. 2. Convergence on neurones mediating disynaptic cortico-motoneuronal excitation. Exp Brain Res 26:521–540

Illert M, Lundberg A, Tanaka R 1977 Integration in descending motor pathways controlling the forelimb in the cat. 3. Convergence on propriospinal neurons transmitting disynaptic excitation from the corticospinal tract and other descending tracts. Exp Brain Res 29:323–346

Illert M, Lundberg A, Padel Y, Tanaka R 1978 Integration in descending motor pathways controlling the forelimb in the cat. 5. Properties of and monosynaptic excitatory convergence on C_3-C_4 propriospinal neurons. Exp Brain Res 33:101–130

Jankowska E, Padel Y, Tanaka R 1976 Disynaptic inhibition of spinal motoneurones from the motor cortex in the monkey. J Physiol (Lond) 258:467–487

Jenny AB, Inukai J 1983 Principles of motor organization of the monkey cervical spinal cord. J Neurosci 3:567–575

Keizer K, Kuypers HGJM 1984 Distribution of corticospinal neurons with collaterals to lower brain stem reticular formation in cat. Exp Brain Res 54:107–120

Kuypers HGJM 1964 The descending pathways to the spinal cord, their anatomy and function. In: Eccles JC, Schadé JP (eds) Organization of the spinal cord. Elsevier, Amsterdam (Prog Brain Res vol 11) p 178–200

Kuypers HGJM 1981 Anatomy of the descending pathways. In: Brooks VB (ed) Motor control, pt 1. American Physiological Society, Bethesda, MD (Handb Physiol sect 1 The nervous system, vol 2) p 597–666

Kuypers HGJM, Brinkman J 1970 Precentral projections to different parts of the spinal intermediate zone in the rhesus monkey. Brain Res 24:29–48

Kuypers HGJM, Lawrence DG 1967 Cortical projections to the red nucleus and the brain stem in the Rhesus monkey. Brain Res 4:151–188

Lawrence DG, Kuypers HGJM 1968a The functional organization of the motor system in the monkey. I. The effects of bilateral pyramidal lesions. Brain 91:1–14

Lawrence DG, Kuypers HGJM 1968b The functional organization of the motor system in the monkey. II. The effects of lesions of the descending brain-stem pathways. Brain 91:15–36

Lemon RN, Mantel GWH, Muir RB 1987 The effects upon the activity of hand and forearm muscles of intracortical stimulation in the vicinity of corticomotor neurones in the conscious monkey. Exp Brain Res 267, in press

Molenaar I 1978 Distribution of propriospinal neurons projecting to different motoneuronal cell groups in cats' brachial cord. Brain Res 158:203–206

Molenaar I, Kuypers HGJM 1978 Cells of origin of propriospinal fibers and of fibers ascending to supraspinal levels. A HRP study in cat and rhesus monkey. Brain Res 152:429–450

Muakkassa KF, Strick PL 1979 Frontal lobe input to primate motor cortex: evidence for four somatotopically organized premotor areas. Brain Res 177:176–182

Pandya DN, Kuypers HGJM 1969 Cortico-cortical connections in the rhesus monkey. Brain Res 13:13–36

Pandya DN, Vignolo LA 1971 Intra- and interhemispheric projections of the precentral, premotor and arcuate areas in the rhesus monkey. Brain Res 26:217–233

Schoen JHR 1964 Comparative aspects of the descending fiber systems in the spinal cord. In: Eccles JC, Schadé JP (eds) Organization of the spinal cord, Elsevier, Amsterdam (Prog Brain Res vol 11) p 203–222

Shinoda Y, Arnold A, Asanuma H 1976 Spinal branching of pyramidal tract neurons in the monkey. Exp Brain Res 26:215–234

Shinoda Y, Yamaguchi T, Futami T 1986 Multiple axon collaterals of single corticospinal axons in the cat spinal cord. J Neurophysiol 55:425–448

Woolsey CN 1958 Organization of somatic sensory and motor areas of the cerebral cortex. In: Harlow HF, Woolsey CN (eds) Biological and biochemical bases of behavior. University of Wisconsin Press, Madison, p 63–81

Functional studies of motor cortex

Robert Porter

John Curtin School of Medical Research, G.P.O. Box 334, Canberra, ACT 2601, Australia

Abstract. Defining functions for neural elements becomes more difficult the more remote they are, in synaptic linkages, from motor neurons. The precentral motor cortex contains a corticomotoneuronal projection system, only one synapse removed from motor neurons. Corticomotoneuronal fibres produce monosynaptic excitation of spinal motor neurons, which is more powerful for those acting distally, innervating extensor muscles of the fingers and intrinsic hand muscles. Latencies and time-course of corticomotoneuronal excitation are defined. Amplitudes of unitary corticomotoneuronal excitatory postsynaptic potentials are very small. Many corticomotoneuronal cells converge on a given motor neuron. Some motor neurons innervating proximally acting muscles appear to receive no corticomotoneuronal excitation. Disynaptic inhibitory actions are produced by corticospinal volleys via the common Ia inhibitory interneuron—possibly reciprocal actions produced over collaterals of corticomotoneuronal fibres. Anatomical divergence of projections of collaterals of an identified corticomotoneuronal fibre is extensive enough to provide both for delivery of synapses to a large number of motor neurons and for the dispersion of specific projections to inhibitory interneurons, to fusimotor neurons and to other interneurons. Functions of corticomotoneuronal elements in motor cortex whose targets have been identified and whose excitatory or inhibitory actions have been specified by cross-correlation have been studied by Fetz & Cheney (J Neurophysiol 1980; 44:751–772).

1987 Motor areas of the cerebral cortex. Wiley, Chichester (Ciba Foundation Symposium 132) p 83–97

Two major approaches are now available which allow functions of neural elements in regions of the brain to be examined. The first involves intracellular microelectrode recordings of the influences exerted on target cells whose function has been established (e.g. motor neurons) by activation of pathways travelling from those regions. The second involves the correlation, in awake, performing animals, of the neuronal discharges of individual cells recorded in conjunction with a defined aspect of behaviour. To be meaningful, the second approach also needs to take account of the anatomical connectivity of the neuron under investigation, a point well understood by the late Ed Evarts, whose carefully planned and insightful pioneering studies were strictly limited to examination of identified pyramidal tract neurons (Evarts 1968, 1969). Evarts' work provides the essential background against which all future advances in analysis of the cortical neural networks operating in control of movement will be made.

Earlier attempts to study motor functions of the cerebral cortex had to rely either on detection of movements produced when regions of the cerebral cortex were stimulated electrically or on deficits of movement performance which could be measured after lesions had been produced in the cerebral cortex. Electrical stimulation and the observation of muscle contractions is a neurophysiological form of cartography which maps the locations from which certain movements and muscles can be activated under the conditions of that experiment and also allows cortical addresses, sometimes multiple, to be specified for particular motor actions. In this sense, functions for the addresses and for the territories in which the addresses are located may be defined. But the 'wrist flexion' territory, for example, also contains addresses of other movements, as re-evaluated recently in a thoughtful review of the representation of movements and muscles within the motor cortex (Humphrey 1986). Moreover, many of the cartographers, finding no convenient way to map simultaneously those addresses which were excitatory and those which could have been as powerfully inhibitory, gave the latter no locations. More recent work, using intracortical microstimulation in conscious animals trained to maintain constant levels of muscle contraction in particular groups of muscles from which electromyograms (EMGs) were simultaneously recorded, makes it clear that the effects obtained from brief, weak microstimulation of any one point in area 4 can be excitatory to some muscles and inhibitory to others. In addition, rebound excitation often follows a period of inhibition of the EMG and could have been interpreted, in palpation of muscle contractions, as a direct excitatory effect from the stimulated cortical locus (Schmidt & McIntosh 1984). The effects produced can be complex and they depend on the phase of the task that the animal is performing when the stimulus is delivered (Cheney & Fetz 1985).

To add to the difficulties of ascribing functions to cortical areas, the removal of a mapped territory by circumscribed cortical lesions in animals, and even in humans, often appears to have little permanent effect on the ability to produce movements whose addresses have been resected. Conversely, lesions in areas of the brain not identified as including the principal addresses of movement can lead to noticeable impairment of movement performance, as occurs when the apraxias result from cortical damage.

If we want to assign a role to a given neural element in the complex network that provides the basis for the initiation and control of movement performance, we should try to define the element's connectivity as well as correlate its discharges with aspects of the movement. This requirement becomes more difficult to achieve the further removed the element under study is, in synaptic linkage terms, from the motor neurons themselves. Yet regional corticocortical connections are being understood in greater and greater

detail. The refinement of modern neuroanatomical methods also allows connections between the cerebral cortex and deep brain structures such as the
thalamus, basal ganglia and cerebellum to be described with precision. So
cell-to-cell connectivity, at least for members of the classes of neural elements
which are sampled in brain regions other than area 4, may soon be available
for examination in conjunction with information about discharge patterns
associated with an aspect of an animal's behaviour. Interpretation of those
discharge patterns will be assisted enormously by knowledge about the connectivity of a particular cell and about the influence (whether excitatory or
inhibitory) that the cell exerts on the neurons it contacts.

It is now well established that there is a class of corticospinal neurons, with
its greatest density in area 4, which makes direct, excitatory monosynaptic
connections with motor neurons (Phillips & Porter 1977). I wish to summarize
the anatomical and physiological descriptions of these corticomotoneuronal
(CM) cells, located as they are only one synapse from the motor neurons. The
factors included in these descriptions make up the passport which specifies
the identity of this class of cortical neuron. The features should be matched,
in as many aspects as possible, when one is detailing functional associations
with the execution of movements attributed to CM discharges in conscious,
performing animals. Observations made on cortical cells whose connectivity
matches that defined for CM projections may be interpreted with considerable confidence. And it must always be remembered that part of the diversity
of response patterns observed in earlier studies by different workers, even for
identified pyramidal tract neurons in area 4, and part of the confusion
generated about coding of force or direction or timing of the initiation of
movement, could have resulted from the fact that pyramidal tract neurons
belong to many different classes having a number of destinations. Area 4 also
contains a majority of non-pyramidal tract neurons projecting to a multitude
of brain targets other than motor neurons, but not necessarily irrelevant to
motor control. Included in these classes are the projections to striatum,
thalamus, pontine nuclei and other cortical areas.

It is important also to bear in mind that the same cortical element, with
fixed connections in a complex network, may behave in a number of different
ways as that brain network changes the particular operation in which it is
engaged. To analyse these different functional relationships of the cortical
element, one must feel secure about the specification of the element's connectivity. Then it is possible to state with great confidence that some CM cells in
the motor cortex, rather than coding for force development in their identified
target muscles in the hand, appear to have a special relationship to the
fractionated use of those muscles in performing the finely adjusted force
development of precision grip activities, for example (Muir & Lemon 1983).

The first requirement in identifying a cell must be its direct monosynaptic
linkage to motor neurons. Intracellular recordings of the monosynaptic

excitatory postsynaptic potentials (EPSPs) generated in motor neurons by weak stimuli delivered to the appropriate territory in area 4 on the cerebral cortex reveal the short latency and characteristic time-course of this CM action (Preston & Whitlock 1961, Landgren et al 1962). The latency of a response in a motor neuron will depend on both the conduction velocity of the CM fibre and the distance to be travelled to the cervical or lumbar enlargement of the spinal cord. It can be stated unequivocally that corticospinal neurons with rapidly conducting axons (50 to 70 m/s) produce monosynaptic CM EPSPs in the cervical motor neurons with very short latencies (1 to 2 ms or less) and in lumbar motor neurons with latencies from 3.5 to 6 ms after a cortical stimulus. It is still not possible to state categorically whether corticospinal neurons with slowly conducting axons contribute direct synapses to motor neurons and whether some truly corticomotoneuronal effects could therefore have much longer latencies.

The time course of CM EPSPs is very similar to that of the monosynaptic EPSPs generated in the same motor neurons by stimulation of group I fibres in the homonymous muscle nerve (Landgren et al 1962, Porter & Hore 1969). Different unitary components of the CM EPSP may have different rise times and durations at half amplitude. But, in general, the characteristic CM EPSP rises to its peak in 1.0 to 2.0 ms and decays rapidly and approximately exponentially thereafter, so that the duration of the CM EPSP at half amplitude is about 6 or 7 ms on average (Porter 1985).

The CM EPSP recorded in a given motor neuron after electrical stimulation of the cerebral cortex or pyramidal tract (Jankowska et al 1975, Shapovalov 1975) may be graded in amplitude, but not significantly in latency or time course, by altering the strength of the stimulus or by moving the stimulating electrode across the surface of the cortex to activate different numbers of CM cells. Each member of the colony of CM cells (so defined because they all contribute excitatory synapses to one motor neuron) makes a very small contribution to the total size of the EPSP that can be generated by simultaneous activation of the colony. Attempts, in incredibly difficult experiments, to measure the size of the unitary excitatory contribution of a single CM fibre have revealed that this will be only 100 microvolts or much less in amplitude (Asanuma et al 1979). This small value is similar to that measured for minimal EPSPs generated by graded stimulation of the cortex or the pyramidal tract (Porter 1985). So, if a given motor neuron exhibits a composite EPSP of 2.0 to 5.0 mV in amplitude when the whole colony is activated, a large number of CM axons (probably at least 50 or 100) must converge onto each such cell.

Although some doubts are raised about the mechanism by which it is produced, temporal facilitation at CM synapses remains a feature of the observations made with surface stimulation of the cortex and intracellular recordings from motor neurons in anaesthetized monkeys (Muir & Porter

1973). Temporal facilitation is also seen when the stimuli are delivered to the pyramidal tract, and one component could certainly be a property of the spinal connections of these fibres. It remains to be demonstrated whether repetitive activation of a single CM fibre reveals temporal facilitation in the excitatory effects at the fibre's synapses. However, cross-correlation studies in conscious animals appear to add to the evidence that temporal facilitation increases the probability of motor unit activation after the discharges of a single CM cell (Fetz & Cheney 1980).

More powerful monosynaptic CM excitatory effects are produced on the motor neurons supplying some muscle groups than are revealed when EPSPs are studied in other motor neurons. The largest EPSPs are recorded in motor neurons supplying muscles which act around the distal joints of the limb. Indeed, in about half of the motor neurons that supply some muscles acting proximally, such as triceps brachii, no measurable CM EPSPs could be recorded even when large stimuli were applied to the cortex. Some of these stimuli produced inhibitory hyperpolarizing potentials in these motor neurons (Phillips & Porter 1964). Clough et al (1968) found that the largest CM EPSPs were recorded in motor neurons supplying the intrinsic muscles of the hand and extensor digitorum communis. Independent confirmation that this differential distribution of CM excitation is strongest to motor neurons supplying hand muscles has recently come from Fritz et al (1985).

Some monosynaptic CM connections are made with fusimotor neurons (Grigg & Preston 1971, Clough et al 1971). At present it is not established whether these fusimotor actions occur by collateral influences of axons which also cause CM EPSPs in alpha motor neurons. This is a theoretical possibility which could be of very great significance if alpha-gamma co-activation occurs automatically as a result of CM activity (Phillips 1969), especially in the light of recent evidence from cross-correlation studies in conscious animals that indicate that CM cells in the cortex may contribute to 'long loop' transcortical reflex activation of muscles subjected to stretch (Cheney & Fetz 1984).

Inhibitory influences on motor neurons have been a feature of all studies using cortical stimulation. IPSPs with latencies consistent with a disynaptic pathway from the cortex to motor neurons were reported in the first studies of CM effects made with intracellular microelectrodes (Preston & Whitlock 1961, Landgren et al 1962). Jankowska & Tanaka (1974) have shown that these disynaptic inhibitory effects on lumbar motor neurons in the monkey are produced over a pathway that utilizes the common Ia inhibitory interneuron. Cross-correlation studies in conscious monkeys show that reciprocal inhibitory actions on antagonistic muscles occur after the individual discharges of single CM cells, making it essential to consider that the common Ia inhibitory interneurons in the cervical spinal cord may be activated by collaterals of CM fibres that excite agonist motor neurons (Cheney et al 1985).

One other influence remains to be considered. Both the magnitude and the duration of some of the post-spike facilitation records generated in cross-correlation studies in conscious animals seem to exceed what would be expected from an influence exclusively of very small unitary CM EPSPs in motor neurons. The possibility exists that, in the conscious monkey, other excitatory actions on the motor neuron are generated by collateral influences of one CM fibre. There could be collateral activation of excitatory proprio-spinal or segmental interneurons. Evidence for such effects is not strong in intracellular records made in anaesthetized monkeys. Perhaps the slightly delayed oligosynaptic excitation is almost completely suppressed by anaesthetic agents. Since a propriospinal system activated by the pyramidal tract provides the pathway for CM excitation of cervical motor neurons in the cat (Illert et al 1976a, b), a similar excitatory pathway may exist in the cervical spinal cord of the monkey.

In addition to making CM contacts with alpha motor neurons innervating one muscle group, individual CM fibres might be able to send collateral branches to motor neurons of other muscles and to fusimotor neurons, inhibitory interneurons and propriospinal or segmental excitatory inter-neurons. As a first step towards evaluating this possibility, Shinoda et al (1981) made intra-axonal injections of horseradish peroxidase (HRP) into corticospinal axons to visualize their terminal and preterminal arborizations. We combined this approach with the intracellular injection of HRP into a few motor neurons innervating intrinsic muscles of the hand (Lawrence et al 1985). This has the advantage that the entire surface membrane of these motor neurons, including virtually the whole dendritic tree, can be visualized. The corticospinal axon can be designated as a CM axon if it can be shown by light microscopy to make synapses on the surface of such a stained motor neuron. The collateral territory of the branches of the CM axon—but not, alas, the other neural elements that are contacted within that territory—can then be described with confidence.

Very few complete observations of the branching patterns of intraspinal collaterals of definitive CM axons have been reported. Shinoda et al (1981) found that a single corticospinal axon distributed boutons in the vicinity of up to four motor nuclei. These boutons could innervate motor neurons of the 'muscle field' of that axon, and those motor neurons could potentially include representatives innervating antagonists as well as agonists. The great capacity for divergence of the influence of the collaterals of individual CM axons, which have been proved to innervate motor neurons supplying the intrinsic muscles of the hand, was revealed in the descriptions published by Lawrence et al (1985). The main collateral branches of such CM axons ending in the lower cervical spinal cord were within a horizontal cylinder 0.5 mm in dia-meter and 1.5 mm in length in lamina IX of the C8, T1 region. A multitude of synaptic boutons or clusters of boutons was evident within this cylinder and these could potentially contact a very large number of dendrites of motor

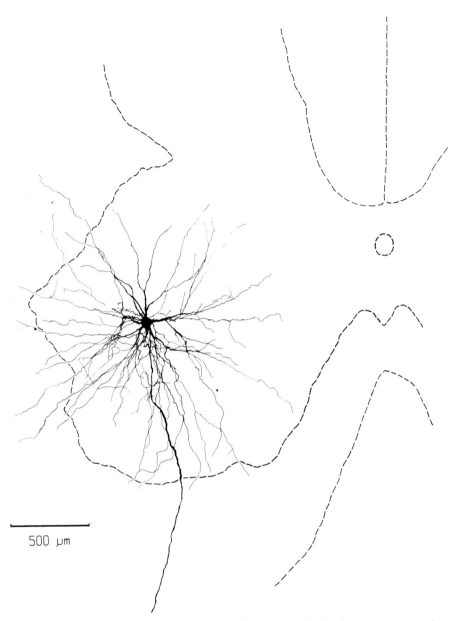

500 μm

FIG. 1. Microscopic reconstruction from serial sections of a lumbar motorneuron in the monkey, illustrating the extent of the dendritic ramifications of this cell in the anterior horn of the spinal cord. This motorneuron had been filled with horseradish peroxidase by ionophoresis from an intracellular microelectrode. The neuron was demonstrated to innervate distally-acting musculature by way of an axon in the lateral popliteal nerve. It was in receipt of a monosynaptic corticomotoneuronal excitatory postsynaptic potential produced by electrical stimulation of the 'leg' area of the contralateral precentral motor area of the cerebral cortex. (Histological reconstruction produced by Dr Wu Chien-ping from superimposed camera lucida drawings of serial sections 80 μm in thickness.)

neurons. Unless the whole dendritic tree of the particular neurons under investigation is visualized, these methods cannot determine whether these motor neurons would then be shown to belong to agonist or antagonist muscles. The range over which the dendrites of a motor neuron spread, and the way in which dendrites from one motor pool intermingle with those from another, serve only to emphasize the difficulty of equating boutons in a particular part of the spinal cord with synapses on the somata that occupy that region (Fig. 1).

But the observation that the collateral of a particular CM axon innervates both of the only two ulnar motor neurons sampled which had dendrites in the vicinity of the collateral arbor must argue for a very high probability of contacts between this axon collateral and a large proportion of the appropriate species of motor neurons in its vicinity. This high probability of contacts would be accompanied automatically by a great convergence of synapses from the CM colony of which this was a single identified example. In one spinal cord preparation in which collaterals of two CM fibres were stained in the same part of the spinal cord as two intrinsic 'hand' motor neurons, each of the cells received synaptic contacts from each of the fibres—an occurrence which would not be predicted for such a tiny sample unless the CM axons destined to end on motor neurons innervating this group of intrinsic hand muscles had a very high probability of contacting most of the appropriate motor neurons.

Although the branches of the CM axon collateral were most profuse within lamina IX, some long-range branches spread much more extensively, ending among motor neurons in the next segment of the spinal cord and delivering boutons to more medial regions. These more extensive branches could conceivably deliver collateral influences to the remote dendrites of other motor neurons, to fusimotor neurons, to the inhibitory interneurons involved in reciprocal innervation and, if they are situated segmentally, to the proposed excitatory interneurons. Certainly the divergence of the collaterals of CM fibres seems to be extensive enough to allow the CM influences to be delivered to a group of cooperating motor neurons and also to be directed to appropriate selected populations of spinal neurons with other functions. This collateral divergence may act in parallel with other pathways which are more predominantly involved in interneuronal control and which do not themselves make CM connections. But the anatomical evidence to date does not preclude a CM axon that innervates 'hand' motor neurons from additionally influencing selected inhibitory interneurons, for example, by means of collateral branches of its own major projection.

Acknowledgements

The work summarized here was initiated by Professor Charles Phillips in Oxford. Over a number of years, others have contributed significant observations. Among these have been a number of postgraduate students, visitors and other colleagues—Jonathan Hore, Murray Lewis, Malcolm Horne, Ray Muir, Jacoba Brinkman, Roger Lemon,

Don Lawrence, Stephen Redman and Wu Chien-ping. I have drawn extensively on their observations. In Australia, the scientific work of the laboratory has been supported by the National Health and Medical Research Council.

References

Asanuma H, Zarzecki P, Jankowska E, Hongo T, Marcus S 1979 Projection of individual pyramidal tract neurons to lumbar motor nuclei of the monkey. Exp Brain Res 34:73–89

Cheney PD, Fetz EE 1984 Cortico-motoneuronal cells contribute to long-latency stretch reflexes in the rhesus monkey. J Physiol (Lond) 349:249–272

Cheney PD, Fetz EE 1985 Comparable patterns of muscle facilitation evoked by individual cortico-motoneuronal (CM) cells and by single intracortical microstimuli in primates: evidence for functional groups of CM cells. J Neurophysiol (Bethesda) 53:786–804

Cheney PD, Fetz EE, Palmer SS 1985 Patterns of facilitation and suppression of antagonist forelimb muscles from motor cortex sites in the awake monkey. J Neurophysiol (Bethesda) 53:805–819

Clough JFM, Kernell D, Phillips CG 1968 The distribution of monosynaptic excitation from the pyramidal tract and from primary spindle afferents to motoneurones of the baboon's hand and forearm. J Physiol (Lond) 198:145–166

Clough JFM, Phillips CG, Sheridan JP 1971 The short latency projection from the baboon's motor cortex to fusimotor neurones of the forearm and hand. J Physiol (Lond) 216:257–279

Evarts EV 1968 Relation of pyramidal tract activity to force exerted during voluntary movement. J Neurophysiol (Bethesda) 31:14–27

Evarts EV 1969 Activity of pyramidal tract neurons during postural fixation. J Neurophysiol (Bethesda) 37:373–381

Fetz EE, Cheney PD 1980 Postspike facilitation of forelimb muscle activity by primate cortico-motoneuronal cells. J Neurophysiol (Bethesda) 44:751–772

Fritz N, Illert M, Kolb FP et al 1985 The cortico-motoneuronal input to hand and forearm motoneurones in the anaesthetised monkey. J Physiol (Lond) 366:20P

Grigg P, Preston JB 1971 Baboon flexor and extensor fusimotor neurons and their modulation by motor cortex. J Neurophysiol (Bethesda) 34:428–436

Humphrey DR 1986 Representation of movements and muscles within the primate precentral motor cortex: historical and current perspectives. Fed Proc 45:2687–2699

Illert M, Lundberg A, Tanaka R 1976a Integration in descending motor pathways controlling the forelimb in the cat. 1. Pyramidal effects on motoneurones. Exp Brain Res 26:509–519

Illert M, Lundberg A, Tanaka R 1976b Integration in descending motor pathways controlling the forelimb in the cat. 2. Convergence on neurones mediating disynaptic cortico-motoneuronal excitation. Exp Brain Res 26:521–540

Jankowska E, Tanaka R 1974 Neuronal mechanism of the disynaptic inhibition evoked in primate spinal motoneurones from the corticospinal tract. Brain Res 75:163–166

Jankowska E, Padel Y, Tanaka R 1975 Projections of pyramidal tract cells to alpha motoneurones innervating hindlimb muscles in the monkey. J Physiol (Lond) 249:637–667

Landgren S, Phillips CG, Porter R 1962 Minimal synaptic actions of pyramidal impulses on some alpha motoneurones of the baboon's hand and forearm. J Physiol (Lond) 161:91–111

Lawrence DG, Porter R, Redman SJ 1985 Cortico-motoneuronal synapses in the monkey: light microscopic localization upon motoneurons of intrinsic muscles of the hand. J Comp Neurol 232:499–510

Muir RB, Lemon RN 1983 Corticospinal neurons with a special role in precision grip. Brain Res 261:312–316

Muir RB, Porter R 1973 The effect of a preceding stimulus on temporal facilitation at cortico-motoneuronal synapses. J Physiol (Lond) 228:749–763

Phillips CG 1969 Motor apparatus of the baboon's hand. Proc R Soc Lond B Biol Sci 173:141–174

Phillips CG Porter R 1964 The pyramidal projection to motoneurones of some muscle groups of the baboon's forelimb. In: Eccles JC, Schadé JP (eds) Physiology of spinal neurons. Elsevier, Amsterdam (Prog Brain Res vol 12) p 222–245

Phillips CG, Porter R 1977 Corticospinal neurones: their role in movement. Academic Press, New York

Porter R 1985 The cortico-motoneuronal component of the pyramidal tract:cortico-motoneuronal connections and functions in primates. Brain Res Rev 10:1–26

Porter, R, Hore J 1969 Time course of minimal cortico-motoneuronal excitatory postsynaptic potentials in lumbar motoneurons of the monkey. J Neurophysiol (Bethesda) 32:443–451

Preston JB, Whitlock DG 1961 Intracellular potentials recorded from motoneurons following precentral gyrus stimulation in primate. J Neurophysiol (Bethesda) 24:91–100

Shapovalov AI 1975 Neuronal organization and synaptic mechanisms of supraspinal motor control in vertebrates. Rev Physiol Biochem Pharmacol 72:1–54

Shinoda Y, Yokota J, Futami T 1981 Divergent projection of individual corticospinal axons to motoneurons of multiple muscles in the monkey. Neurosci Lett 23:7–12

Schmidt EM, McIntosh JS 1984 Microstimulation mapping of precentral cortex in awake behaving monkeys. Soc Neurosci Abstr 10:737

DISCUSSION

Rizzolatti: Is there any evidence that corticospinal fibres terminate on motor neurons in such a way as to control coordinated movements? For example, is there any evidence that a single corticospinal neuron controls the opposition of the thumb and index finger?

Porter: I have no such evidence. It would have to come from the sorts of observations that Roger Lemon and Ray Muir have made. In our experiments we are limited to studying motor neurons sending axons into a peripheral nerve, like the ulnar nerve or the median nerve. It would be technically very difficult to make a dissection that involved backfiring of motor neurons from individual branches of nerves supplying the small muscles of the hand.

Lemon: Two of the muscles important in precision grip are the first dorsal interosseous and the adductor of the thumb. In our work these two muscles were facilitated in combination by the same cortical cell on a remarkably large number of occasions, suggesting that two coordinately acting muscles can be controlled by a single corticospinal neuron (Buys et al 1986).

Strick: I was struck by the disparity between the single fibre filling of corticospinal fibres and Professor Kuypers' observations on termination patterns. The corticospinal termination patterns certainly go to lamina IX but they are most dense outside lamina IX, in the region he terms the spinal cord intermediate zone. The single-fibre data that you illustrated show arborizations in lamina IX, but there must be equally, if not more, extensive projections to the spinal cord intermediate zone.

Porter: Dr Shinoda has studied transverse sections and I think our observations are consistent. I can really only illustrate corticomotoneuronal (CM) intraspinal fibres and their collaterals in the few cases in which we have demonstrated that the collaterals innervate motor neurons supplying the small muscles of the hand. That says nothing about all the other fibres that Hans Kuypers finds by degeneration studies, which may not have anything to do with the innervation of the motor neurons for the intrinsic muscles of the hand.

Shinoda: Our data have shown that there are relatively few fibres to the intermediate zone from the corticospinal axons projecting extensively to motor neurons innervating distal muscles of the arm (Shinoda et al 1981). Most of these axons originate from the rostral bank of the central sulcus. Corticospinal neurons in the rostral part of area 4 might give rise to fibres to the intermediate zone of the cord. Kuypers & Brinkman's data (1970) suggest this possibility.

Kuypers: Your findings suggest that two different types of fibres may exist: those going to the interneuronal area of the intermediate zone and those going to the motor neuronal cell groups. In the chimpanzee a lesion in the rostral bank of the lower third of the central sulcus produced fibre degeneration only in bulbar motor nuclei. However, when the lesion also involved the adjoining convexity of the precentral gyrus, the fibre degeneration to the motor nuclei was accompanied by fibre degeneration to the interneuronal areas of the lateral reticular formation. This means that in the chimpanzee the anterior bank of the central sulcus contains an almost pure culture of corticobulbar neurons projecting only to the bulbar motor nuclei (Kuypers 1958), in keeping with your findings in the spinal cord, Dr Shinoda.

Fetz: The surface stimulation map we have just seen showed some sites in postcentral cortex evoking CM EPSPs. Does your evidence indicate that postcentral corticospinal cells make monosynaptic connections on motor neurons?

Porter: Physical spread of the stimulus from a wide region of cortex can activate a population of motor neurons which may be situated many millimetres away from where the stimulus is delivered. While I understand why people want to study the distribution of the terminal arborizations of corticospinal cells arising in the postcentral gyrus or in the supplementary motor area, I think it will have to be done with the sort of techniques that I have just illustrated and that Dr Shinoda has used. As far as I am aware, that has not yet been done.

Kuypers: Chambers and Liu (personal communications) and I observed that after a lesion of the postcentral gyrus in the monkey a very few degenerating fibres are distributed to the spinal motor neuronal cell groups. Therefore perhaps a very few postcentral fibres to motor neurons exist.

Porter: I am not denying it but I can't say how they are distributed, because we have not studied them.

Lemon: In the very beautiful plot of the motor neuron you showed, some of the dendrites clearly went outside lamina IX. We have seen that the direct connections seem to avoid the more proximal dendrites of the motor neurons. Why is that? Did you see axonal terminations or arborizations close to the cell bodies of motor neurons that you hadn't filled? Why do the CM connections, which we know from experiments in all sorts of different primates to be very powerful, conspicuously avoid the most influential parts of the dendritic tree?

Porter: I don't think they avoid those areas. From measurements of the shape of minimal EPSPs generated by stimulating either the cerebral cortex or group Ia fibres, Jonathan Hore and I concluded that the CM connections were likely to be more remotely situated on the dendritic tree of motor neurons than those from group Ia synapses (Porter & Hore 1969). In these more recent experiments we studied the distribution of a small number of CM boutons that were shown by light microscopy to approximate so closely to the dendrites of motor neurons that they are likely to be synapses. These cover the same extensive territory of the motor neuron surface as the group Ia synapses measured by Stephen Redman and Bruce Walmsley (1981). We don't have enough observations to say whether there is a statistical difference or whether there is, on average, a more remote location of the CM synapses than of the group Ia synapses. Even the synapses involved in the monosynaptic stretch reflex are unevenly distributed over the dendritic surface, being most dense in the middle part of the dendritic tree, with relatively few on the soma or at the terminations of the dendrites (Jack et al 1971). There is a distribution over that dendritic tree and, from the very small number of observations that we made, I cannot claim that, anatomically, the CM synapses are significantly different.

Wiesendanger: I was puzzled by Dr Shinoda's observation that one collateral of a pyramidal tract fibre may innervate up to four motor nuclei. Do you have evidence suggesting that some of the axons are more restricted? Would you consider that these divergent fibres subserve small synergies like the precision grip?

Another possibility, perhaps a particularly interesting aspect of cortical control, is that before a 'start' signal for a movement comes down the spinal cord there is preselection of which neurons should be fired. We know that we can control a few motor units voluntarily. This may mean that the selection of motor units may be finely controlled by presetting and that not all motor neurons monosynaptically connected with the collaterals of pyramidal tract axons are fired.

Porter: There is presumptive evidence from Dr Shinoda's work (Shinoda et al 1981) that terminations of corticospinal fibres occur within the territory of the somata of motor neurons supplying a variety of different muscles. However, when one understands the extent of the dendritic tree and takes into account the observations about the location of many of those CM synapses on rather remote parts of the dendritic tree, it is no longer possible to state categorically that because boutons are seen in and around the somata they end on those somata, rather than on the dendrites of other cells.

Secondly, Roger Lemon's work on post-spike facilitation in different muscles associated with the precision grip suggests that the muscle fields innervated by individual corticospinal fibres may be more restricted for the motor neuron populations that innervate the small muscles of the hand than for those of the wrist, elbow or shoulder. That is consistent with the intraspinal electrical stimulation mapping of the divergence of fibres that has been done by Asanuma, Dr Shinoda and a number of other people (see Asanuma et al 1979). This work showed that great divergence of branching can be detected for a given antidromically identified corticospinal fibre. That divergence may be more restricted for those corticospinal fibres with terminations among the motor neurons supplying distally acting muscles. The onus is on all of us to determine whether studying the descending fibre connections with more rostral regions of the spinal cord where there are motor neurons supplying proximal muscles produces a different anatomical picture.

Fetz: In your experiments in which the amplitudes of CM EPSPs were increased when cortical stimulation was increased, the EPSPs showed remarkably little change in their latency. The EPSPs increased without the dispersion at onset that one would expect if the CM cells had different conduction velocities. Do the CM cells to these motor neurons actually have a very restricted range of conduction velocities, or could there be some mechanism synchronizing the conduction of impulses in the descending volley? Your observations are consistent with recent evidence that ionic and electrical interactions between neighbouring pyramidal tract fibres may synchronize their action potentials (Canedo & Towe 1985, Schmied & Fetz 1987).

Porter: The method of stimulating the cerebral cortex with surface anodal pulses synchronizes the outflow in corticospinal axons, because the impulse-generating region of the cell adjacent to the white matter is the point that is being stimulated, while all the intracortical circuitry is bypassed. Secondly, we know that the rapidly conducting fibres, which have a fairly limited range of conduction velocity in the monkey of between 50 and 70 m/s, certainly contribute to the growth of the amplitude of the compound monosynaptic CM EPSP. I cannot comment about whether more slowly conducting fibres can also depolarize the motor neurons. There could be alternative explanations involving later disynaptic or oligosynaptic events. All I can conclude is that there is a population of corticospinal fibres with rapidly conducting axons which con-

verge onto motor neurons in a way that enables the synaptic excitation produced by those axons to grow.

Shinoda: In some invertebrates, it is known that spike potentials are often
blocked at the branching points of axons, depending on their frequency. Do
you have any evidence that spikes are always conveyed via those fine collateral
branches without failure under physiological conditions?

Porter: In the anaesthetized animal it is difficult to measure the effect on a
motor neuron of an individual impulse in one of those collateral branches. Dr
Wu tried to measure the amplitude of unitary single-fibre EPSPs, but without
success; that was also the experience of Asanuma, Jankowska and others
(Asanuma et al 1979). In many of the motor neurons they studied, even the
population of motor neurons with axons in one peripheral nerve, they found no
EPSPs at all, even though they were triggering off the cell body discharges of a
fibre which clearly innervated that motor pool. If many of the CM contacts are
indeed on dendritic spines, and if only one CM collateral is being activated,
with no supporting activity in other descending fibres, the impulse may remain
confined to the spine and that may be why it is difficult to detect.

There are other possible explanations: there may be a failure of invasion into
those very fine terminals, especially under anaesthesia, when perhaps the
presynaptic receptors on the membranes of those fine terminals are influenced
by GABA or some other inhibitory or depressing compound. It may not be
necessary to demonstrate the presence of axo-axonic terminals in the spinal
cord in order to reveal a phenomenon akin to presynaptic inhibition. So there
are a number of problems to be resolved.

Where an appropriate search has been made, one must conclude that some
of the synapses detected anatomically cannot have their synaptic impacts
measured electrophysiologically under the conditions of activation of a single
local collateral of a CM fibre, even when one is recording in appropriate motor
neurons.

References

Asanuma H, Zarzecki P, Jankowska E, Hongo T, Marcus S 1979 Projection of individual pyramidal tract neurons to lumbar motor nuclei of the monkey. Exp Brain Res
   34:73–89
Buys EJ, Lemon RN, Mantel GWH, Muir RB 1986 Selective facilitation of different
   hand muscles by single corticospinal neurones in the conscious monkey. J Physiol
   (Lond) 381:529–549
Canedo A, Towe AL 1985 Superposition of antidromic responses in pyramidal tract cell
   clusters. Exp Neurol 89:645–658
Jack JJB, Miller S, Porter R, Redman SJ 1971 The time course of minimal excitatory
   post-synaptic potentials evoked in spinal motoneurones by group Ia afferent fibres. J
   Physiol (Lond) 215:353–380
Kuypers HGJM 1958 Some projections from the peri-central cortex to the pons and

lower brain stem in the monkey and chimpanzee. J Comp Neurol 110:221–256

Kuypers HGJM, Brinkman J 1970 Precentral projections to different parts of the spinal intermediate zone in the rhesus monkey. Brain Res 24:29–48

Porter R, Hore J 1969 Time course of minimal cortico-motoneuronal excitatory post-synaptic potentials in lumbar motoneurons of the monkey. J Neurophysiol 32:443–451

Redman SJ, Walmsley B 1981 The synaptic basis of the monosynaptic stretch reflex. Trends Neurosci 4:248–250

Schmied A, Fetz EE 1987 Activity-related changes in electrical thresholds of pyramidal tract axons in the behaving monkey. Exp Brain Res 65:352–360

Shinoda Y, Yokota J, Futami T 1981 Divergent projection of individual corticospinal axons to motoneurons of multiple muscles in the monkey. Neurosci Lett 23:7–12

Functional relations between primate motor cortex cells and muscles: fixed and flexible

E.E. Fetz and P.D. Cheney

Department of Physiology & Biophysics, University of Washington, Seattle, WA 98195, USA

Abstract. In behaving monkeys the effects of motor cortex cells on muscles are inferred from two quite different types of 'correlational' evidence: their co-activation and cross-correlation. Many precentral cells are *coactivated* with limb muscles, suggesting that they make a proportional contribution to muscle activity; however, such coactivation is typically quite flexible, and can be changed by operantly conditioning the dissociation of cell and muscle activity. *Cross-correlating* cells and muscles by spike-triggered averaging of the electromyogram (EMG) shows that certain cells produce short-latency post-spike facilitation of EMG; this correlational linkage is relatively fixed under different behavioural conditions and its time course suggests it is mediated by a corticomotoneuronal (CM) synaptic connection. CM cells typically facilitate a set of coactivated agonist muscles, and some also inhibit their antagonists.

The firing patterns of CM cells can differ significantly from those of their target muscles. During ramp-and-hold wrist responses most CM cells discharge a phasic burst that precedes target muscle onset and that contributes to changes in muscle activity. At low force levels many CM cells are activated without their target motor units. Conversely, many CM cells are paradoxically inactive during rapid forceful movements that vigorously activate their target muscles; they appear to be preferentially active during finely controlled movements. Thus CM cells, with a fixed correlational linkage to their target muscles, may be recruited without their target muscles, and vice versa.

1987 Motor areas of the cerebral cortex. Wiley, Chichester (Ciba Foundation Symposium 132) p 98–117

The classic work of others in this symposium has documented the direct effects that primate motor cortex can exert on motor neurons via the so-called corticomotoneuronal (CM) cells and has established much about their functional organization (Phillips & Porter 1964, 1977, Porter 1985). The size of maximal CM-excitatory postsynaptic potentials (CM-EPSPs) in forelimb motor neurons of the baboon (Clough et al 1968) relative to unitary CM-EPSPs (Asanuma et al 1979, Porter & Hore 1969) suggests that each motor neuron receives convergent monosynaptic input from a colony of 10–50 CM

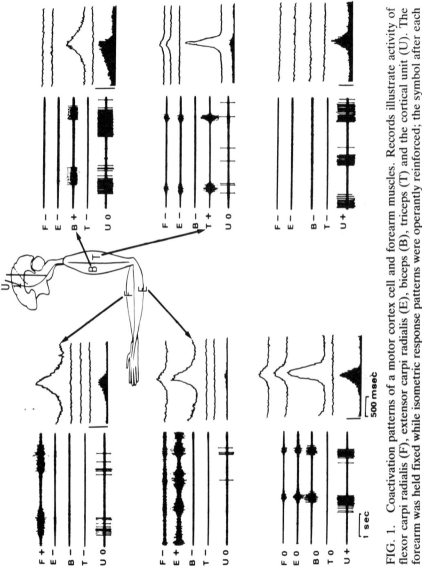

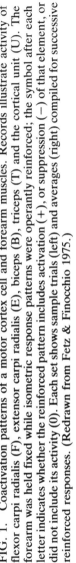

FIG. 1. Coactivation patterns of a motor cortex cell and forearm muscles. Records illustrate activity of flexor carpi radialis (F), extensor carpi radialis (E), biceps (B), triceps (T) and the cortical unit (U). The forearm was held fixed while isometric response patterns were operantly reinforced; the symbol after each letter indicates whether the reinforced pattern includes activation (+), or suppression (−) of that element, or did not include its activity (0). Each set shows sample trials (left) and averages (right) compiled for successive reinforced responses. (Redrawn from Fetz & Finocchio 1975.)

cells. These cells are distributed over relatively wide cortical regions (Landgren et al 1962, Jankowska et al 1975). Extensive divergence of terminals of single corticospinal cells is suggested by anatomical reconstruction (Shinoda et al 1981, Lawrence et al 1985) and electrophysiological evidence (Asanuma et al 1979).

Chronic unit recordings in behaving monkeys have further confirmed the role of motor cortex cells in the control of muscle activity. The close relation between the activity of pyramidal tract neurons and muscle force, first demonstrated by Evarts (1968), is now commonly considered to represent the typical behaviour of motor cortex cells. Further studies, too numerous to cite individually, showed that the activity of motor cortex cells may also be related to various other aspects of movement (cf. Thach 1978). Yet the observation that neuronal activity covaried with force—or any other movement parameter—was soon recognized as inconclusive evidence for a causal relationship between the two.

Coactivation of motor cortex cells and muscles

The question of causal involvement is illustrated by a study designed to determine whether motor cortex cells fired with particular sets of forelimb muscles (Fetz & Finocchio 1975). In these experiments the monkeys were trained to isometrically contract each of four representative forearm muscles in relative isolation. The cell illustrated in Fig. 1 was coactivated with isometric contractions of the flexors of the wrist and elbow (top left and right), but not the extensors of these joints (middle left and right). This neuron was also coactivated with the flexor muscles during active elbow flexion, and under isometric conditions when the monkey was rewarded for firing the cell in bursts (bottom left). Such consistent coactivation under different behavioural conditions would seem to suggest some sort of functional relationship. Yet when the monkey was preferentially rewarded for activating the cell without the muscles it readily dissociated their activity (bottom right). These results are representative of similar findings with other precentral neurons, and they illustrate two features of cell–muscle coactivation patterns: single motor cortical neurons were typically coactivated with multiple muscles, and their coactivation was quite flexible, subject to dissociation. Whether these cells had any causal effect on the associated muscles is not established by their coactivation (nor disproved by their dissociation).

Correlational linkages between cells and muscles

An independent means of confirming a causal relation between motor cortex cell and muscle activity is provided by the cross-correlation technique. Spike-triggered averages of forelimb muscle activity can detect the average post-

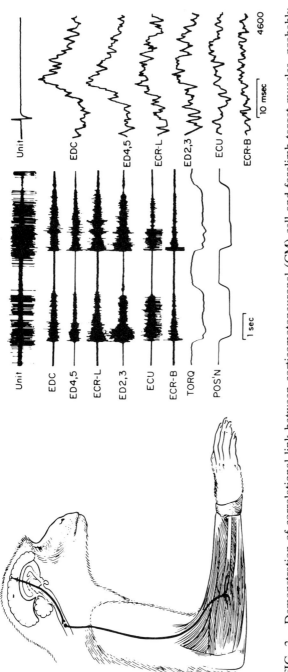

FIG. 2.   Demonstration of correlational link between corticomotoneuronal (CM) cell and forelimb target muscles, probably mediated by corticomotoneuronal connections, as schematized at left. Responses of an extension-related CM cell during wrist movements against an elastic load (middle) show coactivated extensor muscles of the wrist (ECR-L; ECR-B; ECU) and the digits (EDC; ED4,5; ED2,3). Spike-triggered averages of rectified EMG (right) show post-spike facilitation in several target muscles. (Redrawn from Fetz & Cheney 1978.)

spike effects of certain motor cortex neurons on muscle activity (Fetz et al 1976, Fetz & Cheney 1978, 1980, Muir & Lemon 1983). Some neurons produce post-spike facilitation (PSF) whose magnitude and time course is consistent with mediation by monosynaptic connections (Fig. 2). Such cells may be identified as CM cells, where CM can be taken to imply an underlying corticomotoneuronal connection, or simply to identify a 'corticomotor cell' with a correlational linkage to its target muscles.

Single CM cells typically facilitate one or more of the coactivated forelimb muscles. The set of facilitated muscles, or *muscle field*, is usually a subset of the muscles that are coactivated synergistically during a movement. Monitoring six flexor and six extensor muscles of the wrist and fingers during alternating ramp-and-hold wrist movements, we found the average muscle field of extensor CM cells (2.5 muscles) to be slightly greater than that of flexor CM cells (2.1) (Fetz & Cheney 1980). Monitoring intrinsic hand as well as forearm muscles during a precision grip task, Buys et al (1986) found that their CM cells facilitated about 20–30% of the independent synergists. Their findings further suggested that distal muscle fields may be more restricted than proximal.

In contrast to the flexibility of the broad unit-muscle coactivation patterns, the correlational linkages revealed by spike-triggered averaging are relatively fixed. Spike-triggered averages compiled separately during the phasic and static component of a ramp-and-hold movement show PSF in the same muscles (Fetz et al 1976, Lemon et al 1986). Averages compiled during precision grip and power grip responses also reveal PSF in the same muscles, although their amplitudes were sometimes lower during the power grip (Buys et al 1986). To test for modulation of the PSF we trained monkeys to make alternating wrist movements in the horizontal plane with the wrist held in different postures (R.M. Martin & E.E. Fetz, unpublished work). With the wrist semi-prone the flexors and extensors were reciprocally activated as antagonists; with the wrist in a prone or supine position the ulnar flexors and extensors were synergistically coactivated, as were the radial flexors and extensors. Under these different movement conditions, CM cells continued to facilitate the same target muscles, with the same relative amplitudes.

These observations suggest that PSF is mediated by relatively direct synaptic linkages. Although the occurrence of PSF in a muscle is repeatable, its amplitude may change under different conditions. This modulation is understandable in terms of the underlying mechanisms. For multi-unit EMG recordings the PSF represents the net result of all the facilitated motor units. Any one motor unit would contribute in proportion to its post-spike firing probability convolved with its rectified action potential. The post-spike firing probability in turn is a function that is largely proportional to the derivative of the postsynaptic potential produced in the motor neuron (Fetz & Gustafsson 1983, Cope et al 1987). Thus the PSF amplitude could be modulated by recruitment of different motor units, which have different post-spike firing probabilities and whose action potentials contribute differently to the net PSF. Therefore, changes in PSF amplitude are consistent with monosynaptic connections, and do not necessarily indicate the presence of a modulating interneuron. It seems relevant to note a case in which PSF appeared in new muscles: this was observed under the special conditions produced by a small, brief perturbation (Cheney & Fetz 1984); spike-triggered averages selectively compiled during the stretch-evoked muscle response revealed a significant increase in the PSF of target muscles, and additional PSF in muscles that showed no facilitation during the static hold period. These results may be explained by recruitment of higher threshold target motor units, or by enhanced postsynaptic potentials mediated disynaptically via spinal interneurons that are facilitated by synchronous input.

The question of synchrony between cortical neurons can be raised in conjunction with the wide muscle fields of CM cells. Could some of their postspike effects be mediated by synchronous firing with other CM cells? Direct evidence on the degree of synchrony has been obtained by cross-correlating the activity of simultaneously recorded neighbouring neurons. The cross-correlation peaks between motor cortex cells, when present, are typically broad (mean width:18 ms) (Smith & Fetz 1986). Cross-correlation peaks between pairs of CM cells with common target muscles can be somewhat sharper, but are still wider than required to mediate the post-spike effects (Cheney & Fetz 1985, W.S. Smith & E.E. Fetz, unpublished work). Thus, the clear PSF with sharp post-spike onsets can be confidently attributed to the output effects of the triggering cell rather than to its synchrony with other output cells.

In addition to post-spike facilitation, spike-triggered averages have also revealed post-spike suppression of muscles. In some cases the cell was coactivated with the muscles to which it had an inhibitory correlational linkage (Cheney et al 1985). More often, during ramp-and-hold responses cortical cells are reciprocally activated with the inhibited muscles, precluding spike-triggered averages. To reveal the correlational linkage of CM cells to antagonists of their target muscles, Kasser & Cheney (1985) used glutamate to generate spikes during the phase of movement in which the cell was normally inactive. This technique revealed that 40% of extensor CM cells and 18% of flexor CM cells had reciprocal inhibitory effects on the antagonists of their target muscles. The remaining CM cells had purely excitatory effects, and with one exception, facilitated only their coactivated target muscles.

Response patterns of CM cells and target muscles

The ability to identify CM cells in awake monkeys provides a model system in which the relative activation of connected elements can be compared under normal behavioural conditions. During active movements CM cell activity

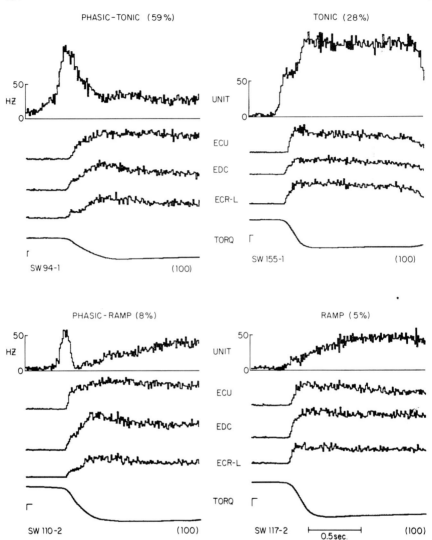

FIG. 3. Response patterns of CM cells during generation of isometric ramp-and-hold torque responses. Each set shows the time histogram of CM cell activity, averages of synergistic muscle activity and isometric torque. Titles give name and relative frequency of each type of CM cell. (From Cheney & Fetz 1980.)

does not simply mirror the activity of its target muscles. The differences in their discharge patterns reveal some significant distinctions between CM cells and motor units.

During simple ramp-and-hold wrist responses most of the CM cells exhibit

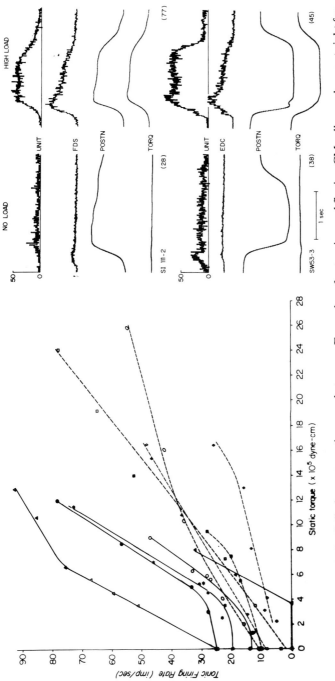

FIG. 4. Relation of CM cell discharge to active muscle torque. Examples of extension and flexion CM cells are shown at right for responses at two torque levels. Plot of tonic firing rate versus torque at left shows higher rate-torque slopes for extensor CM cells (solid lines) than flexor CM cells (dotted lines). (Graphs redrawn from Cheney & Fetz 1980.)

a phasic burst of discharge at the onset of muscle activity (Cheney & Fetz 1980) (Fig. 3). Such high frequency firing helps to bring the motor neurons to threshold. For those cells with inhibitory links to antagonist muscles this phasic discharge would simultaneously help to turn the antagonists off, and to inhibit their activation by stretch reflexes. Thus the cortical discharge pattern has a strong *phasic* component representing a *change* of muscle force. Physiologically this is dictated by the requirements for activating the relatively inert motor neurons, which require substantial input current to prod them to discharge. Interestingly, the firing patterns of rubromotoneuronal cells emphasize the phasic components of movement even more than CM cells (Cheney et al 1987).

During the static hold period of ramp-and-hold movements, when the force is maintained at a steady level, most CM cells (87%) fire at a constant rate; this *tonic* firing rate is an increasing function of the static *force* (Fig. 4). A small proportion of CM cells (13%) exhibit a gradually incrementing discharge frequency during the hold. These firing patterns of CM cells contrast with those of forearm motor units under the same conditions. Fifty-six per cent of motor units also fire tonically during the hold period, at rates proportional to static force, but 39% exhibit decrementing discharge (Palmer & Fetz 1985). It seems reasonable to speculate that the incrementing discharge of CM cells functions to counter the adaptation of motor neurons to steady input. Thus the contrast between the discharge patterns of CM cells and motor neurons can be understood in terms of the physiological properties of motor neurons and the inputs required to make them discharge appropriately.

It seems worth noting parenthetically that the representation of active force in CM cells is similar to the representation of peripheral stimuli in many sensory cortex cells. A passive ramp-and-hold joint rotation or cutaneous pressure typically evokes a phasic–tonic discharge in postcentral cortex cells. Thus, both motor and sensory cortex cells show an initial phasic component of discharge that codes a change in the peripheral event and a tonic discharge which codes its sustained intensity. The muscle field of CM cells is also obviously analogous to the receptive field of sensory cortex cells, in that both kinds of cortical cells represent the activity of a set of peripheral elements. Even the inhibitory component of the receptive field has its analogue in the reciprocal inhibitory linkages of CM cells to antagonists of their target muscles.

Dissociated activation of CM cells and target muscles

In addition to the differences in the response patterns of CM cells and their target motor units, there are circumstances in which each can be activated without the other. In general, CM cells appear to have a lower threshold for activation and they fire without their target muscles in three situations. First, during ramp-and-hold movements most CM cells begin to increase their discharge well before the onset of activity in their target muscles. The mean onset time of phasic–tonic CM cells was 71 ms before their target muscles, and some began several hundred milliseconds earlier. As noted, this initial CM cell discharge would help to bring their target motor neurons to threshold. Secondly, during the static hold at low force levels, many CM cells are recruited into tonic activity without their target motor units. Whereas CM cells typically discharge at the lowest levels of active force, the motor units are recruited over a wider range of forces. Thirdly, many CM cells can be driven by adequate natural stimulation, which does not evoke responses in their target muscles (Cheney & Fetz 1984). Most CM cells respond to passive joint rotation that stretches their target muscles, and some respond to cutaneous stimulation. All these examples are of course consistent with the fact that CM-EPSPs are too small to produce obligatory responses in motor neurons, and they indicate that in the conscious primate motor cortex cells undergo a wider range of activities than is reflected peripherally in the muscles.

Perhaps more interesting is the evidence for the reverse dissociation: activation of target muscles without activation of the CM cells that facilitate them. Again three examples can be cited. During the ramp-and-hold movements some CM cells, particularly those without an initial burst, begin firing after their target muscles. For example, the mean onset time of the ramp cells was 100 ms after their target muscles. Secondly, during the static hold, a few CM cells were recruited at levels higher than their target muscles (Fig. 4); however, such high-threshold CM cells are seen rarely.

The most interesting case of muscle activation without CM cells occurs with rapid forceful movements. CM cells that fired strongly with moderate, well-controlled ramp-and-hold movements showed paradoxically meagre activity in relation to rapid alternating shaking of a manipulandum (Cheney & Fetz 1980). The latter ballistic movements involved considerably more intense activity of the cells' target muscles. This phenomenon has also been clearly demonstrated by Muir & Lemon (1983) for CM cells related to intrinsic hand muscles. When the monkey performed a precision grip response with thumb and forefinger, related CM cells were strongly activated; when the monkey performed a power grip task, involving even greater activity in the target muscles, the cells were relatively inactive.

Further evidence of such dissociation was obtained in studies in which CM cells were documented during both alternating ramp-and-hold movements and power grip responses (R.J. Kasser & P.D. Cheney, unpublished work). The CM cell in Fig. 5 facilitated several extensor muscles and fired with wrist extension during alternating ramp-and-hold responses, in which flexors and extensors were reciprocally activated. When the monkey performed a power grip by squeezing a pair of nylon bars, the extensors and

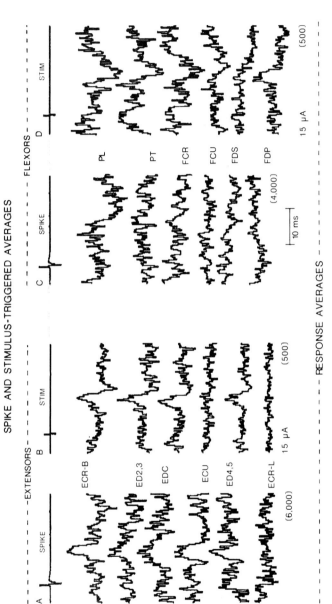

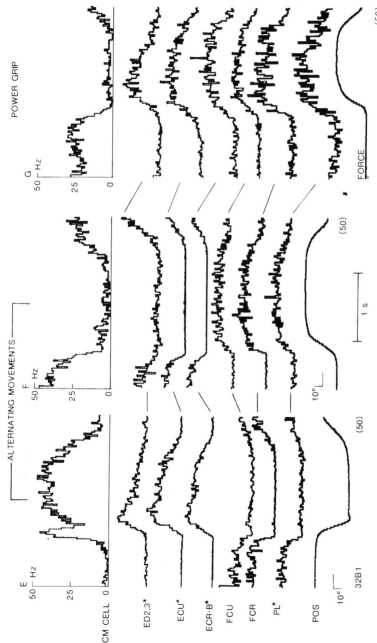

FIG. 5. Relation of a reciprocal CM cell to alternating wrist movements and power grip. Top records show reciprocal correlational linkages of the cell: post-spike facilitation of extensor muscles (A) and post-spike suppression of flexors (C). These reciprocal effects are further demonstrated by similar post-stimulus effects in averages triggered from single-pulse microstimuli delivered at the site of this CM cell (B,D). Response averages show that the CM cell was coactivated with its target muscles during alternating movements (E,F), and was suppressed during co-contraction of extensors and flexors in the power grip (G). Target muscles are indicated by asterisks. (From Cheney et al 1985.)

flexors co-contracted; during these co-contractions the activity of the CM cell dropped sharply, while its target muscles were vigorously active (bottom right). Such dissociation of CM cell and target muscle activity was observed in 14/23 of the CM cells tested under both conditions. An additional property of this cell provides a possible functional rationale for its behaviour: it had an inhibitory linkage to the flexor muscles, as revealed by spike-triggered averages of flexor EMG (top). Since the suppression of flexors is incompatible with their coactivation in the power grip, the neural mechanisms generating co-contraction of antagonists may exclude activation of such reciprocal CM cells. Support for this hypothesis can be found if one compares the correlational linkages of the CM cells to flexors and extensors with their relation to reciprocal responses versus co-contraction of these muscles. The reciprocal CM cells, which suppressed the antagonists of their target muscles, were less likely to be active during the power grip (4 of 13 cases) than the CM cells that produced pure facilitation (5 of 10 cases). It seems significant that the neural mechanisms that produce co-contraction of antagonists forgo the use of the reciprocal CM cells rather than inactivate the inhibitory interneurons.

Functional implications

The flexibility between CM cells and their target muscles allows a more extensive repertoire of responses than would be available with obligatory linkages. For example, the subthreshold effects of CM cells allow movements to be more specific than the muscle fields of the participating CM cells. A single muscle could be activated in isolation if its entire aggregrate of CM cells was recruited; even though many of these cells facilitate additional muscles, these wider effects would be more sparsely distributed and could remain subthreshold. Similarly, a movement involving coactivation of a group of muscles is unlikely to depend only on CM cells whose muscle fields match the activated muscles. *A priori*, the number of possible motor combinations clearly exceeds the number of CM cells available for each. It seems likely that a coordinated movement recruits a population of CM cells whose muscle fields include the activated muscles, but which may also include additional muscles. However, the above experiments suggest that significant constraints may pertain to the coactivation of physiological antagonists; CM cells with reciprocal correlational linkages seemed to be less involved in coactivation of antagonist muscles during performance of the power grip. Whether this observation is more related to the strength of the movement than to coactivation of the muscles remains to be determined by future experiments.

Acknowledgements

This work was supported in part by NIH grants NS 12542, RR 00166, NS 5082 and NSF grant BNS 82–16608. We thank our colleagues for permission to cite unpublished observations.

References

Asanuma H, Zarzecki P, Jankowska E, Hongo T, Marcus S 1979 Projections of individual pyramidal tract neurons to lumbar motor nuclei of the monkey. Exp Brain Res 34:78–89

Buys ER, Lemon RN, Mantel GWH, Muir RB 1986 Selective facilitation of different hand muscles by single corticospinal neurones in the conscious monkey. J Physiol (Lond) 381:529–549

Cheney PD, Fetz EE 1980 Functional classes of primate corticomotoneuronal cells and their relation to active force. J Neurophysiol 44:775–791

Cheney PD, Fetz EE 1984 Corticomotoneuronal cells contribute to long-latency stretch reflexes in the rhesus monkey. J Physiol (Lond) 394:249–272

Cheney PD, Fetz EE, Palmer SS 1985 Patterns of facilitation and suppression of antagonist forelimb muscles from motor cortex sites in the awake monkey. J Neurophysiol 53:805–820

Cheney PD, Kasser RJ, Fetz EE 1985 Motor and sensory properties of primate corticomotoneuronal cells. Exp Brain Research Suppl 10:211–231

Cheney PD, Mewes K, Fetz EE 1987 Encoding of motor parameters by corticomotoneuronal and rubromotoneuronal cells producing post-spike facilitation of forelimb muscles in the behaving monkey. Brain Behav, in press

Clough JFM, Kernell D, Phillips CG 1968 The distribution of monosynaptic excitation from the pyramidal tract and from primary spindle afferents to motoneurones of the baboon's hand and forearm. J Physiol (Lond) 198:145–166

Cope TC, Fetz EE, Matsumura M 1987 Cross-correlation assessment of synaptic strength of single Ia fibre connections with triceps surae motoneurons in the cat. J Physiol (Lond) in press

Evarts EV 1968 Relation of pyramidal tract activity to force exerted during voluntary movement. J Neurophysiol 31:14–27

Fetz EE, Cheney PD 1978 Muscle fields of primate corticomotoneuronal cells. J Physiol (Paris) 74:239–245

Fetz EE, Cheney PD 1980 Postspike facilitation of forelimb muscle activity by primate corticomotoneuronal cells. J Neurophysiol 44:751–772

Fetz EE, Finocchio DV 1975 Correlations between activity of motor cortex cells and arm muscles during operantly conditioned response patterns. Exp Brain Res 23:217–240

Fetz EE, Gustafsson B 1983 Relation between shapes of post-synaptic potentials and changes in firing probability of cat motoneurones. J Physiol (Lond) 341:387–410

Fetz EE, Cheney PD, German DC 1976 Corticomotoneuronal connections of precentral cells detected by post-spike averages of EMG activity in behaving monkeys. Brain Res 114:505–510

Fromm C, Evarts EV 1977 Relation of motor cortex neurons to precisely controlled and ballistic movements. Neurosci Lett 5:259–266

Jankowska E, Padel Y, Tanaka R 1975 Projections of pyramidal tract cells to α-motoneurones innervating hindlimb muscles in the monkey. J Physiol (Lond) 249:637–667

Kasser RJ, Cheney PD 1985 Characteristics of corticomotoneuronal postspike facilitation and reciprocal suppression of EMG activity in the monkey. J Neurophysiol 53:959–978

Landgren S, Phillips CG, Porter R 1962 Cortical fields of origin of the monosynaptic
  pyramidal pathways to some alpha motoneurones of the baboon's hand and forearm.
  J Physiol (Lond) 161:112–125
Lawrence DG, Porter R, Redman S 1985 Corticomotoneuronal synapses in the
  monkey: light microscopic localisation upon motoneurons of intrinsic muscles of the
  hand. J Comp Neurol 232:499–510
Lemon RN, Mantel GWH, Muir RB 1986 Corticospinal facilitation of hand muscles
  during voluntary movement in the conscious monkey. J Physiol (Lond) 381:497–527
Muir RB, Lemon RN 1983 Corticospinal neurons with a special role in precision grip.
  Brain Res 261:312–316
Palmer SS, Fetz EE 1985 Discharge properties of primate forearm motor units during
  isometric muscle activity. J Neurophysiol 54:1178–1193
Phillips CG, Porter R 1964 The pyramidal projection to motoneurones of some muscle
  groups of the baboon's forelimb. In: Eccles JC, Schadé JP (eds) Physiology of spinal
  neurones. Elsevier, Amsterdam (Prog Brain Res vol 12) p 222–242
Phillips CG, Porter R 1977 Corticospinal neurones: their role in movement. Academic
  Press, London (Monogr Physiol Soc 34) p 158–161
Porter R 1985 The corticomotoneuronal component of the pyramidal tract: corticomotoneuronal connections and functions in primates. Brain Res Rev 10:1–26
Porter R, Hore J 1969 The time course of minimal cortico-motoneuronal excitatory
  postsynaptic potentials in lumbar motoneurons of the monkey. J Neurophysiol 32:
  443–451
Shinoda Y, Yokota J-I, Futami T 1981 Divergent projection of individual corticospinal
  axons to motoneurons of multiple muscles in the monkey. Neurosci Lett 23:7–12
Smith WS, Fetz EE 1986 Task-related synchronization of primate motor cortex cells
  during active movement. Soc Neurosci Abstr 12:256
Thach WT 1978 Correlation of neural discharge with pattern and force of muscular
  activity, joint position and direction of intended next movement in motor cortex and
  cerebellum. J Neurophysiol 41:654–676

DISCUSSION

*Goldman-Rakic:*You said that the corticomotoneuronal (CM) cells were in clusters. There is some evidence that callosum columns alternate with intra-hemispheric (associational) columns in the cortex. Have you tested whether anything different is being coded in the callosum as opposed to adjacent associational columns?

Fetz: Ours were all layer V cells and many were tested for corticospinal projections by pyramidal tract stimulation. I'm not sure how these CM cells would be distributed relative to callosal neurons. We did not stimulate the corpus callosum or the contralateral hemisphere to determine the response properties of callosal cells.

Thach: Fromm & Evarts (1981) attributed a fixed size principle to CM cells. They suggested that smaller cells are first recruited in movements of increasing power and larger ones are only added at the top. This and Roger Lemon's evidence shows that with certain kinds of power grip a cell that is recorded at smaller levels of force for other kinds of grip drops out. This would seem to be a dramatic exception to the small-to-large recruitment order of the size principle.

Fetz: Yes, I agree that this property of CM cells is inconsistent with a size principle of recruitment for these cells. Fromm & Evarts (1981) did not really characterize the target projections of their precentral cells. So the cells that were preferentially recruited with the higher-force movements could also have been involved in activating peripheral or postural muscles that were activated only with the more intense movements.

Freund: Is there evidence for specialized task groups in the motor cortex? Thomas et al (1986) studied the selective activation of motor units located in different compartments of the first dorsal interosseous muscle during different mechanical requirements, such as stretching or adducting the forefinger.

Fetz: That hasn't been looked at directly, to my knowledge.

Porter: Some of the cells that Muir & Lemon (1983) recorded from need not have been activated at all in the tasks your monkeys were performing. Muir & Lemon were particularly interested in the use of individual digits and in the fractionation of muscle contraction associated with that.

Georgopoulos: Did you record any cells that would be activated specifically by co-contraction?

Cheney: We recorded from identified CM cells in monkeys during two tasks—alternating wrist movements and power grip. The alternating movement task involves a reciprocal pattern of activation of wrist flexor and extensor muscles whereas the power grip task involves coactivation of antagonist muscles. Of 51 CM cells for which we computed spike-triggered averages of both flexor and extensor muscles, only one cell, so far, has convincingly co-facilitated both flexors and extensors. However, in recordings from rubromotoneuronal cells under similar conditions we have found a significant population of co-facilitation cells (12 of 53 cells tested).

Georgopoulos: How then can you explain Dr Humphrey's observations?

Cheney: Humphrey & Reed (1983) found a class of cells in the convexity of the precentral gyrus (anterior MI) that were poorly modulated in relation to reciprocal patterns of flexor and extensor muscle activity associated with wrist movements but showed sustained increases in background discharge during coactivation of wrist flexor and extensor muscles. Coactivation was associated with stiffening at the wrist joint to oppose displacements produced by a continuous 1 Hz sinusoidal torque perturbation applied to the wrist. In addition, Humphrey and Reed were able to evoke co-excitation of flexor and extensor muscles by repetitive microstimulation applied to the cortical sites where these co-contraction related cells were found. On the basis of these findings they postulated that such cells may send excitatory terminals to motor neurons of both flexor and extensor muscles. Given the ubiquitous occurrence of antagonist muscle co-contraction, the existence of a unique class of cells specifically organized for co-contraction would seem to have considerable potential utility. However, microstimulation excites multiple corticospinal cells, not just one cell, so the specific pattern of stimulus-evoked motor output that is observed is not necessarily characteristic of any individual cell. The existence of a zone in motor cortex containing cells that individually co-facilitate flexor and extensor muscles remains to be demonstrated at the level of single CM cells. We have found little evidence that individual CM cells are organized to produce co-facilitation. However, our recordings have been largely from the bank of the precentral gyrus, whereas Humphrey's co-contraction zone was on the convexity of the gyrus; so this issue needs to be examined further.

Calne: How stable is the system when you are recording from a cell, Dr Fetz?

Fetz: The monkeys make these movements under relatively stable conditions. The one disruption of input we studied involved torque perturbations of the wrist. We have not used interventions like cooling.

Thach: In those reaction-time experiments Meyer-Lohman et al (1977) showed that cooling the dentate delayed the onset of motor cortex activation of CM cells and also the onset of movement, as shown in the electromyogram (EMG). Presumably the motor cortex–motor neuronal linkage stays fixed and even if the activation of motor cortex and subsequently the EMG was delayed in time, that linkage would remain tight.

Would post-spike facilitation be a useful technique for looking at linkages further into the motor system—for example, at the potentially tight linkage between a cerebellar unit and a motor cortex unit via the thalamus?

Fetz: The probability of detecting post-spike enhancement through a disynaptic link is the product of the probabilities of the two monosynaptic links. Statistically, this tends to be extremely small. Nevertheless, the post-spike suppression indicates that disynaptic links *can* generate detectable effects. Several factors can raise the relative strength of disynaptic mediation: a large number of mediating interneurons, the fact that interneurons are fired more readily than motor neurons, and the enhancement of inhibitory postsynaptic potentials near firing threshold. Disynaptic mediation of *excitatory* effects from cortex to motor neurons in the primate is less probable. If this were a prominent pathway, we should see disynaptic EPSPs in the intracellular recordings. The synaptic potentials in thalamocortical cells from cerebellar nuclear cells are so large that this link should be detected by cross-correlation, if the connected units can be found and recorded simultaneously.

Calne: Rather than cooling the central nucleus, would it be easier to use a drug that takes the striatum out?

Porter: When the drug dose is high enough to abolish transmission through the system it often prevents movement.

Kuypers: You are dealing with cells concerned with movement, not with muscles, aren't you?

Fetz: One could interpret the function of the CM cells as facilitating movements that involve their target muscles. A common question is whether the CM cells are specifically related to those movements that are produced by coactivation of their target muscles. It seems unlikely that they would be exclusively involved in those particular movements and no others. Presumably they would also be active in movements that engage only subsets of their target muscles. Strictly speaking, the empirical evidence indicates that their role is to facilitate activity of their target muscles, and this may occur with a variety of movements.

Kuypers: If I transect the pyramidal tract the precision grip cannot be made, although the power grip can be executed. So I still tend towards the idea that the cells are dealing with movements rather than with muscles.

Fetz: Yes, the evidence suggests that the CM cells are preferentially active in fine movements, and less involved in powerful, rapid movements, although both engage their target muscles.

Rizzolatti: What is the definition of movement in this case? What is lacking for what you saw to be defined as movement?

Fetz: There *is* a wrist movement. I didn't mean to say that it is not a coordinated movement. The question is what is represented by the CM cells. One can interpret the experimental evidence either way. Single CM cells facilitate individual muscles or, more often, a group of target muscles, so in their correlational linkages they clearly represent muscles. When those target muscles are coactivated in a movement, you could also say the cell's activity represents the movement. I'm not sure how useful this distinction really is under these conditions.

Cheney: The issue of whether muscles or movements are represented by CM cells suffers from the implication that one or the other, but not both, must be represented. To the extent that every CM cell has an identifiable set of target muscles, one can argue that muscles are represented by individual cortical cells. It seems to me that the question of whether movements are also represented depends on whether the combinations of muscles facilitated by single cells (the cell's muscle field) form synergies that are functionally meaningful in the sense that activation of the synergy yields a purposeful movement or a distinct part of a purposeful movement. In this sense, cells with reciprocal or co-facilitation patterns of output effects on agonist and antagonist muscles might be thought of as representing movements. In addition, neurons that show strong modula-tion for one type of movement, for example, precision grip, but not another type, despite a similar pattern of activation of the cell's target muscles in the two movements, should also be considered as representing movements, since the neuron's discharge, in this case, would be movement-dependent. To test this issue further will require tasks that fractionate muscles into functionally meaningful combinations (synergies).

Lemon: An even better test might be to test two different fractionated movements which are different both in form and in the goal they are designed to achieve. If you could then see a difference in the activity of the population of CM cells projecting to the muscles of the hand, you would perhaps be nearer to an answer. The patterns of connectivity which you see by averaging should not be confused with the behavioural relationship of the cell's activity to the activity of the muscles. One often finds muscles which are coactivated in a particular movement with a particular corticomotor cell, but the cells have no connection with these muscles. One has to be careful about drawing direct parallels between behaviour and connectivity in this kind of study.

Kuypers: If one cell is involved in that movement and the same muscle makes another movement, would you say that the cell is then probably not involved?

Cheney: I think we are finding that although a descending neuron's connections with motor neurons are relatively fixed, its activity must be considered movement- or task-dependent and not always predictable on the basis of the activity of its target muscles.

Porter: But is there any problem about that? Everyone seems to be saying that an instruction set generated somewhere in the brain selects from the motor cortex, and maybe from many other regions as well, certain descending connections that are to be activated. Their multiple innervation of a whole set of neuronal elements in the spinal cord leads to an output from the spinal cord. That output may be as limited, at least in the human hand muscles, as the activation under voluntary control of a single motor unit. Under other circumstances that output is directed to a wide population of muscles which are activated in what Paul Cheney called synergies. A given cortical cell may or may not be involved in the operation of that system, depending on what its contribution is to the total activation of the spinal cord.

Fetz: The movement may also be very specific and still involve CM cells whose output effects are less specific. For example, contracting a single muscle in isolation may recruit many CM cells with large muscle fields. Since their effects on additional target muscles can be subthreshold, the actual movement can be more specific than the muscle fields of the cells involved.

Strick: One can ask whether there is a CM cell branching pattern for every possible movement. Based on existing data, the answer would have to be no, there is not. Radial and ulnar deviations, for example, require coactivation of wrist flexors and extensors. However, no single cortical cells have been observed that branch to both wrist flexors and extensors.

Lemon: But if you don't search the cortex while the monkey is making this movement you may not find the cell that is related to the movement.

Porter: Pronation and supination are also complex movements involving many muscles, and these movements seem to be very dependent on the operation of corticospinal controls. I presume that another set of activations is required for the use of the muscles in pronation and supination.

Freund: This idea fits fairly well with the general scheme that the further upstream one looks, the more selective is the involvement of the neurons for certain aspects of the movement. If you cut the peripheral nerve no movement will be possible at all. If you cut the pyramidal tract or ablate the precentral motor strip, fractionated movements will disappear but some synergistic movements will recover. In other areas further upstream (premotor, parietal) only some aspects of motor behaviour may be disturbed.

Porter: Dr Fetz, what are the likely conduction velocities of the fibres you studied? This might partly tell us whether slow as well as fast pyramidal tract axons can be involved in this sort of activity. Or are slow pyramidal tract axons, as many people earlier believed, innervating only the parts of the spinal cord that are concerned with activation in proximal muscles?

Fetz: The antidromic latencies of some of the CM cells in our studies were as long as 3.5 ms, representing the slowly conducting pyramidal tract fibres.

Porter: Yet you are confident that the latency of those post-spike facilitations is consistent with a monosynaptic action of those slow-conducting fibres?

Fetz: Yes, the slowly conducting CM cells produced post-spike facilitation at longer latencies—about 15–19 ms. Some of this delay must also represent longer conduction times in smaller motor neurons. We also saw some 'complex' facilitations that began too early to be mediated by monosynaptic action of the recorded cell.

References

Fromm C, Evarts EV 1981 Relation of size and activity of motor cortex pyramidal tract neurons during skilled movements in the monkey. J Neurosci 1:453–460

Humphrey DR, Reed DJ 1981 Separate cortical cell systems for the control of joint movement and of joint stiffness. Soc Neurosci Abstr 7:740

Humphrey DR, Reed DJ 1983 Separate cortical systems for control of joint movement and joint stiffness: reciprocal activation and coactivation of antagonist muscles. In: Desmedt JE (ed) Motor control mechanisms in health and disease. Raven Press, New York (Adv Neurol 9) p 347–372

Meyer-Lohman J, Hore J, Brooks VB 1977 Cerebellar participation in generation of prompt arm movements. J Neurophysiol 40:1038–1050

Muir RB, Lemon RN 1983 Corticospinal neurons with a special role in precision grip. Brain Res 261:312–316

Thomas CK, Ross BH, Stein RB 1986 Motor-unit recruitment in human first dorsal interosseous muscle for static contractions in three different directions. J Neurophysiol 55:1017–1029

General discussion 1

Porter: We have covered a range of observations, from gross anatomical connectivity and the revelations that come from electrical or magnetic stimulation of the brain output system to more refined considerations of what individual elements within those systems may be contributing to the total output when a conscious animal is making some sort of learnt movement. A number of questions have not yet been answered. For example, one issue is the minute organization of the motor areas and whether the radial arrays of cells which are so evident in everyone's anatomical observations really have within them some sort of functional columnar organization. Or will the wide-ranging collaterals of the output cells from those radial arrays make us revise our views of columnar organization and vertical interactions within a radial column?

Lemon: The corticomotoneuronal (CM) projection to the hand muscles is relatively restricted. In our recently published study (Buys et al 1986), we recorded from a total of 58 identified CM cells, together with electromyograms (EMGs) from up to 10 muscles. All the muscles acted on the hand and fingers. Most of these cells showed facilitation in only two or three of the ten sampled muscles. Although the spike-triggered averaging technique is very good for this type of connectivity study, it is very difficult to make precise measures of amplitude and latency from averages of multi-unit EMG. A second problem is that the duration of post-spike facilitation (PSF) in such averages is much longer (mean 14 ms) than might be expected from a brief monosynaptic input to the motor neuron pool and, with durations of this order, oligosynaptic influences can certainly not be ruled out (Lemon et al 1986).

Recently Geert Mantel and I have been trying to get round this problem by making cross-correlations between spikes from single CM cells and the activity of single motor units from thenar muscles (mainly abductor pollicis brevis: AbPB). Recordings were made while the monkey carried out a precision grip movement.

Fig. 1 shows the set of results for one corticospinal cell. This cell discharged before the onset of the precision grip movement (arrowed in Fig. 1F) and it was at least partly coactivated with discharges of a single adductor pollicis (AdP) motor unit that became active during the hold phase of the grip (Fig. 1F). The spike-triggered averages of the rectified AdP surface EMG showed a clear PSF (Fig. 1A). Fig. 1B shows the result of the cross-correlation of 20 000 pyramidal tract neuron (PTN) spikes with discharges of the motor unit. The correlogram shows a clear peak, with a latency of 17.4 ms and a half-width of 1.5 ms. The form and size of the correlation peak are strongly suggestive of monosynaptic

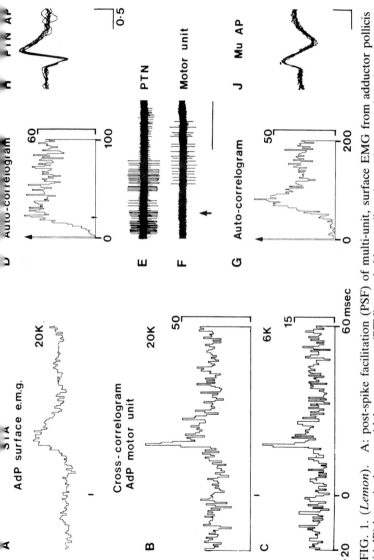

FIG. 1. (*Lemon*). A: post-spike facilitation (PSF) of multi-unit, surface EMG from adductor pollicis (AdP) by a single pyramidal tract neuron (PTN) revealed by a spike-triggered average (STA) of rectified EMG with respect to 20 000 PTN spikes. Spike discharges occurred at time zero (small vertical line). B: cross-correlogram of the same 20K PTN spikes (at time zero) with discharges of a single motor unit recorded from AdP. Bin width 500 μs. Bar at the right indicates number of motor unit discharges per bin. C: as in B, but with the exclusion of PTN trigger spikes preceded or succeeded by interspike intervals of < 20 ms. Note that the principal peak is still present in the correlogram. D and G: autocorrelograms of PTN and motor unit discharges respectively; bin width 1 ms and 2 ms respectively. E and F: recording of PTN and motor unit discharges during a single trial; PTN activity preceded the onset of precision grip (arrowed). Time bar 1s. H and J: superimposed plots of PTN and motor unit action potentials (Mu AP) respectively. Voltage calibrations are 100 μV in H and 200 μV in J.

action and, as far as we are aware, this represents the first direct experimental evidence for a CM input to a single motor unit in a conscious, moving monkey (Mantel & Lemon 1987). Most of the peaks we have observed were very brief (mean 1.9 ms); a few showed a 'tail' after the principal peak (e.g. Fig. 1B). The amplitude of the correlogram peak is usually expressed as the 'k factor': the height of the peak divided by the baseline count. The k factors we have obtained from 30 correlograms with 12 different CM cells ranged from 1.2 to 3.0. Work in which both EPSPs and correlogram peaks have been studied (Gustafsson & Macrea 1984, Cope et al 1987) makes it possible to predict that peaks of this size probably originate from CM EPSPs with peak amplitudes of between 50 and 200 µV. The work by Redman & Walmsley (1983) on Ia synapses indicates that EPSPs of this magnitude could be produced by single synaptic contacts, as described by Lawrence et al (1985).

If a correlation peak was found between a given cortical cell and one motor unit in AbPB, a peak was generally found with most AbPB motor units. An example is shown in Fig. 2. This PTN produced PSF in the averaged surface EMG of AbPB (Fig. 2A), and correlation peaks were seen in correlograms made with all three discriminable motor units recorded in this muscle (Fig. 2B–D). Superimposed action potentials are shown in Fig. 2F–H. Inspection of the motor unit recordings showed that these potentials came from three *different* motor units, and this was confirmed by constructing motor unit-triggered averages (M.u.TA) of unrectified surface EMG; the resulting averages were all clearly different in form and amplitude (Fig. 2J–L).

The range of latencies for onset of correlation peaks in AbPB was 8.1–16.3 ms (mean 12.1 ms, $n = 27$). Different motor units, correlated with the same CM cell, had peaks with latencies varying by as much as 4 ms. This is probably due to differences in the conduction velocity of different motor units. This factor, combined with the temporal dispersion of the motor unit action potential in the surface EMG (compare Fig. 2F–H with J–L), probably explains the long duration of the facilitation observed in spike-triggered averages of surface EMG compared with the correlation peaks of individual motor units.

The motor neuron pools of the thenar muscles are arranged in long narrow columns in the C_8 and Th_1 spinal segments. Since we find positive correlations between single CM cells and most of the sampled AbPB motor units, we infer a longitudinal collateralization of corticospinal axons such as that described by Lawrence et al (1985).

Cheney: I would like to mention some of our recent work on the rubromotoneuronal system which is relevant to the issues we have considered here. Muir & Lemon (1983) reported that some corticospinal cells discharge intensely for precision grip but are relatively unmodulated for power grip, which involves all the fingers acting in concert. We have observed a similar specialization among some cells in the rubromotoneuronal system. Based on discharge relations to movement, we can define two populations of rubromotoneuronal cells: one is strongly modulated during a simple alternating wrist movement

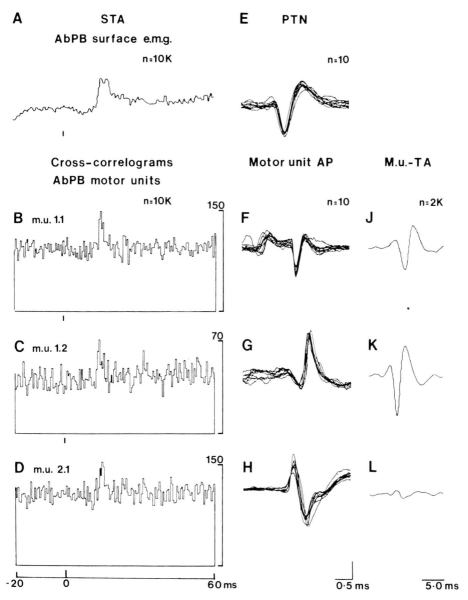

FIG. 2 (*Lemon*). A: spike-triggered average of abductor pollicis brevis (AbPB) surface EMG with respect to 10K spikes from a PTN. B–D: cross-correlograms between the same 10K PTN spikes (discharge at time zero) and discharges of three different motor units recorded from AbPB. E and F–H: 10 superimposed plots of action potentials recorded from the PTN and the three motor units respectively. Voltage calibration: 200 µV (F,G) and 500 µV (H). J–L: averages of unrectified, surface EMG of AbPB made with respect to 2000 action potentials of each individual motor unit. Note the differences in form of the resulting motor unit-triggered averages (M.u.TA).

task; the other shows little or no modulation during this task, despite producing strong post-spike facilitation of the forearm muscles involved in the task. On further testing, we found that the unmodulated cells were, in fact, strongly modulated in relation to a different task involving precision grip of a piece of food using the index finger and thumb. This represents another case in which target muscle activity was dissociated from that of the corresponding descending neuron, and again emphasizes that activation of descending neurons is dependent not only on muscle activity but also on the particular task being executed by those muscles.

Porter: Presumably those cells are being driven by some sort of descending connections with the red nucleus. Have you tried to see what happens to the discharges of rubromotoneuronal fibres when the cortex isn't driving them?

Cheney: The modulation of these rubromotoneuronal cells must be derived from either the cortex or the cerebellum, since those are the two major inputs to red nucleus. But we do not know which input is dominant under the conditions of our behavioural task.

Kuypers: The fibres from the motor cortex to the magnocellular or rather the rubrospinal red nucleus are limited in number, compared to the very large number of cerebellar interpositus fibres that terminate on those same neurons. Further, the cortical fibres have a tendency to terminate on the periphery of the dendritic tree, while the cerebellar fibres end on the dendrites and directly on the neuronal cell bodies. Therefore, the cerebellum must represent a very important driving source for these neurons.

Porter: Do you think the cerebellum takes the decision to move?

Kuypers: I do not know.

Marsden: One of the assumptions about the dissociation between firing of a pyramidal tract neuron and muscle activity under certain conditions is that exactly the same piece of muscle is involved in two separate movements. There is a good precedent for caution about that. Breakdown of the recruitment order and the size principle has been claimed to be demonstrated using the first dorsal interosseous muscle of the human hand as either an abductor or a flexor of the first finger. Reversal of recruitment order of motor units in the first dorsal interosseous can be demonstrated for those two movements and it was assumed that there was a breakdown in the size principle. It has been pointed out that different parts of that muscle are used to undertake that movement. Measurement of the activity of the whole muscle may be giving an incorrect answer if mechanically different parts of the muscle are being used. I don't know how you sort that out.

Kuypers: That is a very interesting observation. It would indicate that a muscle as defined anatomically is perhaps not a true muscle, and that an anatomical muscle actually consists of several 'functional muscles' which are used in different movements. Under such circumstances cortical neurons may be dealing with movements which are brought about by different 'functional muscles'.

Goldman-Rakic: I wonder whether you are really testing the essential function which the cortex has been specialized to do? The motor cortex is probably involved in fine digit control, but is it engaged at a monitoring level, as opposed to performing its quintessential function of integrating information from the environment and deciding to perform an action? The behavioural tests that we neuroscientists have to use to study cortical function in animals sometimes seem to bypass the voluntary aspect.

Thach: As you say, most of our monkeys are over-trained on the simple movement that we study. It becomes very stereotyped and automatic. The cerebellum plays a role in initiating these movements; whether it does so when the movement is less trained and more 'elective' is open to question.

Calne: Beevor has used an analogy between motor control in a ship and motor control in the brain. Everybody knows where the engine room is but nobody knows where the captain is. It seems to me that we have a lot of good engineers and people who understand the mechanism for turning the rudder but this is all execution. We still don't know anything about where or how the captain makes decisions. If one gets back to the concept of parallel processing in relation to control, some decision-making is still needed to integrate the parallel processing. Why is the cortex regarded as having the quintessential role of decision-making?

Lemon: I wish I knew the answer. The studies related to connectivity are only useful in the sense that they allow us to look at the cortical output. Beyond that you might say that studies of functional connectivity are not much use at all. However, if we are to understand which functions are localized in the cortex, we must first decide to study a particular group of cells which have a particular target in the animal's limb. Until we have made that step we cannot hope to see exactly what those particular cells are contributing to *their target muscles and to movement.* To poke an electrode into the cortex and see how the activity of a completely unidentified cell changes with a particular type of movement or whatever function you decide to study is, in my view, a lost cause.

Calne: What you are studying is what you are able to study—if an experiment to analyse the function of the cerebral cortex is possible, that is the experiment you do. That still leaves this big gap of the quintessential role of the motor cortex and its relationship with other components of the motor system. There has been major emphasis on cortical function but not so much on cortical relationships with other parts of the brain. From clinical evidence we know that these other parts clearly have an important role to play in both the execution and the initiation of movement.

Porter: We may come back to some of those matters later. We know what the motor neuron does. We are working towards an understanding of the way in which signals directed to the motor neuron, to make it do what it does, are organized in the brain. One of the output systems that is approachable by the electrophysiologists and that has some relevance to the clinical questions must be the part of the cortex that is most directly connected to the motor neuron population. Tom Thach will tell us later about some of the other connections that are of interest clinically.

References

Buys EJ, Lemon RN, Mantel GWH, Muir RB 1986 Selective facilitation of different hand muscles by single corticospinal neurones in the conscious monkey. J Physiol (Lond) 381:529–549

Cope TC, Fetz EE, Matsumura M 1987 Cross-correlation assessment of synaptic strength of single Ia fibre connections with triceps surae motoneurones in cats. J Physiol (Lond) 390:161–188

Gustafsson B, McCrea D 1984 Influence of stretch-evoked synaptic potentials on firing probability of cat spinal motoneurones. J Physiol (Lond) 347:431–451

Lawrence DG, Porter R, Redman SJ 1985 Cortico-motoneuronal synapses in the monkey: light microscopic localization upon motoneurones of intrinsic muscles of the hand. J Comp Neurol 232:499–510

Lemon RN, Mantel GWH, Muir RB 1986 Corticospinal facilitation of hand muscles during voluntary movement in the conscious monkey. J Physiol (Lond) 381:497–527

Mantel GWH, Lemon RN 1987 Cross-correlation reveals facilitation of single motor units in thenar muscles by single corticospinal neurones in the conscious monkey. Neurosci Lett 77:113–118

Muir RB, Lemon RN 1983 Corticospinal neurons with a special role in precision grip. Brain Res 261:312–316

Redman SJ, Walmsley B 1983 Amplitude fluctuation in synaptic potentials evoked in cat spinal motoneurones at identified group IA synapses. J Physiol (Lond) 343:135–146

Cortical mechanisms subserving reaching

Apostolos P. Georgopoulos

The Philip Bard Laboratories of Neurophysiology, Department of Neuroscience, The Johns Hopkins University, School of Medicine, 725 North Wolfe Street, Baltimore, Maryland 21205, USA

Abstract. The generation and control of reaching in space is a function of several structures, cortical and subcortical. This paper summarizes some principles of the cortical mechanisms subserving this function, as revealed by recording the impulse activity of neurons in motor cortex and area 5 of the posterior parietal cortex in behaving monkeys. Large populations of neurons in these cortical areas are engaged in reaching. This engagement is early in time; for example, cell activity in the motor cortex begins to change 60–80 ms after target onset, and slightly later in area 5. The time course of cell recruitment in the active population is very similar for reaching movements of equal amplitude directed to different targets. In contrast, the intensity of cell discharge in both motor and parietal cortex is clearly modulated with respect to the direction of reaching. Typically, the firing rate is a cosine function of the direction of the movement in space. An unambiguous distributed code for the direction of reaching exists in neuronal populations in the cortical areas studied. The outcome of this population code can be visualized as a vector in neural space that points in the direction of the upcoming movement.

1987 Motor areas of the cerebral cortex. Wiley, Chichester (Ciba Foundation Symposium 132) p 125–141

How is the direction of reaching represented in motor cortex and parietal cortex (area 5)? We studied this problem by recording the impulse activity of single neurons in these cortical areas of rhesus monkeys while the animals reached towards visual targets. In some experiments the monkeys moved a handle towards target lights on a planar working surface (Georgopoulos et al 1982, 1983, Kalaska et al 1983); in others, they reached out freely and touched targets in three-dimensional (3-D) space (Georgopoulos et al 1986). The behavioural, surgical and electrophysiological techniques, as well as the methods used to analyse the results, are described in the aforementioned publications.

Directional tuning

Of the cells activated during reaching, about 80% are tuned around a preferred direction. The frequency of impulse activity is highest with movements in

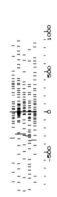

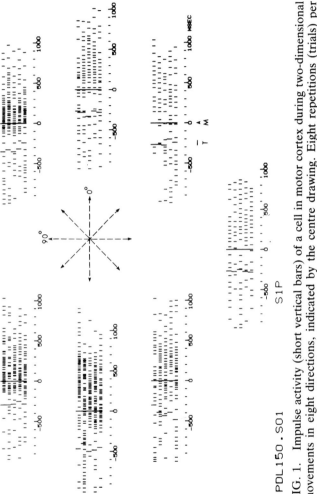

PDL150.SO1   S1P

FIG. 1. Impulse activity (short vertical bars) of a cell in motor cortex during two-dimensional movements in eight directions, indicated by the centre drawing. Eight repetitions (trials) per direction are shown aligned to the onset of movement (M). Longer vertical bars preceding the onset of movement indicate the onset of the target light (T). The animal held the manipulandum at the centre of the working surface for a period of time, and then moved toward a peripheral light when it came on in a reaction-time task (Georgopoulos et al 1982).

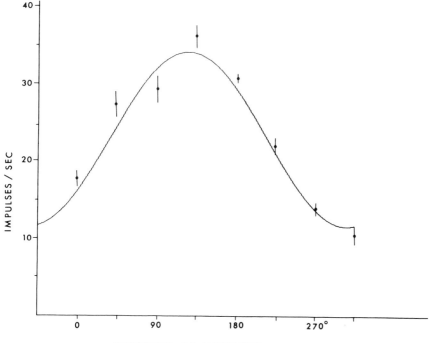

FIG. 2.   Directional tuning curve of the same cell as in Fig. 1. The data points are the mean (± SEM) frequency of discharge from the target onset until the end of the movement. (From Georgopoulos et al 1982. Reproduced by permission of the publisher.)

the neuron's preferred directions and decreases progressively with movements made at larger angles from that preferred direction. The directional tuning is illustrated in Fig. 1 for a motor cortical neuron. The tuning is broad and can be described by a cosine function, which is plotted in Fig. 2. The same broadly tuned cosine function holds for the direction of reaching in 3-D space (Georgopoulos et al 1986).

   It is remarkable that neurons from motor and parietal cortex have similar directional tuning properties (Kalaska et al 1983). This suggests that these interconnected cortical areas (Strick & Kim 1978, Caminiti et al 1985) interact, with respect to the control of reaching, within a common spatial framework.

Latency of change in neuronal activity

Neurons in both motor cortex and area 5 change activity well before the onset of movement. Fig. 3 shows that activity in the motor cortical population

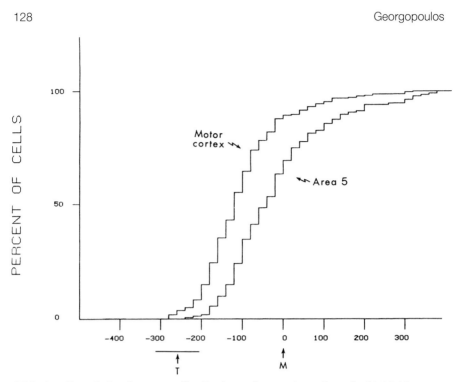

FIG. 3.   Cumulative frequency distributions of onset times (in ms) of initial increase in discharge rate in cells in motor cortex ($n = 216$) and area 5 ($n = 141$). M, T, as in Fig. 1. (From Kalaska et al 1983. Reproduced by permission of the publisher.)

changes about 60 ms before that in area 5. These findings indicate that both structures participate in the generation of reaching. Moreover, the lag of the responses of the neuronal populations in area 5 is consistent with the hypothesis that this area probably receives an efferent copy of the motor command from the motor cortex.

   It is noteworthy that in both cortical areas the time course of cell recruitment in the active population is similar for movements in different directions. This suggests that the neural process subserving the time course of the movement is independent of the movement's spatial characteristics, and that a common process may subserve this time course for reaching movements in any direction. This idea corresponds to the behavioural finding that the bell-shaped velocity profile of reaching movements is independent of the trajectory of the movement (see Georgopoulos 1986 for a review of the subject).

Motor command for reaching in space: coding of the direction of reaching by neuronal populations

It follows from the broad tuning function (Fig. 2) that (a) individual neurons

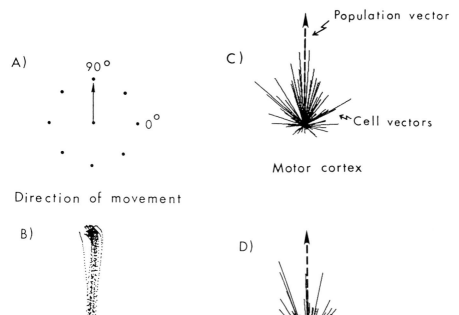

FIG. 4.   Population vector analysis. See text for explanation. The motor cortex ensemble consists of 241 cells (Georgopoulos et al 1982) and the area 5 ensemble of 151 cells (Kalaska et al 1983). (A–C from Georgopoulos et al 1984; D, from Kalaska et al 1983. Reproduced by permission of the respective publishers.)

are active with movements in many directions, and (b) a movement in a particular direction engages many neurons. This suggests that the whole neuronal ensemble is involved in generating the reaching movement. The hypothesized operation by the neuronal ensemble can be visualized in the following way (Georgopoulos et al 1983, 1986). Assume that each neuron in the ensemble exerts a directional influence along the axis of its preferred direction; that is, let an individual neuron be represented as a vector. Assume also that the length of this vector is proportional to the change in the neuron's discharge rate from a certain point. This results in a representation of the neuronal ensemble as a cluster of neuronal vectors. This vectorial ensemble yields a unique and unambiguous directional outcome, the 'population vector', which is the weighted vector sum of the individual neuronal contributions. We found that the population vector points in the direction of the reaching movement. This is illustrated in Fig. 4 A–D. The direction of movement on the planar working surface was toward 12 o'clock (Fig. 4A). Fig. 4B

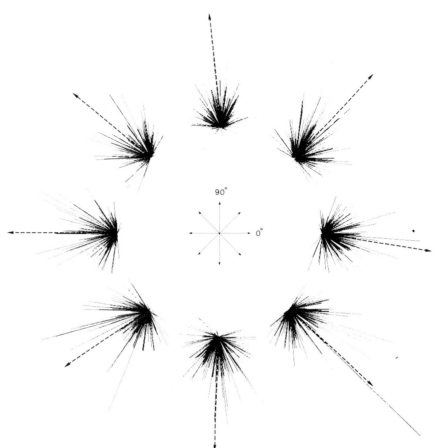

FIG. 5. The same motor cortical population (n = 241 cells) yields eight population vectors (thick interrupted lines) that point in the direction of movement (thin interrupted lines at centre). (From Georgopoulos et al 1983. Reproduced by permission of the publisher.)

shows trajectories of a well trained monkey. Fig. 4 C and D show the results obtained from motor cortex and area 5, respectively. Fig. 5 shows the result for all eight movement directions studied.

Visualizing the motor command in time: the population vector as a predictor of the upcoming movement direction

It is remarkable that the population vector predicts the direction of movement well before the movement begins. This is illustrated in Fig. 6 for the motor cortex and area 5. The population vector shown in the middle trace was calculated every 20 ms from ensembles of motor cortical (n = 241) and area

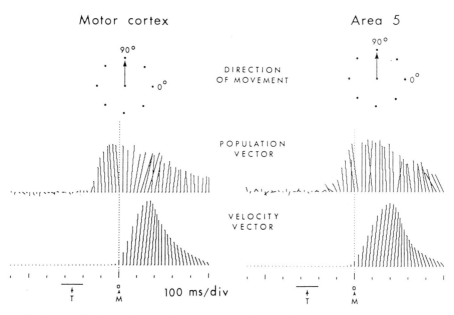

FIG. 6.   Prediction in time of the movement direction by the population vector. See text for explanation. (Motor cortex data from Georgopoulos et al 1984; reproduced by permission of the publisher. Area 5 data are from unpublished observations by A.P. Georgopoulos, J.F. Kalaska and R. Caminiti.)

5 (n = 151) neurons. The velocity vector shown in the lower trace was calculated from the average trajectories of movements of trials from which the respective population vector was derived. It can be seen that long before the onset of movement the population vector lengthens and points in the direction of the upcoming movement. This suggests that the population vector can serve as a neural probe to forecast the direction of movement in space. In fact, we found that the population vector in motor cortex predicts the direction of movement during a waiting period, when the movement is delayed by 0.5–3.2 s (Crutcher et al 1985).

Conclusions

The results summarized above suggest that the motor cortex and area 5 are intimately involved with the generation of reaching in space. The directional properties of single neurons and the coding of the direction of reaching by the respective neuronal ensembles are similar in these areas. This is noteworthy because the motor cortex has traditionally been associated with the control of muscles, whereas area 5 has been regarded as a somatosensory association cortex. Therefore, even if these areas are immediately concerned with different aspects of bodily function, they seem to communicate using the same 'language' in the directional domain. This domain transcends both of the specific functions above and provides the common framework within which generation and control of reaching in space takes place.

Acknowledgements

This work was supported by USPHS Grant NS17413.

References

Caminiti R, Zeger S, Johnson PB, Urbano A, Georgopoulos AP 1985 Corticocortical efferent systems in the monkey: a quantitative spatial analysis of the tangential distribution of cells of origin. J Comp Neurol 241:405–419
Crutcher MD, Schwartz AB, Georgopoulos AP 1985 Representation of movement direction in primate motor cortex in the absence of immediate movement. Soc Neurosci Abstr 11:1273
Georgopoulos AP 1986 On reaching. Annu Rev Neurosci 9:147–170
Georgopoulos AP, Kalaska JF, Caminiti R, Massey JT 1982 On the relations between the direction of two-dimensional arm movements and cell discharge in primate motor cortex. J Neurosci 2:1527–1537
Georgopoulos AP, Caminiti R, Kalaska JF, Massey JT 1983 Spatial coding of movement: a hypothesis concerning the coding of movement direction by motor cortical populations. Exp Brain Res (Suppl) 7:327–336
Georgopoulos AP, Kalaska JF, Crutcher MD, Caminiti R, Massey JT 1984 The representation of movement direction in the motor cortex: Single cell and population studies. In: Edelman GM et al (eds) Dynamic aspects of neocortical function. Wiley, New York, p. 501–524
Georgopoulos AP, Schwartz AB, Kettner RE 1986 Neuronal population coding of movement direction. Science (Wash DC) 233:1418–1419
Kalaska JF, Caminiti R, Georgopoulos AP 1983 Cortical mechanisms related to the direction of two-dimensional arm movements: Relations in parietal area 5 and comparison with motor cortex. Exp Brain Res 51:247–260
Strick PL, Kim CC 1978 Input to primate motor cortex from posterior parietal cortex (area 5). I. Demonstration by retrograde transport. Exp Brain Res 157:325–330

DISCUSSION

Thach: To what extent is the population vector related to the direction of the fingertip trajectory, independently of the movements of joints or the actions of muscles? Might the population discharge occur in response to a specific muscle pattern?

Georgopoulos: All the work I discussed was based on the direction of the hand. We have not seen any clear relationships to particular aspects of joint movement. We recorded from the proximal muscles and the muscles acting on the upper arm. In the two-dimensional task, the electromyographic (EMG) activity was broadly tuned, relative to the direction of the movement. We did not record EMGs simultaneously with neural recordings. We have not used other measures to see whether there is any relationship between particular muscle fibres and cell patterns.

Wu: Do these cells respond to peripheral stimuli?

Georgopoulos: In this area of the motor cortex very few cells respond to peripheral stimulation. In more lateral regions of the motor cortex, in which cell activity relates to the hand and fingers, there are clear responses to peripheral stimulation.

Rizzolatti: Are these neurons bilateral? Since they code such an abstract characteristic as direction of movement, one would expect them to fire in relation to movements of both arms.

Georgopoulos: We tested both arms at the beginning of this study but the driving was nearly always contralateral so we did not continue testing both arms. We usually restrain the other arm so that the animal performs the task with the contralateral hand.

Fetz: It seems remarkable at first sight that you can derive such a close correlate of movement direction from the activity of cortical cells without dealing with all the complex intervening mechanisms. But wouldn't the vector hypothesis produce this result for *any* large population of cells having preferred directions of firing? If you add the cells' vector contributions according to this hypothesis, the cells whose preferred direction coincides with the movement direction would add the most towards the net population vector. The cells whose preferred direction is opposite to the movement direction would add very little, and in fact if you take their relative activity as a negative amplitude, their vectors would even make a positive contribution. The off-axis vector components of the other cells would cancel out for a large enough population. Thus, the vector hypothesis inevitably leads to a population vector that points in the movement direction, whether the cells are causally involved or not.

Georgopoulos: You seem to have restricted your question to two opposite directions. In our experiments we deal with directions in all two- or three-dimensional space. Now, the answer to your question is 'no': the vector hypothesis would *not* hold for *any* population of cells with a preferred direction. Consider for example a population consisting of cells with preferred directions *only* towards 12 or 6 o'clock: this population would never give you a vector pointing in any other direction than towards 12 or 6 o'clock; even if you were making a movement towards 2, 4 or 9 o'clock, you would not get a population vector pointing in those directions. The reason is simple: the vector hypothesis assumes that a cell makes a vectorial contribution *in its own preferred direction*; therefore, if these preferred directions are arbitrarily restricted to certain directions, the hypothesis may not work. In the example above, the population vector will work only for the directions toward 12 or 6 o'clock but not for other directions in the two-dimensional space, and this result is independent of the number of cells in the population: even if you have a million cells, you cannot get a population vector pointing towards 3 o'clock if all your cells have preferred directions only towards 12 or 6 o'clock. The population vector hypothesis works *not* because any population of cells with a preferred direction will do, nor because any large number of cells will automatically give the appropriate result, due to their sheer number. It works, rather, for the following three reasons. First, the directional tuning functions of the constituent cells are radially symmetrical around their preferred direction. Secondly, these preferred directions are distributed throughout the three-dimensional directional space. And thirdly, the peak-to-peak tuning amplitude is independent of the preferred direction. Under these conditions, even a relatively small number of cells (e.g. 100–200) yields a population vector that points in the direction of movement (Schwartz et al 1986).

Therefore, our hypothesis works not because of some arbitrary theoretical reason, or a 'law of large numbers', but because the *experimentally observed* distributions are what they are in the actual data. In fact, it can be shown analytically that the conditions above are sufficient for our model to work.

Fetz: Granted that all these directions are represented in the activity of enough task-related cells, the question is whether the nervous system is really using this activity in the way the vector hypothesis proposes. As demonstrated by Humphrey et al (1970), one can derive population functions that match a variety of movement parameters, but this does not prove that these population functions are actually used to control those parameters, nor does it explain the underlying neural mechanisms.

Georgopoulos: Yes, the question is open on how that information is used; we are beginning to study the local cortical mechanisms that may subserve this directional information processing. I think you were right to put the question in an information context. Our population vector hypothesis has been successfully applied to the analysis of results from other cortical areas and from different experiments, including area 5 (this paper, and Kalaska et al 1983) and recently area 7 of the posterior parietal cortex (Steinmetz et al 1987). In the latter study the direction of a visual stimulus in space was successfully predicted by the population vector of directionally selective (in the visual space) cells of area 7. Therefore, our hypothesis should properly be regarded in the context of information processing, with the motor cortex data as one particular application.

Kuypers: I have a little trouble with the interconnections between the frontal and the parietal areas as you show them. I would expect the frontal area in question to be connected with at least the banks of the interparietal sulcus (Pandya & Kuypers 1969, Jones & Powell 1969, 1970).

Georgopoulos: We defined the arm area of area 5 purely by finding where the cells are that relate to proximal arm movements. That area extends over about the upper third of the interparietal sulcus but we did not explore further down.

Marsden: What happens when the animal has been trained to delay the response?

Georgopoulos: About 70% of the cells in the motor cortex respond after the cue.

Marsden: Does restraining the monkey's arm make any difference?

Georgopoulos: We have not done that experiment.

Thach: Again with respect to whether it is purely the abstract factor of direction that engages cortical discharge: have you tried loading the arm? This would alter muscle activity while keeping trajectory direction constant. If cortical discharge remained the same, then you could say it was indeed coded purely for direction.

Georgopoulos: Not yet.

Kalaska: We have done that experiment and the result depends on which neuron you are recording from. The results of many experiments suggest that the 'typical' motor cortex neuron is a cell that encodes the level of muscle force or torque at a particular angle across a joint. You can interpret the preferred direction vector as somehow corresponding to the angle for which that cell is controlling force or torque across the shoulder joint, so causing the limb to move along a particular path. If you apply a load which pulls the limb in a direction opposite to the preferred direction you should therefore see an enhancement of cell discharge, if the load parallels the preferred direction you should see a reduction, and with intermediate directions of load you should see continuous gradations of discharges. Essentially this experiment is a repetition of the studies done by Evarts in the 1960s, but in two dimensions instead of one. When we do this we see the predicted effect for many cells in the motor cortex—large changes in discharge with different directions of movement and with different directions of applied loads. Some neurons, however, are very directional for movement but show no effects in response to load direction, and one can see a continuum of cells with properties between these two extremes.

We are currently investigating what properties might determine where a cell lies along this continuum, but it is too early to say much on that question. However, I can say that the cells which show the largest load effects are the neurons with large-amplitude spikes, located in the intermediate layers. Again we have not confirmed whether these are corticospinal neurons. This work has been published in preliminary form (Kalaska & Hyde 1985).

We did the same study in area 5 and saw little load effect. The cells in area 5 seem to encode exclusively the spatial aspect of movement, whether joint angles, movement direction, or some other related factor. They show virtually no reflection of the muscle activity required to produce the movement.

Georgopoulos: In the usual task we use, when the signal comes the animal makes a movement. In the delayed task (Crutcher et al 1985) the light comes on and there is a delay before the dimming of the light that triggers the movement. The monkeys are trained not to move until the light dims. Even a very small change in muscle activity would take the monkey out of the small positional window within which the animal has to keep the handle. The delay is randomized and we have not observed any changes in muscle activity during that period. But 70% of the cells in the motor cortex show changes early in the delay period.

Goldman-Rakic: How long was the delay?

Georgopoulos: It varied from 0.5 to 3.2 s and it was randomized so that the animal could not predict when the light would dim. Consistent changes in cell activity were observed about 60–80 ms after the onset of the cue. If we do the population analysis after the onset of the cue, the population vector predicts the direction of the upcoming planar movement.

Porter: You made the recordings and then looked back at the population, rather than looking at the population while the animal was doing the test and predicting the direction then?

Georgopoulos: Yes. I believe that if we were making simultaneous recordings from 200 cells we would observe the same result.

Marsden: Does the population vector start off as though the movement was going to occur and then continue during the delay period?

Georgopoulos: Yes. The length of that vector is less than the length we see after the go signal. Whether that is transmitted downstream and is not enough to drive the spinal neuronal pools, or whether it is being gated somewhere else, we don't know, but the information is there.

Deecke: The oculomotor system has some formal similarity with the system you have investigated. There are cells in PPRF or tectum which are organized analogously in that they code the direction of saccadic eye movements in their firing characteristics. Would you like to expand a little on this analogy?

Georgopoulos: There are three points here. One concerns the tuning function, another the representation of the amplitude (i.e. extent) of the movement, and the third the population coding in the oculomotor system.

Concerning the directional tuning function, a cosine function similar to those described here has been used to describe the relations between the direction of saccadic eye movements and the frequency of discharge of cells in the pontine reticular formation (Henn & Cohen 1976). However, the preferred directions ('reference directions') of Henn & Cohen (1976, p 322) of those cells coincided with the pulling directions of the eye muscles, whereas in our case the preferred directions of the motor cortical and area 5 cells were distributed throughout the whole directional continuum.

Concerning the coding of the amplitude of the movement by the frequency of discharge of motor cortical cells, we first did experiments in which the movement amplitude was 8 and 16 cm. In that study we did not observe significant relations between movement amplitude and discharge rate during the reaction time, and only a few cells showed such relations during the movement time (A.P. Georgopoulos, J.F. Kalaska & R. Caminiti, unpublished work). In a second series of experiments (A.P. Georgopoulos & A.B. Schwartz, unpublished work) we tried four movement amplitudes in a logarithmic scale (1.5, 3.0, 6.0, 12.0 cm). In that case, several cells showed a weak but statistically significant relation to the amplitude of the movement. Of course, the amplitude of the movement could also be represented as a population parameter, for example, total number of impulses, total number of cells active, etc.

A third point of comparison with the oculomotor system is the population idea. Studies by McIlwain (1975) have shown that in the superior colliculus one is also dealing with coding in terms of neuronal populations.

Porter: But for the colliculus the population appears to code for the extent as well as the direction of the saccade that the eyes make to fixate a peripheral object.

Calne: In a sense, loading or restraining the limb is a perturbation of the normal behaviour of the cells from the periphery. Have you looked at the effect of a more confusing signal, such as two lights, one being a signal for initiating movement and the other for determining the direction?

Georgopoulos: Yes. When two or more lights were presented simultaneously, the animals tended to choose one while ignoring the others (A.P. Georgopoulos, J.F. Kalaska & J.T. Massey, unpublished work). When two lights were presented in quick succession, monkeys (Georgopoulos et al 1981) and human subjects (Massey et al 1986) moved the hand first towards the first light for a period of time that was proportional to the time for which the first light stayed on, and then changed direction and moved to the second light (Georgopoulos et al 1981; under those conditions saccadic eye movements recorded simultaneously were full to the first and second lights). Cells in the motor cortex (Georgopoulos et al 1983) and in area 5 (Kalaska et al 1981) showed successive changes in activity related to the first and the second target. We are currently trying central perturbations that we would rather call mental operations. We train monkeys to move at an angle from a stimulus direction. For example, we present the light at 12 o'clock and they have to move 90° counterclockwise, towards 9 o'clock; in the next trial the light is presented at a different location, e.g. 7 o'clock, and the animals have to move again 90° counterclockwise, towards 4 o'clock. Therefore, they have to make an angular transformation. Under those conditions, the reaction time of human subjects increases in a linear fashion with the amplitude of the angle: this suggests a mental rotation of an imagined movement vector (Georgopoulos & Massey 1987). Could one visualize this hypothesized operation as a rotation of the population vector? We hope that the current experiments may answer this question.

*Roland:*You and John Kalaska have now shown very nicely that you find a population of neurons in area 5 coding for a certain direction of movement.

Here you have a population of neurons in area 6 or 4 also coding for the direction of movement. How does the motor cortex know in what direction to move? You have shown that the area 5 cells fire *after* the motor cortex cells start to fire. Is this coding laid down during learning or is it a kind of hard-wiring of the premotor or motor cortex that was there all the time?

Georgopoulos: I don't think we know. We see very early engagement of the motor cortex, though, at 60 or 80 ms after a visual cue.

Roland: If you knock out area 5, you certainly get great deficits in reaching movements.

Georgopoulos: It depends how you grade the effect. It may be more a lack of motor planning than inaccuracy. The parietal cortex may provide the background for spatial operations. For that function, it does not have to be activated before the motor cortex: it can still provide the spatial framework for motor operations in space.

Porter: But both these groups of cells may be being driven by some other source of information.

Strick: I have two comments. First, the neural responses to the cue seemed remarkably early in some cases. You showed changes in activity that were 30–50 ms after the onset of the visual stimulus. Since it can take some time for the process of transduction to occur in the retina, 30–50 ms seems very early for a visual response to occur in the primary motor cortex.

Second, it is important to determine whether the change in activity you observed with the onset of the instruction is really dissociated from a change in tonic EMG activity. How confident are you that muscle activity was constant during the instruction period?

Georgopoulos: Murphy et al (1982, 1985) also recorded short latencies (≈ 50 ms) for arm-related cells in the motor cortex. Very short latencies could be due to anticipation of some sort by the animals.

The EMG traces showed no change in activity during the delay period. On the other hand there was no loading of the arm. In our system the plane is tilted 15° towards the animal. There is almost no friction and very little inertia. The animal exerts a force of about 40 g against gravity and there is a 10 mm positional window within which the animal has to hold the handle. The movement involves two joints (shoulder and elbow). To get tensing of muscles and still be within that window under these very light conditions the animal has to make a co-contraction in all possible muscles acting on these joints. It takes the animal about 10–15 days to learn the task—that is, to learn to hold still. They are simply trained not to move, and tensing their muscles will most probably take the hand away from the positional window.

Calne: As we learn movements and become very experienced with them, they become almost automatic. They might therefore be operated at a lower level of the nervous system. This also gets back to what is the quintessential function of the cortex and to the point about whether the pyramidal cells are simply output neurons. What happens if the monkeys are trained to move repeatedly so that the action becomes virtually automatic, like changing gears on a car?

Georgopoulos: We did a slightly different experiment using two tasks. In one task the target was presented in a random sequence and in the other the same target was presented again and again after the animal had already learnt the task. The variability in the direction of the trajectory was less when the same movement was being repeated. Under these conditions, the variability of the population vector was also significantly decreased, as compared to the random presentation of targets.

It takes about 30–40 days to train the animals to do the two-dimensional task with one hand. At first the animal makes haphazard movements but with time the trajectories become very tight. Then we train an animal to use the other hand for exactly the same task. The animal knows what the lights are—that is, it knows the cognitive part—but it has as much trouble performing the task as it had with the original hand in the first place. After four or five days, however, it can do the task perfectly well, so something is being transferred (Georgopoulos et al 1981). We plan to make recordings throughout this short period of rapid motor learning.

Lemon: Old experiments on people writing with hand and arm movements of different sizes tell us that parts of our motor system transcend the problem of which muscles and which joints to operate, and you seem to have found a population of cells which behave in this way. Is the tuning of the muscular system you are studying very different to that of the cells? If the tuning of the muscular system is also very broad, we have not yet found the population of cells that transcends the mechanical concept of movement.

Georgopoulos: In the two-dimensional task the EMG activity of muscles acting on the shoulder was broadly tuned (Georgopoulos et al 1984); in the three-dimensional task the results were unclear. However, the tuned muscles define a limited set of preferred directions (as many as the muscles), whereas the preferred directions of the cells were not clustered around those of the muscles but extended throughout the directional continuum; therefore, muscles and cells are dissociated with respect to the preferred directions in that task.

In fact, it may be unrealistic to think of strict one-to-one connections between single cells in the proximal arm area of the motor cortex and single proximal muscles because, in any case, these cells do not seem to make monosynaptic connections to motor neurons. Our working hypothesis is that through interneuronal systems single motor cortical cells from the proximal arm area influence several motor neuronal pools in a weighted fashion. Even for a small number of muscles, the number of their weighted combinations can be large, and such weighted combinations can effect a variety of spatial trajectories of the arm. I believe that the motor cortical cells reflect precisely this rich variety of spatial trajectories, on the input side, and the various combinations of muscles, on the output side. The association between the two may be hard-wired but it should also be subject to modification and adaptation according to changing external loads.

Porter: You are looking at individual muscles and their tuning, whereas when you study the cerebral cortex you have a conglomerate of units in the cortex. To answer Roger Lemon's question, surely you should really be adding together the components of all the activities of all the muscles that are modified during a movement such as pointing to a particular place?

Georgopoulos: Yes; that is correct.

References

Crutcher MD, Schwartz AB, Georgopoulos AP 1985 Representation of movement direction in primate motor cortex in the absence of immediate movement. Soc Neurosci Abstr 11:1273

Georgopoulos AP, Massey JT 1987 Cognitive spatial-motor processes. 1. The making of movements at various angles from a stimulus direction. Exp Brain Res 65:361–370

Georgopoulos AP, Kalaska JF, Massey JT 1981 Spatial trajectories and reaction times of aimed movements: effects of practice, uncertainty, and change in target location. J Neurophysiol 46:725–743

Georgopoulos AP, Kalaska JF, Caminiti R, Massey JT 1983 Interruption of motor cortical discharge subserving aimed arm movements. Exp Brain Res 49:327–340

Georgopoulos AP, Kalaska JF, Crutcher MD, Caminiti R, Massey JT 1984 The representation of movement direction in the motor cortex: single cell and population studies. In: Edelman G et al (eds) Dynamic aspects of neocortical function. Wiley, New York, p 501–524

Henn V, Cohen B 1976 Coding of information about rapid eye movements in the pontine reticular formation of alert monkeys. Brain Res 108:307–325

Humphrey DR, Schmidt EM, Thompson WD 1970 Predicting measures of motor performance from multiple cortical spike trains. Science (Wash DC) 179:758–762

Jones EG, Powell TPS 1969 Connexions of the somatic sensory cortex of the rhesus monkey. I. Ipsilateral cortical connexions. Brain 92:477–502

Jones EG, Powell TPS 1970 An anatomical study of converging sensory pathways within the cerebral cortex of the monkey. Brain 93:793–820

Kalaska JF, Hyde ML 1985 Area 4 and area 5: differences between the load direction-dependent discharge variability of cells during active postural fixation. Exp Brain Res 59:197–202

Kalaska JF, Caminiti R, Georgopoulos AP 1981 Cortical mechanisms of two-dimensional aimed arm movements. III. Relations of parietal (areas 5 and 2) neuronal activity to direction of movement and change in target location. Soc Neurosci Abstr 7:563

Kalaska JF, Caminiti R, Georgopoulos AP 1983 Cortical mechanisms related to the direction of two-dimensional arm movements: relations in parietal area 5 and comparison with motor cortex. Exp Brain Res 51:247–260

Massey JT, Schwartz AB, Georgopoulos AP 1986 On information processing and performing a movement sequence. Exp Brain Res Suppl 15:242–251

McIlwain JT 1975 Visual receptive fields and their images in superior colliculus of the cat. J Neurophysiol 38:219–230
Murphy JT, Kwan HC, MacKay WA, Wong YC 1982 Precentral unit activity correlated with angular components of a compound arm movement. Brain Res 246:141–145
Murphy JT, Wong YC, Kwan HC 1985 Sequential activation of neurons in primate motor cortex during unrestrained forelimb movement. J Neurophysiol 53:435–445
Pandya DN, Kuypers HGJM 1969 Cortico-cortical connections in the rhesus monkey. Brain Res 13:13–36
Schwartz AB, Kettner RE, Georgopoulos AP 1986 Population coding of 3-dimensional movement direction in primate motor cortex: confidence intervals, robustness, and evolution in time of the population vector. Soc Neurosci Abstr 12:256
Steinmetz MA, Motter BC, Duffy CJ, Mountcastle VB 1987 Functional properties of parietal visual neurons: radial organization of directionalities within the visual field. J Neurosci 7:177–191

Neuronal activity in the primate non-primary cortex is different from that in the primary motor cortex

Jun Tanji

Department of Neurophysiology, Brain Research Institute, Tohoku University, School of Medicine, Seiryo-machi, Sendai 980, Japan

Abstract. This paper describes differences in the properties of single-cell activity in the primary and non-primary motor cortex of behaving monkeys (*Macaca fuscata*). New findings were obtained in relation to two different behavioural paradigms. First, we found that a large number of non-primary motor cortex neurons exhibit selective or preferential relationships to either signal-triggered or self-paced movement. In the second series of experiments, monkeys were trained to press a small key with the right or left hand, or with both hands. Most primary motor cortex neurons behaved like muscles in the contralateral hand. In contrast, a number of non-primary motor cortex neurons exhibited a selective relationship to the movement (right or left key press, or bilateral key press). The differences suggest the different roles of these two areas in motor control. Studies of this sort seem to start providing answers to the old question of why the non-primary motor cortex exists.

1987 Motor areas of the cerebral cortex. Wiley, Chichester (Ciba Foundation Symposium 132) p 142–150

Although the existence of cortical non-primary motor fields has long been known and their roles in different aspects or conditions in the motor control of primates have been inferred (Wiesendanger 1981, Wise 1985), it is only recently the differences in neuronal activity in these fields have been studied (Brinkman & Porter 1979, Kubota & Hamada 1978, Tanji & Kurata 1982, Kurata & Tanji 1986, Weinrich et al 1984). In this article, I shall refer to the medial portion of the frontal non-primary field in *Macaca fuscata* as the supplementary motor area (SMA), its lateral portion as the premotor area (PM) and the primary motor area as the precentral motor cortex (PCM). When these areas are studied in simple reaction-time paradigms where monkeys responded to visual or auditory signals and started simple limb movements, the following differences have appeared. (1) The magnitudes of activity changes are generally smaller but their onsets are earlier in the non-primary fields. (2) Some SMA and PM neurons exhibited modality-specific premovement activity; that is, they respond to either a visual or an auditory signal but not to both. (3) Some SMA and PM neurons exhibited responses tightly coupled in time to visual or auditory signals. Although these neurons were active in relation to the initiation of movement, neuronal activity appeared to be evoked by sensory signals. These findings suggest that the SMA and PM are more remote from the peripheral motor apparatus than the PCM and that they are involved in relatively earlier stages of information processing where these sensory signals are converted into signals that command the initiation of movement. We have further studied neuronal activity in different behavioural paradigms and found other properties of non-primary motor cortex neurons suggest that their roles differ from those of primary neurons in motor control.

Neuronal activity preceding visually triggered and self-paced movement

In order to examine whether separate groups of cortical neurons are involved in sensory-triggered and self-initiated movements, we examined single-cell activity in the three motor fields. In one behavioural mode, monkeys performed a key-press movement triggered by a visual signal presented on a panel in front of the animal. In the other mode the key-press movement was self-initiated. Electromyographic studies made it clear that muscle activity was limited to the distal forelimb and that the magnitudes of premovement activities in the triggered key press did not differ from those in the self-paced key press.

One hundred and fifty-five PCM neurons changed their activity before movement onset. In 86% of them the activity changes were classified as the short-lead type, observed up to 480 ms before movement onset. In five neurons the activity changes started more than 1s before movement onset and were classified as the long-lead type. The remaining 17 neurons exhibited both the long-lead and short-lead types of activity changes. In most of the short-lead as well as the long-lead neurons the magnitudes of activity changes preceding both signal-triggered and self-paced movement were similar. All of the small number of neurons exhibiting a preferential relation to either the triggered or self-paced movement were recorded outside the cortical fifth layer.

The non-primary motor area contained a large number of neurons related differentially to one or the other of the differently initiated key-press movements. One hundred and fifty-one neurons recorded from PM changed their activity before the key press. Of these, 132 neurons exhibited the short-lead type of activity changes, four exhibited the long-lead type and 15 exhibited both types of activity. In 53 PM neurons, the magnitudes of the short-lead activity changes were similar before the signal-triggered and self-paced movement, just as in the majority of PCM neurons. However, in 49 neurons the magnitudes were greater before triggered than before self-paced movement. Forty-three neurons exhibited only short-lead activity changes before triggered movement. In two neurons the activity changes were greater before self-paced movement. In another two neurons, the activity increased before triggered movement but decreased before self-paced movement. As for the long-lead activity changes, they were similar in five neurons but preferential in 14 neurons.

Of 217 task-related neurons recorded from SMA, 107 neurons showed the short-lead and 58 the long-lead activity changes. The remaining 52 neurons showed both. In 93 of these 217 neurons the magnitudes of the short-lead activity changes were similar before signal-triggered and self-paced movements. However, in 17 neurons the short-lead activity changes were more closely related to self-paced movement and in 10 neurons they were exclusively related to it. Conversely, seven neurons were more closely related to triggered movement and 21 neurons were exclusively related to this type of movement. Of interest was the presence of 11 neurons exhibiting a reciprocal relationship. In six neurons the activity increased before self-paced movement but decreased before triggered movement. In five neurons the relationship was reversed. Long-lead activity changes were observed in 110 SMA neurons. Of these, 79 neurons exhibited activity changes only before self-paced movement. In 23 neurons the activity changes were greater before self-paced than before triggered movement. In three neurons the magnitudes were similar and in another five the relationship was reciprocal.

These results indicate that in many non-primary motor cortex neurons premovement activity can vary greatly, depending on how a particular movement is initiated. This property is rare in PCM, providing additional support for the view that the primary motor cortex is situated at a later stage of information processing, closer to movement initiation (Tanji & Kurata 1982, Lamarre et al 1983).

One of the hypotheses on the possible functional differentiation between the SMA and PM has been that SMA takes part in self-initiated movement whereas PM is involved in movements guided or triggered by sensory signals (Eccles 1982, Evarts & Wise 1984, Goldberg 1985, Rizzolatti et al 1983). This view is based on phylogenetic study (Sanides 1964), on histological studies employing tracer techniques, on clinical observations on local cerebral lesions (Goldberg 1985), and on studies utilizing measurements of cerebral motor potentials (Deecke & Kornhuber 1978, Libet et al 1983) as well as regional cerebral blood flow (Roland et al 1980a, b). The results presented above do not support the hypothesis in its simplest form, since both SMA and PM neurons were active in either visually triggered or self-paced movement. However, PM neurons show relatively more prominent responses to the visual trigger signal and SMA neurons are intimately related to a long-lasting process leading to initiation of the self-paced movement. It is entirely possible that neuronal activity in the two areas is grossly different, depending on whether a certain movement paradigm calls for more sophisticated use of sensory signals to guide its execution.

Neuronal activity preceding single and bilateral hand movements

Another series of experiments was performed in order to learn the extent to which neuronal premovement activity in the primary and non-primary motor cortex deviates from that observed in skeletal muscle (Phillips 1975). Monkeys were trained to perform a key-press movement with the right or left hand, or with both hands, according to instruction signals displayed on a lamp panel. The keys were designed to fit the second to fourth digits and to be pressed with only a small amount of force. The instructions were given 2.6–5.4 s before a movement–trigger signal, also given on the lamp panel. Great care was taken to train the animal to use only the required part of the limb, including careful fixation of the palm, wrist, elbow and shoulder. After extensive training, electromyographic studies revealed that muscle activities before the key press were limited to the digit and forearm muscles of the limb instructed to move.

The great majority (83%) of the PCM neurons recorded from the digit area of the motor cortex (mostly limited to the anterior bank of the central sulcus) exhibited a contralateral relation, namely an increase or decrease in activity before the onset of the contralateral and bilateral key-press movement. In all except six neurons the magnitudes of the changes in activity preceding contralateral and bilateral movement were similar. Of interest was the presence of 9% of neurons whose activity changes were limited only before ipsilateral and bilateral movement. This indicates that, even if the movement is limited to the distal part of the forelimb, a certain group of PCM neurons exhibit the ipsilateral relationship. The remaining neurons showing atypical relationships were all recorded outside the cortical fifth layer (where the cells of origin of descending outputs are located). Most of the remaining neurons were related to all three types of movement in various degrees. Thus, although exceptions may not be rare, the activity of a majority of PCM neurons appeared to be akin to that of hand muscles.

The most striking finding in the non-primary motor cortex was the presence of a large number of non-primary neurons whose relationships to the task were never or only rarely observed in the primary motor cortex. Of particular interest was the exclusive relationship observed in 28% of SMA and 16% of PM neurons. Some of these neurons were active before the key-press movement with the right hand but not with both hands. Others were active before the left keypress but not the bilateral key press. Still others were active before the bilateral key press but not before the right or left key press. Furthermore, there were even examples whose activity changed before either the right or left key press but not before the bilateral key press. In separate groups of neurons (37% of SMA and 61% of PM) the activity changes were always observed before all types of key-press movements. Among the non-primary motor cortex neurons the contralateral relationships most frequently observed in PCM neurons were in the minority.

In addition to the period immediately preceding movement onset, activity changes were also observed in the period after the instruction signals. In the PCM, the instruction-induced activity changes were mostly related to the contralateral key press. This is not the case in the non-primary motor cortex. In both SMA and PM, the instruction-induced activity was most frequently observed non-selectively after all the instructions. In 18% of SMA and 6% of PM instruction-related neurons, the relationship was exclusive—for example, only after the instruction for the right key press.

These findings indicate that the majority of non-primary motor cortex neurons do not seem to be coding the muscle or muscles that are to be activated in a motor task. A considerable number of these neurons seem to be related to the movement the animal is performing. This deviation of neuronal activity from that of skeletal muscle, and the closer relationship of such neuronal activity to the movement itself (in this particular paradigm the usage of the right or left hand, or both hands), are characteristic properties of the non-primary motor fields.

Acknowledgement

This research was supported in part by a Grant-in Aid for Special Project Research on Plasticity of Neural Circuits from the Japanese Ministry of Education, Science and Culture.

References

Brinkman C, Porter R 1979 Supplementary motor area in the monkey. Activity of neurons during performance of a learned motor task. J Neurophysiol 42:681–709

Deecke L, Kornhuber HH 1978 An electrical sign of participation of the mesial 'supplementary' motor cortex in human voluntary finger movements. Brain Res 159:473–476

Eccles JC 1982 The initiation of voluntary movements by the supplementary motor area. Arch Psychiatr Nervenkr 231:423–441

Evarts EV, Wise SP 1984 Basal ganglia outputs and motor control. In: Functions of the basal ganglia. Pitman, London (Ciba Found Symp 107) p 83–96

Goldberg G 1985 Supplementary motor area structure and function: review and hypothesis. Behav Brain Sci 8:567–615

Kubota K, Hamada I 1978 Visual tracking and neuron activity in the post-arcuate area in monkeys. J Physiol (Paris) 74:297–313

Kurata K, Tanji J 1986 Premotor cortex neurons in macaques: activity before distal and proximal forelimb movements. J Neurosci 6:403–411

Lamarre Y, Busby L, Spidalieri G 1983 Fast ballistic arm movements triggered by visual, auditory and somesthetic stimuli in the monkey. I. Activity of precentral cortical neurons. J Neurophysiol 50:1343–1358

Libet B, Wright EW, Gleason CA 1983 Preparation—or intention—to act, in relation to pre-event potentials recorded at the vertex. Electroencephalogr Clin Neurophysiol 65:367–372

Phillips CG 1975 Laying the ghost of 'muscles versus movements'. Can J Neurol Sci 2:209–218

Roland PE, Larsen B, Lassen NA, Skinhoj E 1980a Supplementary motor area and other cortical areas in organization of voluntary movements in man. J Neurophysiol 43:118–136

Roland PE, Skinhoj E, Lassen NA, Larsen B 1980b Different cortical areas in man in organization of voluntary movements in extrapersonal space. J Neurophysiol 43:137–150

Rizzolatti G, Matelli M, Pavesi G 1983 Deficits in attention and movement following the removal of postarcuate (area 6) and prearcuate (area 8) cortex in macaque monkeys. Brain 106:655–673

Sanides F 1964 The cyto-myeloarchitecture of the human frontal lobe and its relation to phylogenetic differentiation of the cerebral cortex. J Hirnforsch 6:269–282

Tanji J, Kurata K 1982 Comparison of movement-related activity in two cortical motor areas of primates. J Neurophysiol 48:633–653

Weinrich M, Wise SP, Mauritz K-M 1984 A neurophysiological study of the premotor cortex in the rhesus monkey. Brain 107:385–414

Wiesendanger M 1981 Organization of secondary motor areas of cerebral cortex. In: Brooks VB et al (eds) Motor control, part 2. American Physiological Society, Bethesda, MD (Handb Physiol sect 1 The nervous system vol 2) p 1121–1147

Wise SP 1985 The primate premotor cortex: past, present and preparatory. Annu Rev Neurosci 8:1–19

DISCUSSION

Kalaska: You presented data from a neuron recorded during a 'cued-delay' task. In one trial the neuronal activity was markedly different to that in the other trials, and in that trial the monkey made a mistake. Did the preparatory activity in that trial predict the erroneous response?

Tanji: Yes, we can always predict when the monkey is going to make a mistake, just by watching the neuronal activity.

Jones: You showed neuronal activity related to movements that you might not predict to be related to neurons in the primary motor cortex, such as ipsilateral movement, and in your data the level of spontaneous neuronal activity was always higher in those circumstances than with the more predictable pattern. This may also apply to similar responses in the SMA. Are you uncovering a latent neuronal response here?

Tanji: In that example the baseline activity was high but there are many cases where it is almost zero.

Porter: Studies on the human cerebral cortex by Goldring & Ratcheson (1972) revealed some ipsilateral relationships of cellular discharge to hand movements. There are other observations that suggest that a component of neuronal activity, even in area 4, may be related to ipsilateral movements.

Roland: Does tactile instruction to SMA neurons give rise to higher frequency firing than auditory instruction?

Tanji: No; we have many examples of the reverse.

Roland: With your new knowledge of the SMA, can you formulate a kind of population coding, so that we can understand the function of the SMA more clearly?

Tanji: One type of neuron which shows a distinct property is intermingled with other very different types of neurons, so population studies may not be very meaningful.

Strick: There has been a great deal of controversy about whether the premotor areas, including the SMA and the arcuate premotor area, contain representations of distal musculature. I think there is a growing body of evidence that the premotor areas are concerned, in part, with the control of distal movements. Your observations of significant changes in neural activity in premotor areas when animals are making only finger movements appear to support this conclusion. Can you comment on this issue?

Tanji: We have studied that problem. In one paradigm the monkey has to make a distal movement with the fingers and in other situations the monkey has to make proximal limb movements. Neuronal activity related to distal movement appears in a very small area caudal to the arcuate sulcus. A group of neurons related almost exclusively to proximal movements are found in the more dorsomedial area and some are also found close to the precentral sulcus. In the SMA there are both distally related neurons and proximally related neurons. They are distributed in rostral and caudal parts of forelimb SMA but there is some overlap.

Rizzolatti: We also find that in the postarcuate cortex 90% of neurons are related to distal movement and only about 10% to proximal movement.

Freund: You showed us the recordings made once the monkey was trained to do the specific task. Did you ever record from cells during the training process?

Tanji: No, but I would like to do that in the future.

Goldman-Rakic: Where are you recording within the SMA?

Tanji: I do not think there is enough evidence to distinguish different subareas within the SMA. There certainly is a somatotopy organized in the anterior–posterior direction but I do not think there is any need to divide the SMA into anterior and posterior parts.

Strick: You would agree that the neurons related to arm movement are located just caudal to the posterior extent of the arcuate sulcus?

Tanji: Yes.

Goldman-Rakic: Is there any evidence that cells in the SMA are coded for direction?

Tanji: We compared the neuronal activity in two regions, SMA and the postarcuate area, and they were quite similar in their responses to directional cues.

Lemon: The three areas you mention have been distinguished by some investigators on the basis of cell size, which is clearly very different in the premotor area and in the caudal parts of area 4. Christoph Fromm has pointed out that some of the physiological differences between areas may be due to sampling of different cell sizes, rather than true areal differences. Some years ago there was a report that rapidly conducting pyramidal tract axons showed a better relationship to ipsilateral movements than did more slowly conducting axons (Matsunami & Hamada 1980). Have you checked that your samples are not simply influenced by cell size?

Tanji: In area 4 we sampled a large number of neurons in layers superficial to the pyramidal tract layer. Even in these superficial layers, there were plenty of contralateral relationships and others were quite rare. In layer 5 most of the neurons are related to the contralateral hand with the exception of ipsilateral neurons: no neurons have exclusive relationships in that layer. In area 6, both in the deep (layers 5 and 6) and the superficial layers, we recorded many neurons exhibiting the preferential relationship or a relationship to all three types of movement. Concerning the slowly conducting neurons, we identified seven pyramidal tract neurons related to ipsilateral movement and three of them were slowly conducting neurons. But others were fast-conducting.

Shinoda: Some single corticospinal neurons in the monkey project extensively to intrinsic muscle motor neurons contralaterally and at the same time have axon collaterals crossing the midline and terminating ipsilaterally at lamina VII medial to lamina IX, although the number of such neurons is small. I was a bit surprised to find those cells, as I did not expect that corticospinal neurons innervating distal hand muscles would have bilateral projections.

Kalaska: Dr Tanji, you have these examples of cells discharging in a test environment in which the monkeys are making arbitrary and complex stimulus–response transformations. An important question to resolve is whether this activity is related more to the arbitrary stimulus–response transformation or to the ultimate selection and initiation of the motor response. What do these neurons do in a more freely behaving animal under more natural behavioural conditions?

Tanji: That is a difficult question to answer. The trouble is that if you let the monkey make free and uncontrolled movements, it is hard to analyse what the cells are doing.

Wiesendanger: Did you say that you find these cells everywhere within the SMA, including the medial bank and the roof of the cingulate sulcus? Are they clustered together?

Tanji: Yes, we found them in the medial surface of the hemisphere as well as the upper bank of the cingulate sulcus. Neurons with similar properties were clustered. Quite often, if you keep recording from one type of neuron for some time, you suddenly get a signal from a different type of neuron.

Kuypers: When you move from the hand representation in area 4 rostrally towards area 6 the spinal projections gradually change from being mainly contralateral to being mainly bilateral.

Rizzolatti: But Dr Tanji is recording from neurons controlling distal movements as well. The bilateral system you described, Professor Kuypers, is related to axial and proximal movements (Kuypers 1973). Dr Tanji's results and those from my laboratory (Rizzolatti et al 1987) show that there is a bilateral control of finger movements.

Porter: The recordings of neuronal responses show bilateral associations but they do not show that the cells from which you are recording project bilaterally.

Rizzolatti: You are right.

References

Goldring S, Ratcheson R 1972 Human motor cortex: sensory input data from single neuron recordings. Science (Wash DC) 175:1493–1495

Kuypers HGJM 1973 The anatomical organization of the descending pathways and their contributions to motor control especially in primates. In: Desmedt JE (ed) New developments in electromyography and clinical neurophysiology. Karger, Basel, p 38–68

Matsunami K, Hamada I 1980 Antidromic latency of the monkey pyramidal tract neuron related to ipsilateral hand movements. Neurosci Lett 16:245–249

Rizzolatti G, Gentilucci M, Fogassi L, Luppino G, Matelli M, Ponzoni Maggi S 1987 Neurons related to goal-directed motor acts in inferior area 6 of the macaque monkey. Exp Brain Res, in press

Two cortical systems for directing movement

R.E. Passingham

Department of Experimental Psychology, University of Oxford, Oxford OX1 3UD, UK

Abstract. It is argued that the cortical premotor areas are concerned with the conditions for action. Actions are based both on facts about the outside world and about the actions of the animal itself. Observations on monkeys (*Macaca fascicularis, Macaca mulatta*) suggest that the arcuate premotor area directs actions on the basis of visual cues about the outside environment and that the supplementary motor area directs actions on the basis of proprioceptive cues concerning the animal's own actions.

1987 Motor areas of the cerebral cortex. Wiley, Chichester (Ciba Foundation Symposium 132) p 151—164

The motor cortex is under the direction of several premotor areas. Four regions of frontal cortex send projections to the arm area of the primary motor cortex (MI) in monkeys (Muakkassa & Strick 1979). These regions are the supplementary motor cortex, the cortex in the lower bank of the cingulate sulcus, the cortex in the precentral sulcus, and the cortex in and behind the arcuate sulcus (the arcuate premotor area).

Why should there be several independent cortical premotor areas? This is much the same as asking why there are so many visual areas. One way of answering such questions is to record the activity of cells in the different regions. Thus it turns out that the different visual areas are specialized for the analysis of colour, movement and so on (Cowey 1985); and reasons can be given why it would be inefficient to analyse all aspects of vision in a single mapped area (Cowey 1979).

Visual cues

The strategy of recording cell activity has not been as helpful in distinguishing between the functions of the different premotor areas. For example, in both supplementary motor cortex and the arcuate premotor area there are cells that fire differentially according to whether an animal has received a visual instruction to pull a handle or push it (Tanji et al 1980, Wise & Mauritz 1985, Godschalk et al 1985). This might tempt one to believe that both areas play a crucial role in the direction of movement according to visual cues.

But recordings from single cells may be misleading as to function. It will not always be possible to establish the function of a population of cells just by measuring the activity of cells in that population one at a time. For example, in motor cortex the whole population of cells can code for very specific directions even when no single cell does so with much accuracy (Georgopoulos et al 1986).

If the question is the function of an area rather than its mode of action, there are better methods than single-cell recording. The study of functional anatomy can be pursued by determining the activity of a whole area. This can be done be measuring the metabolic requirements of the area when it is active, as is done in studies of cerebral blood flow. The alternative is to measure the behaviour of the whole animal after removing the relevant area; the effect of the lesion reflects the contribution of the whole population of cells. The advantage of the first method is that it is possible to study the contribution of several areas at the same time. One advantage of the lesion method is that it is possible to be precise about the exact boundaries of the different functional areas.

We have used the lesion method to examine the role of premotor and supplementary motor areas in directing movement on the basis of visual cues. We train monkeys (*Macaca fascicularis*) to operate a handle. As in the study of Tanji et al (1980) the instruction as to which movement to make is given by an aribitrary colour cue; if this is blue the handle must be pulled, if red the handle must be turned. When the monkeys have learnt the task we remove the relevant cortical area bilaterally. The monkeys are then retrained on the task until their performance returns to the required level.

We have already established that when we remove the arcuate cortex on both sides, monkeys do not easily relearn this visual conditional motor task (Passingham 1985). They can readily make either of the movements but they are slow to relearn which movement to make in response to the colour cues, as shown in Fig. 1.

We recently trained six more monkeys of the same species on an automated version of this task, in which they move a joystick, either by pulling it or turning it to the right. When the monkeys had learnt the task we removed the supplementary motor area bilaterally from three animals; all the animals were then retrained. The operated monkeys relearnt the task with as few errors as the three control animals. (Fig. 1).

These results strongly suggest that visual cues instruct motor cortex via premotor cortex and not via supplementary motor cortex. Why, then, is it

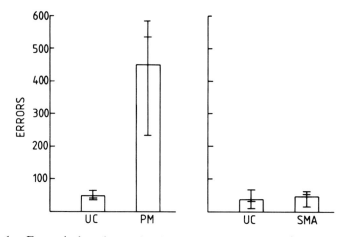

FIG. 1.   Errors in learning a visual conditional motor task (operating a handle in response to a colour cue). The data on the left are from Halsband & Passingham (1982). The histograms give the means and the bars the scores for individual monkeys (three in each group). UC, unoperated control animals; PM, animals with premotor lesions; SMA, animals with supplementary motor lesions.

possible to record cells in supplementary motor cortex that respond when visual cues give instructions about the response to be made (Tanji et al 1980)? We are often talking loosely when we claim that a cell in a motor area has a 'visual' property. That the activity of the cell is well locked in time with the presentation of the visual cue shows only that when the area acts the cue has already been analysed in the brain. There is direct evidence that the cell may be quite ignorant of the visual properties of the cue. Godschalk et al (1985) tested cells in the arcuate premotor area that responded on presentation of a visual cue directing the movement to be made. The correct direction could be specified either by the sight of the correct location or by an arbitrary visual cue. These authors found cells that responded in the same way irrespective of whether the cue was spatial or arbitrary, so long as the two cues both specified the same movement. Furthermore, Weinrich & Wise (1982) have reported cells in the arcuate premotor area that responded similarly when the animal was instructed to reach for a location, irrespective of whether the instruction was a light or a sound.

    The results of recording from single cells late in the hierarchy of cortical processing may be quite misleading as to the function of the area. The inputs to a visual area early in the system can be reliably studied using electrophysiological recording. A cell may respond only when the animal is shown a spot in a particular part of the visual field or when a spot moves in a particular direction. The conditions under which cells respond in a premotor area are much more complex and much less specific.

Proprioceptive cues

Sequences

The same arguments apply when we consider the use of proprioceptive cues
to direct movement. Again we might draw different conclusions about the
function of the different premotor areas depending on whether we attend to
the evidence of electrophysiological studies or behavioural studies. Wiesendanger et al (1985) have shown that in monkeys both supplementary motor
cortex and the arcuate premotor cortex receive a proprioceptive input. These
authors recorded from cells while displacing the arm of the animal; 15% of
cells responded in supplementary motor cortex and 25% in premotor cortex.
It might be tempting to conclude that both areas direct movement on the basis
of proprioceptive cues.

   However, the effects of removing the two areas separately suggest otherwise. We have taught monkeys (*Macaca fascicularis*) to perform a sequence
of three movements; they must operate a catch by first pushing it up, then
twisting it, and finally lifting it to uncover a food well (Halsband & Passingham 1982). After the monkey has made each movement the apparatus is
withdrawn to allow the catch to return to its resting position. Thus the monkey
is unable to see by the position of the catch which movement to make next.
The cue to which movement to make is provided by the previous movement.

   After the arcuate premotor cortex was removed, the monkey had no
difficulty in relearning the task (Halsband & Passingham 1982). Yet two of
the three animals that had supplementary motor cortex removed from both
sides failed to relearn the task in 1000 trials (Fig. 2) (Halsband 1987). The
third monkey also made many errors (Fig. 2), although in this animal the
lesion included only the anterior part of the supplementary motor area.

Reaching

We have also taught monkeys (*Macaca fascicularis*) to reach out to a position
specified by proprioceptive cues. The monkey sits at the front of a cage in the
dark. If it reaches out of the cage to a position at roughly eye-level, its hand
interrupts an invisible infrared beam. When the beam is interrupted the
monkey wins a peanut. The monkey has 65 peanuts to earn in a session and
works at its own rate, raising its arm to the correct position whenever it wants
a peanut.

   David Thaler and I have studied the effects of removing the supplementary
motor cortex bilaterally. Fig. 3 presents the results for the last four sessions
before and the first four sessions after surgery. Retraining began two weeks
after the operation to allow the animals to recover from the immediate effects

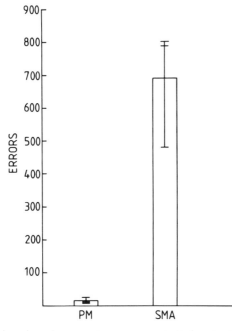

FIG. 2. Errors in relearning a motor sequence task (see text). The histograms give the means and the bars the scores for individual animals (three in each group). PM, animals with premotor lesions; SMA, animals with supplementary motor lesions. In one SMA animal the lesion included only the anterior part of the SMA; this animal is one of the two animals described by Halsband (1987) as having a medial prefrontal lesion.

of surgery. After surgery the monkeys made few successful movements. From films made with an infrared camera we could see that the monkeys still made movements but were inaccurate in finding the target zone.

That the animals could make the required movement is evident from their performance in another session when the lights were turned on and they were required to reach for a peanut placed at the same height as the beam. When an animal reached for the peanut its arm intercepted the beam. The monkeys with supplementary motor lesions were as quick and accurate in reaching for the peanut as the unoperated control animals (Fig. 3). They could reach accurately for targets they could see but not for a position specified by proprioceptive cues.

There is additional evidence that these monkeys could move rapidly if the movement was triggered by a visual cue. Before surgery we had taught all monkeys to operate two levers. We trained them to hold the lower of the two levers. When a light went off they released the lower lever and then pressed the upper one. We could thus measure the reaction time to release the lower

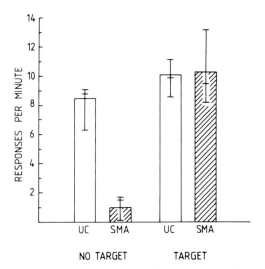

FIG. 3. Successful responses (per minute) on an arm-raising task. The histograms give the means and the bars the scores for individual animals (three in each group). The scores for the no-target condition are based on 260 trials (4 days) and the scores for the target condition are 65 trials (1 day). UC, unoperated control animals; SMA, monkeys with supplementary motor lesions; no target, in dark; target, reaching for peanut in the light.

lever and the movement time in reaching up to the lever 20 cm above it. The monkeys performed at their own speed; we imposed no penalty for slow performance. After surgery the monkeys with supplementary motor lesions reacted and moved as quickly as they had before surgery (Fig. 4). Their performance was also no different from that of the three control monkeys (Fig. 4).

Proprioceptive conditional motor task

The next step will be to examine whether monkeys from which the arcuate premotor cortex has been removed can reach out on the basis of proprioceptive cues. We have not yet done this. However, we have other results that strongly suggest that animals with arcuate premotor lesions can use proprioceptive cues. We have trained six monkeys (*Macaca mulatta*) to squeeze or rotate a handle. We then taught them to make the movement on the basis of a proprioceptive cue. The animal is unable to see the handle. It reaches for the handle through a hole and finds that it is locked in such a way that only one movement is possible: the handle can be either squeezed or rotated. Five seconds later the animal again reaches for the handle and now it has a free choice as to which movement to make. The rule is that if the animal was

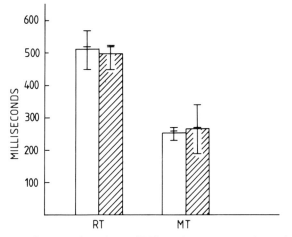

FIG. 4. Postoperative reaction times (RT) and movement times (MT) in milliseconds. The histograms give the means and the bars the scores for individual animals (three in each group). Clear histograms, unoperated control animals; hatched histograms, monkeys with supplementary motor lesions.

forced to squeeze it 5 s before, it must now squeeze the handle again; and, if it was forced to rotate the handle, then it must now rotate the handle again. After we had trained monkeys on this difficult task we made bilateral lesions, including premotor cortex. Two of the animals relearnt the task with little difficulty, making only 20 and 32 errors (Passingham 1986, 1987). The third animal had more trouble, making 176 errors; but in this animal there was a large left frontal infarct.

The experiments described here strongly suggest that supplementary motor cortex is specialized for directing movement on the basis of proprioceptive cues and that the arcuate premotor cortex is specialized for directing movement on the basis of visual rather than proprioceptive cues. Electrophysiological studies show that there is proprioceptive input to the arcuate premotor area (Wiesendanger et al 1985), but these studies do not necessarily indicate the use to which the information is put. There may be many reasons why the arcuate premotor area requires information about the animal's own movements in order to carry out its functions. The available evidence suggests that the information is not used for directing which movement is to be performed.

Discussion

There are two major influences on our actions. First, we take account of facts about the outside world, of the circumstances around us as we know them from the evidence of our eyes and ears. Second, we take account of facts about ourselves, about what we are doing or have done in the past. Our actions must be decided in the context not only of external events but also of the history of our own actions.

The evidence reviewed above suggests that the premotor areas are concerned with the conditions for action, and that the different areas are concerned with different conditions. The arcuate premotor area lies on the lateral surface and it appears to play a role in the direction of action based on information provided by the eye and ear about the outside world. The supplementary motor area lies on the medial surface and it appears to play a role in the direction of action based on information provided by proprioception about the animal's own actions.

The suggestion that the medial and lateral systems might be distinguished in this way is not novel (Goldberg 1985). Roland and colleagues have used measures of cerebral blood flow to compare the functions of the supplementary motor area and the lateral premotor cortex in humans. They find that the supplementary motor area is active when a person performs a predetermined sequence of finger movements, but that there is little change in the activity of the lateral premotor area (Roland et al 1980, 1982). If, however, the person must direct the movements of a finger according to external instruments given verbally, the activity of the lateral premotor cortex increases (Roland et al 1980).

In this paper I have argued that there are separate premotor areas because there are different conditions on which actions may be based. Information about the animal directs its influence via dorsomedial frontal cortex; there is a direct input to supplementary motor cortex from the somatosensory areas and from superior parietal association area 5 (Powell 1977, Petrides & Pandya 1984). Visual information about the external environment is processed both in inferior parietal association area 7 and in temporal association cortex (Mishkin et al 1983). In turn, parietal area 7 projects to the arcuate premotor area (Petrides & Pandya 1984) and temporal association cortex may influence the arcuate premotor cortex via projections to ventral prefrontal cortex (Pandya & Yeterian 1985).

This general organization holds not only for the limbs as represented in supplementary motor cortex but also for the eyes and vocal cords. The supplementary frontal eye field lies in dorsomedial frontal cortex, and here many units change activity before the animal moves its eyes spontaneously (Shlag & Shlag-Rey 1985). In contrast, the primary frontal eye field lies in ventrolateral frontal cortex and here most units only respond before eye movements when a visual target is presented (Bruce & Goldberg 1985).

There is a similar organization for the direction of speech in people. The supplementary speech area lies in dorsomedial frontal cortex whereas Broca's area is located in ventrolateral premotor cortex (Penfield & Roberts 1959). When a person recites a preprogrammed series, such as the days of the week, the supplementary speech area is active but Broca's area is not (Ingvaar &

Schwartz 1974, Larsen et al 1978). On the other hand Broca's area is activated when a person operates on an external input, as in reading or conversing (Ingvaar & Schwartz 1974, Lassen et al 1978).

In normal life these areas operate together. Thus, when Broca's area is active so is the supplementary speech area (Ingvaar & Schwartz 1974, Lassen et al 1978). Similarly, when someone moves a finger in a maze as instructed verbally there is an increase in blood flow not only in the lateral premotor cortex but also in supplementary motor cortex (Roland et al 1980). There are close interconnections between these two premotor areas (Kunzle 1978).

However, to some extent each area can function independently. This can be established by studying the contribution of one area after removing the influence of the other. Thus in the laboratory we can establish that supplementary motor cortex plays no essential role when an animal reaches for a visual target (Fig. 3) or in directing movements according to arbitrary visual cues (Fig. 1). In monkeys with supplementary motor lesions the lateral premotor cortex is intact. We must conclude that premotor cortex can perform its normal functions independently of the supplementary motor area.

Sometimes nature runs the experiment. There are reports of patients who have suffered infarcts of the medial frontal cortex, including the supplementary speech area and cingulate gyrus. These patients may be mute at first and yet, remarkably, may be able to speak when prompted by questions, repeating words they hear and naming objects they see (Laplane et al 1977, Jonas 1981, Damasio & Van Hoesen 1983). Understanding how this might happen becomes possible if we assume that the supplementary speech area is specialized for the spontaneous production of speech and that Broca's area is specialized for the production of speech on the basis of visual or auditory cues. In such patients Broca's area is intact, lying as it does in ventrolateral premotor cortex. Presumably when the patients speak it is Broca's area speaking.

Acknowledgements

This research was funded by MRC Grant 971/1/397/B and Wellcome Grant G8122258N. I am grateful to David Thaler for his helpful comments on an earlier draft.

References

Bruce CJ, Goldberg ME 1985 Primate frontal eye fields: I. Single neurons discharging before saccades. J Neurophysiol 53:603–635

Cowey A 1979 Cortical maps and visual perception: the Grindley memorial lecture. QJ Exp Psychol 31:1–17

Cowey A 1985 Aspects of cortical organization related to selective attention and selective impairments of visual perception: a tutorial review. Attention Performance 11:41–62

Damasio AR, Van Hoesen GW 1983 Emotional disturbances associated with focal lesions of the limbic frontal lobe. In:Heilman K, Satz P (eds) Neuropsychology of human emotion. Guildford Press, New York, p 85–110

Georgopoulos AP, Schwartz AB, Kettner RE 1986 Neuronal population coding of movement direction. Science (Wash DC) 233:1416–1419

Godshalk M, Lemon RN, Kuypers HGJM, van der Steen J 1985 The involvement of monkey premotor cortex neurones in preparation of visually cued arm movements. Behav Brain Res 18:143–158

Goldberg G 1985 Supplementary motor area structure and function: review and hypotheses. Behav Brain Sci 8:567–588

Halsband U 1987 Higher disturbances of movement in monkeys (Macaca fascicularis). In: Jantchev CN et al (eds) Motor control. Plenum, New York, p 79–87

Halsband U, Passingham RE 1982 The role of premotor and parietal cortex in the direction of action. Brain Res 240:368–372

Ingvaar DH, Schwartz MS 1974 Blood flow patterns induced in the dominant hemisphere by speech and reading. Brain 97:273–288

Jonas S 1981 The supplementary motor region and speech emission. J Commun Disord 14:349–373

Kunzle H 1978 An autoradiographic analysis of the efferent connections from premotor and adjacent prefrontal regions (areas 6 and 9) in Macaca fascicularis. Brain Behav Evol 15:185–234

Laplane D, Talairach J, Meininger V, Bancaud J, Orgogozo JM 1977 Clinical consequences of corticectomies involving the supplementary motor area in man. J Neurol Sci 34:301–314

Larsen B, Skinhoj JE, Lassen NA 1978 Variations in regional blood flow in the right and left hemispheres during automatic speech. Brain 101:193–209

Lassen NA, Ingvaar DA, Skinhoj E 1978 Brain function and blood flow. Sci Am 239:50–59

Muakkassa KF, Strick PL 1979 Frontal lobe inputs in primate motor cortex: evidence for four somatotopically organized 'premotor' areas. Brain Res 177:176–182

Mishkin M, Ungerleider LG, Macko KA 1983 Object vision and spatial vision: two cortical pathways. Trends Neurosci 6:414–417

Pandya DN, Yeterian EH 1985, Architecture and connections of cortical association areas. In: Peters A, Jones EG (eds) Cerebral cortex, vol 4: association & auditory cortices. Plenum, New York, p 3–61

Passingham RE 1985 Premotor cortex: sensory cues and movement. Behav Brain Res 18:175–186

Passingham RE 1986 Cues for movement in monkeys (Macaca mulatta) with lesions in premotor cortex. Behav Neurosci 100:695–703

Passingham RE 1987 Premotor cortex and the retrieval of movement. Brain Behav Evol, in press

Penfield WP, Roberts L 1959 Speech and brain mechanisms. Princeton University Press, New Jersey

Petrides M, Pandya DN 1984 Projections to the frontal cortex from the posterior parietal region in the rhesus monkey. J Comp Neurol 228:105–116

Powell TPS 1977 The somatic sensory cortex. Br Med Bull 33:129–135

Roland PE, Larsen B, Lassen NA, Skinhoj E 1980 Supplementary motor cortex and other cortical areas in organization of voluntary movements in man. J Neurophysiol 43:118–136

Roland PE, Meyer E, Shibasaki T, Yamamoto YL, Thompson CJ 1982 Regional cerebral blood flow changes in cortex and basal ganglia during voluntary movements in normal human volunteers. J Neurophysiol 48:467–480

Schlag J, Schlag-Rey MJ 1985 Unit activity related to spontaneous saccades in frontal
  dorsomedial cortex of monkey. Exp Brain Res 58:208–211
Tanji J, Taniguchi K, Saga T 1980 The supplementary motor area: neuronal responses
  to motor instructions. J Neurophysiol 43:60–68
Weinrich M, Wise SP 1982 The premotor cortex of the monkey. J Neurosci 2:1329–
  1345
Wiesendanger M, Hummelsheim H, Bianchetti M 1985 Sensory input to the motor
  fields of the agranular frontal cortex: a comparison of the precentral, supplementary
  motor and premotor cortex. Behav Brain Res 18:89–94
Wise SP, Mauritz K-H 1985 Set-related neuronal activity in the premotor cortex of
  rhesus monkeys: effects of changes in motor set. Proc R Soc Lond B Biol Sci
  223:331–354

DISCUSSION

Calne: Where the monkey had to twist the handle and pull it out, was each component intact? Was it just the sequencing that could not be accomplished?

Passingham: That is our impression.

Calne: The clinical analogy is ideational apraxia. A patient may not be able, for example, to open a box of matches, take out a match and strike it. All these actions may have been learnt well in the past and each can be executed in isolation but when put together as a task the patient cannot do them. The implication is that a complex dyspraxic problem arises from a lesion of the SMA.

Passingham: I would prefer not to talk about apraxia because clinicians disagree so much about it. Some people regard ideational apraxia as a problem in sequencing; others regard it as a problem in actually dealing with objects. We will probably not be helped by saying that what we have seen is the same as a clinical syndrome. Clinicians tend to think that apraxia is the result of damage to the parietal cortex but computerized tomography scanning shows that such people often have deep lesions of the white matter. It would be rash to make an analogy.

Calne: The terminology is unfortunate; one should not use 'akinesia' if one is not prepared to use 'apraxia', because all the same arguments apply.

Passingham: We are claiming that there is a higher disorder of movement but that the individual movements are normal.

Roland: Metabolic studies show that Broca's area in humans is active even when there are no external cues and someone is just talking with his or her eyes closed. Broca's area, however, is also metabolically active during sensory tasks such as tone discrimination and probably during tasks such as repeating the names of the days of the week (Roland et al 1981, 1985).

Passingham: I unwisely used the word 'internal' at one point. It is a dangerous term because it does not distinguish between, say, proprioceptive instructions and visual instructions in memory. These are both in the head and therefore get called internal. Broca's area may operate not only on cues in the external world but also on visual or auditory memory.

Roland: You may be right. Broca's area is active when patients imagine they are in their living rooms and describe the rooms in fluent descriptive speech, without any external cues (Roland et al 1985).

We should be cautious about what medial infarctions really damage in the cerebral cortex in humans. There are some important areas for the overall regulation of behaviour in front of the SMA on the medial side in the human cerebral cortex and these areas are often also damaged when there are infarctions in the anterior cerebral artery domain, so there is not a clear SMA lesion.

Your findings seem to fit in with the idea that whenever the premotor area is active, SMA is also active. However, the reverse is not true: SMA can be active without the premotor area being active. Even the arm-raising experiment supports this view.

Passingham: With the arm-raising task we have so far only considered supplementary motor cortex. We have not yet studied premotor cortex in relation to this task.

Freund: Two important issues are involved in your tests. One is sensory guidance of the movement and the other is learning. Do your tests reveal that the premotor areas are important for the sensory guidance of movements or rather for the learning part of it?

Passingham: We are interested in learnt associations between cues and movements. The animals have no general problems in sensory guidance in the sense of reaching for things. The stress has to be on the learning. The cues we use are deliberately arbitrary. We chose them because Drs Tanji and Evarts set up their motor cortex experiments with colours for cues. Colours have no meaning for movement other than learnt meanings.

Kuypers: How long does the defect last after this kind of lesion?

Passingham: We retested the animals on arm-raising five weeks after surgery. They were less impaired than at first but were still markedly impaired compared with normal monkeys. If we trained animals day after day on that task I believe they would regain the normal level of performance. If we waited six months and then trained them for the first time I think they would be impaired.

Kuypers: The striking thing with all these defects is that the testing is also learning. When our animals with parietal lesions (Haaxma & Kuypers 1975) were tested once a week the deficit remained clear. If we tested them every day the deficit became gradually less pronounced.

I was glad you mentioned Broca's area. I believe Dr Pandya and I were the first to see a very heavy projection from the posterior bank of the arcuate sulcus and the adjoining convexity to the rostral bank of the central sulcus in the hand area and in the upper parts of the face area (cf. Pandya & Vignolo 1971). At that time we referred to this area as the writing centre.

Goldman-Rakic: The animals are spared by the SMA lesion in one task and impaired in the other. Since one task is visual and the other is kinaesthetic, don't they differ also with respect to external cues versus internally generated cues?

Passingham: We also compare a sequence with a conditional task.

Goldman-Rakic: But the animal is just raising its hands, so there isn't much of a sequence there. Is the deficit related to kinaesthetic versus visual or to internally versus externally driven responses? The distinction is crucial.

Passingham: What do you mean by internal and external?

Goldman-Rakic: In the visually guided task a stimulus elicits a response. In the other task the animal moves its hand spontaneously and generates the cues for movement. There is no imperative stimulus in the situation which elicits the response. It is a genuinely self-produced response.

Passingham: There are no problems about triggering. The animals know when to respond.

Deecke: Masdeu et al (1978) investigated lesions in the left hemisphere that were clearly restricted to the SMA, such as blocked branches of the anterior cerebral artery. The patients were described as having a 'global aphasia' but maybe it was more a lack of motivation to speak. Some people say that we have three speech centres, two pre-rolandic and one post-rolandic. Speech loses its fluency only when Broca's area and the SMA are destroyed. When we have a lesion of the retro-rolandic area (Wernicke's area), there is an increase in fluency rather than a decrease. If the left SMA in humans is a third speech centre, why is 'aphasia' so transient? After four weeks the patients seem to be normal again. There are two possible explanations. One is that we have two SMAs and if one is damaged the other takes over. The other possibility is that not everything is completely normal again. F. Duffy (personal communication, 1985) said that even in the long term these patients were 'unwilling' to speak. If a patient had been a fluent speaker, loved to speak and had a ready tongue in the pre-morbid state, he or she became rather lazy afterwards. The same was true for reading or writing. Thus, again it is the motivational aspects of SMA function that are uncovered by such observations in the long follow-up of patients with SMA lesions.

Passingham: There are two aspects: internal triggers to get us to move, and instructions based on our movements. I should have restricted myself to the latter. In the arm-raising test the problem was not one of reaching spontaneously but of reaching a target zone accurately.

References

Haaxma R, Kuypers HGJM 1975 Intrahemispheric cortical connections and visual guidance of hand and finger movements in the rhesus monkey. Brain 98:239–260

Masdeu JC, Schöne WC, Funkenstein H 1978 Aphasia following infarction of the left supplementary motor area. Neurology 28:1220–1223

Pandya DN, Vignolo LA 1971 Intra- and interhemispheric projections of the precentral, premotor and arcuate areas in the rhesus monkey. Brain Res 26:217–233

Roland PE, Skinhoj E, Lassen NA 1981 Focal activations of the human cerebral cortex during auditory discrimination. J Neurophysiol 45:374–386

Roland PE, Friberg L, Lassen NA, Olsen TS 1985 Regional cortical blood flow changes during production of fluent speech and during conversation. J Cereb Blood Flow Metab 5(suppl 1):S205–S206

General discussion 2

Pandya: Motor cortex has traditionally been equated with the precentral gyrus (area 4) and subdivided functionally along the dorsoventral axis according to the classical concept of the motor homunculus. Other physiological and anatomical studies, however, have shown that the rostrocaudal dimension may also be relevant to understanding the functional organization of the motor cortex. Thus the rostral portion of area 4 seems to be involved mainly in control of trunk, head and neck movement, while caudal portions of the precentral gyrus are involved mainly in governing muscular activity of the extremities (Woolsey 1958, Kuypers 1981). Adding to this complexity is the fact that more recent studies (Muakkassa & Strick 1979) have shown that several other motor representations exist within the frontal lobe, aside from the traditional precentral (MI) and supplementary (MII) motor regions.

I wish to present here a unified organizational schema, based on cytoarchitectonics and neural connections, that may account for all these proposed divisions of the cortical motor system. This schema stems from the hypothesis that the cerebral cortex has evolved from two so-called prime moieties, or regions of primitive undifferentiated cortex, namely archicortex (hippocampus) and palaeocortex (olfactory cortex) (Sanides 1970). According to this notion, subsequent pathways of cortical differentiation from these two regions lead through periallocortex (PA11) and proisocortex (Pro) to the development of true six-layered isocortex (Fig. 1A,B). From the hippocampal moiety may be traced the proisocortex of the cingulate gyrus (area 24), while the olfactory region leads to insular proisocortex. Fig. 1C shows the subsequent architectonic steps which continue from these two proisocortices to premotor and precentral cortex. The dorsal trend leads from cingulate gyrus to MII and the dorsal portion of the premotor cortex (area 6) as well as dorsal motor cortex. The ventral trend, by contrast, progresses from insular proisocortex to area ProM (area ProM seems to be equivalent to MII of the dorsal trend) and to the ventral portion of the premotor cortex (area 6) as well as ventral motor cortex. Fig. 2 shows the cytoarchitectonic patterns of subregions within these two trends.

The different architectonic regions of the dorsal and ventral frontal trends have systems of intrinsic or local connections that parallel the architectonic sequences (Fig. 3). Thus the rostral cingulate gyrus (area 24) projects to the supplementary motor area and dorsal area 6. The supplementary motor area in turn projects on the one hand to dorsal area 6 and area 4 and, on the other hand, to area 24 (Damasio & VanHoesen 1980). The dorsal portion of premotor cortex (area 6), and particularly its caudal subdivision, projects to dorsal area 4

165

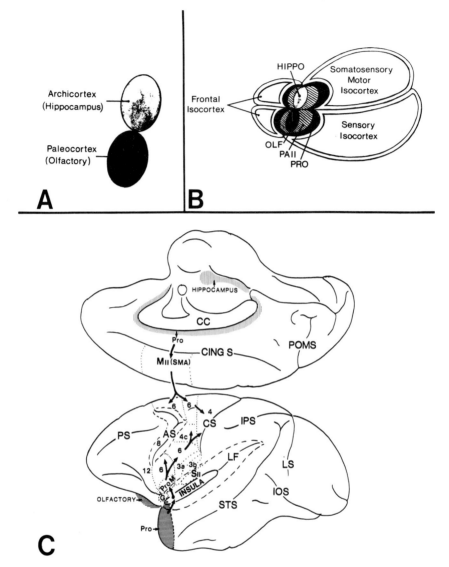

FIG.1 (*Pandya*). A–B: evolutionary development of cortical areas from two moieties, the archicortical (hippocampal) and the palaeocortical (olfactory). C: dorsal (hippo-campal–cingulate) and ventral (olfactory–insular) architectonic trends, showing prog-ressive architectonic steps leading to dorsal and ventral sectors of premotor (area 6) and motor (area 4) cortices in *Macaca mulatta*. AS, arcuate sulcus; CC, corpus callosum; CF, calcarine fissure; CING S, cingulate sulcus; CS, central sulcus; G, gustatory area; IOS, inferior occipital sulcus; IPS, intraparietal sulcus; LF, lateral fissure; LS, lunate sulcus; MII (SMA), supplementary motor area; OTS, occipito-temporal sulcus; POMS, parieto-occipito-medial sulcus; PAll, periallocortex; Pro, proisocortex; ProM, pre-motor area; PS, principal sulcus; SII, second sensory area; STS, superior temporal sulcus.

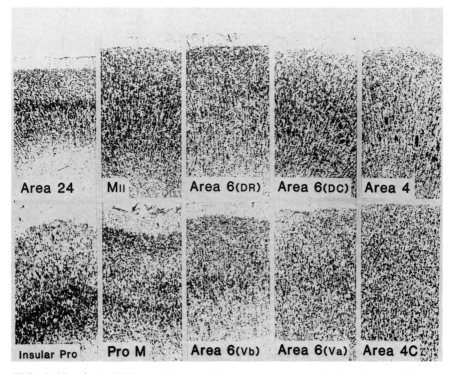

FIG. 2 (*Pandya*). Differential cytoarchitectonic patterns of subregions within two motor trends. The dorsal trend consists of area 24, MII, rostral and caudal dorsal area 6, dorsal area 4. The ventral trend consists of insular cortex, ProM, ventral area 6 and area 4c.

(MI) as well as to MII and area 24 (Barbas & Pandya 1987). Indeed most of these connections are reciprocal. A similar situation exists for ventral regions. Thus, the insular cortex projects to area ProM in the frontal operculum and ventral area 6 (Mesulam & Mufson 1982). Area ProM sends projections back to the rostral insula and also projects to ventral area 6. Ventral area 6, in turn, projects back to area ProM and the ventral precentral motor area. Many of these connections are reciprocal; and there are also interconnections at several points between areas in the dorsal and ventral pathways.

Thus there appears to be a dual organization of motor-related cortex. The dorsal region, related to the hippocampus and rostral cingulate region, includes the supplementary motor area (MII), dorsal premotor cortex (area 6), and dorsal motor cortex (MI, area 4). The ventral division, related to the rostral insula, includes area ProM in the frontal operculum, the ventral premotor region (area 6) and ventral motor cortex (MI, area 4). These two major divisions of motor-related cortex have different patterns of long corticocortical connections. The dorsal region has connections with the dorsal parietal and prefrontal regions, whereas the ventral region is connected preferentially with

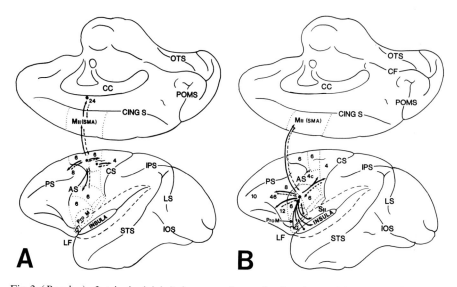

Fig.3 (*Pandya*). Intrinsic (vicinity) connections of subregions within dorsal (A) and ventral (B) motor trends.

ventral parietal and prefrontal regions. These differential connections of the two divisions suggest different functions. In view of the progressive trends outlined above, the multiple representations reported in the premotor region (Muakkassa & Strick 1979) are not surprising. They can be viewed as reflecting successive steps in the development of the motor system from proisocortex to its present form as area 4.

Up to now it has been customary to focus on motor, premotor and supplementary motor areas as well as their immediately related regions when studying the cortical components of the motor system. It may, however, be more meaningful to include all related areas from which cortical motor areas have sequentially evolved. A consideration of dorsal and ventral evolutionary pathways may provide a valuable context for understanding certain basic aspects of motor function, even though the older regions of these pathways (cingulate and insular cortices) do not appear to have a motor role in the strictest sense. It is possible that these regions do influence motor behaviour at a broader, more fundamental level. Thus, the cortical components of the dorsal pathway may be engaged in providing a spatial context for motility, while the ventral motor pathway may provide emotional input which influences motor activity. According to this view it is the combined contributions from different regions of these two motor pathways which result in fully integrated motor behaviour.

Wiesendanger: What are your cytoarchitectonic criteria for SMA? Do you place it within mesial area 6?

Pandya: The main difference between area 6 and SMA is that in SMA there is still emphasis on infragranular layers (i.e. layers V and VI). Area SMA is located medial to area 6 (Fig. 2). There is a subtle difference between MII and area 6. The main difference is that layers V and VI are more dense in MII than in area 6 (Fig. 2).

Wiesendanger: So it is still area 6 but has some special features?

Pandya: Yes.

Kuypers: I was surprised that your lesions in the frontal lobe did not show any projection into the parietal lobe.

Pandya: I have described only local projections within premotor, motor and nearby medial and ventral regions. Undoubtedly there are projections to the parietal lobe, as has been described previously.

Marsden: No one has mentioned Glickstein et al's (1980) work on how visual information from parieto-occipital areas gets to the motor cortex. Is it through corticocortical connections or down to pons and thence to cerebellum and back again? This is relevant to Dick Passingham's view about visual input via corticocortical connections into lateral premotor cortex as the crucial pathway. Or is it the descending pathway via cerebellum going back to motor cortex that is important in a visually guided task?

Kuypers: Our findings (Haaxma & Kuypers 1975) after transection of the parietal white matter combined with a commissurotomy demonstrated that corticocortical connections are very important in the visual guidance of hand and finger movements. I am convinced, however, that in the brain there are always several parallel systems which deal with a certain item, and that is probably also the case here. The possible involvement of the cerebellum was suggested by the following findings, obtained by Dr L. Moll and myself. After frontal lesions involving the postarcuate area, the area above the arcuate sulcus, including the rostral part of the motor cortex and the area of the SMA, showed a deficit in visually guided hand and finger movements similar to that after transection of the parietal white matter. However, the frontal deficit was much less long-lasting than the parietal one, unless the commissurotomy was extended to involve the decussations of the tectospinal and rubrospinal tracts. There might, therefore, be a certain cerebellar back-up through the red nucleus since, presumably, the rubrospinal neurons are under the dominance of the cerebellum.

Roland: Charles Kennedy and his collaborators (1980) did an autoradiographic study in a monkey that had to reach out and press a button every time the button lit up. Metabolic activity during this task was increased in the premotor cortex, in the SMA and in the primary motor cortex. In addition, the basal ganglia were bilaterally active. There was activity in the grey matter of the pons and bilaterally in the cerebellum, with some preponderance in one hemisphere. There also seemed to be some kind of population coding in the spinal cord. All the cervical segments in the anterior horn region of the spinal cord were metabolically active during this reaching task. Single-cell studies may not be suitable for investigating these questions. Does anyone know whether a very restricted movement, for instance of a single finger in a monkey, excites all the segments of the cervical cord?

Goldman-Rakic: I don't think that has been done with 2-deoxyglucose.

Lemon: I would challenge anybody to get a monkey to move one finger *and nothing else!*

Thach: Mark Schieber at Washington University, St. Louis, has trained two monkeys to make independent movements of the thumb. Movements of the index and the little finger are independent of each other, but each is accompanied by movement of the third and fourth finger at their present level of training. Whether the fingers can be made to go in combinations and sequences is another question that he is addressing.

As to the effect of cerebellar lesions on visually guided reaching tasks, Goldberger & Growdon (1973) felt that the task could still be performed, albeit with some inaccuracy due to tremor or ataxia, which would be consistent with clinical dogma.

References

Barbas H, Pandya DN 1987 Architecture and frontal cortical connections of the premotor cortex (area 6) in the rhesus monkey. J Comp Neurol 256:211–228

Damasio AR, Van Hoesen GW 1980 Structure and function of supplementary motor area. Neurology 30:359

Glickstein M, Cohen JL, Dixon B et al 1980 Cortico-pontine visual projections in Macaque monkeys. J Comp Neurol 190:209–229

Goldberger ME, Growdon JH 1973 Pattern of recovery following cerebellar deep nuclear lesions in monkeys. Exp Neurol 39:307–322

Haaxma R, Kuypers HGJM 1975 Intrahemispheric cortical connections and visual guidance of hand and finger movements in the rhesus monkey. Brain 98:239–260

Kennedy C, Miyaoka M, Suda S et al 1980 Local metabolic responses in brain accompanying motor activity. Trans Am Neurol Assoc 105:13–17

Kuypers HGJM 1981 Anatomy of the descending pathways. In: Brooks VB (ed) Motor control, pt 1. American Physiological Society, Bethesda, MD (Handb Physiol sect 1 The nervous system, vol 2) p 597–666

Mesulam MM, Mufson EJ 1982 Insula of the old world monkey. III. Efferent cortical output and comments on function. J Comp Neurol 221:38–52

Muakkassa KF, Strick PL 1979 Frontal lobe input to primate motor cortex: evidence for four somatotopically organized premotor areas. Brain Res 177:176–182

Sanides F 1970 Functional architecture of motor and sensory cortices in primate in the light of a new concept of neocortex evolution. In: Nobaek CR, Montagna W (eds) Advances in Primatology. Appleton-Century-Crofts, New York, p 137–208

Woolsey CN 1958 Organization of somatic sensory and motor areas of cerebral cortex. In: Harlow HF, Woolsey CN (eds) Biological and biochemical basis of behaviour. University of Wisconsin Press, Madison, p 63–81

Functional organization of inferior area 6

Giacomo Rizzolatti

Istituto di Fisiologia Umana dell'Università di Parma, via Gramsci 14, 43100 Parma, Italy

Abstract. The rostral part of the agranular frontal cortex (area 6) of the monkey consists of two large sectors: a superior sector lying medial to the spur of the arcuate sulcus (superior area 6) and an inferior sector lying lateral to it (inferior area 6). Single neurons have been recorded from inferior area 6 in behaving monkeys (*Macaca nemestrina*). The results were: (a) Proximal movements are essentially represented caudally in the histochemically defined area F4. Neurons related to these movements respond strongly to tactile and visual stimuli. Visual receptive fields are located in the space around the animal's body (peripersonal space) and their location does not change with eye movements. The direction of movements effective in triggering the neurons is congruent with the position of their visual receptive field. (b) Distal movements are represented rostrally in the anterior part of F4 and in F5. Neurons related to these movements discharge vigorously during motor acts that have a precise aim. The neurons were subdivided into four classes: grasping-with-the-hand neurons, grasping-with-the-hand-and-mouth neurons, holding neurons, and tearing neurons. Regardless of the class they belong to a large number of neurons show specificity for different types of object prehension—discharging, for example, during precision grip but not during whole-hand prehension. It is proposed that inferior area 6 contains a vocabulary of motor acts related to hand–mouth movements. The motor acts can be retrieved by visual and somatosensory stimuli. The possibility is discussed that a series of vocabularies where movements of various complexity are stored represents the neural basis of cortical motor organization.

1987 Motor areas of the cerebral cortex. Wiley, Chichester (Ciba Foundation Symposium 132) p 171–186

The largest portion of the agranular frontal cortex of primates is formed by cytoarchitectonic area 6 (see Blinkov & Glezer 1968). Structurally this area is not uniform and by taking into account small histological differences it can be subdivided into several subareas. The non-homogeneity of area 6 is confirmed by histochemical studies. Matelli et al (1985), using the cytochrome oxidase method (Wong-Riley 1979), described five histochemically defined areas in the agranular cortex which roughly correspond to the cytoarchitectonic areas of von Bonin & Bailey (1947). The location of these areas is shown in Fig. 1. F1 corresponds to the precentral motor cortex (area FA), whereas F3 should correspond to the supplementary motor area, which lacks a

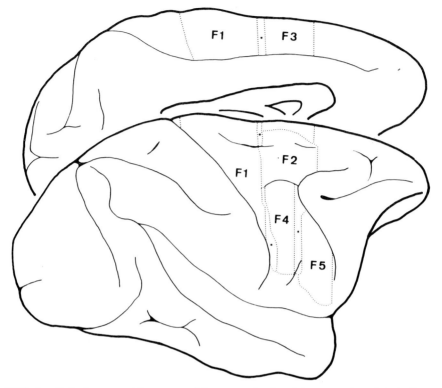

FIG. 1.   Cytochrome oxidase map of the agranular frontal cortex. Asterisks indicate transition zones and zones that were impossible to define because of the sulcal pattern. The spur of the arcuate sulcus sets the limit between superior and inferior area 6. For the correspondence between the cytochrome oxidase and cytoarchitectonic subdivision see text.

histological counterpart in von Bonin & Bailey's maps. Finally F2, F4 and F5 match well with von Bonin & Bailey's areas FB, FBA and FCBm, respectively. In this review I will summarize our new findings on the properties of neurons in areas F4 and F5 (inferior area 6) of the macaque monkey (*Macaca nemestrina*). The relevance of these findings to area 6 function and organization is discussed.

F4 neurons

General characteristics

The neurons recorded from area F4 can be subdivided into two main groups. The first is formed by cells highly responsive to somatosensory stimuli and, in most cases, related to proximal and facial movements. These neurons represent the great majority of units encountered in a region of F4 which extends rostrally from the border of F1 almost to the border of F5 and laterally from the spur of the arcuate sulcus for about 4 mm. They will be referred to as F4 neurons.

The second group is formed by neurons mostly related to distal movements. These neurons fire strongly during specific active movements and are usually less responsive than those of the first group to passive stimulation. They are located in a rostral strip near the border of F5. Since their properties are indistinguishable from those of F5 neurons they will be discussed with those neurons.

Neuronal responses to somatosensory and visual stimuli

F4 neurons responded well to tactile stimuli. When the agranular cortex was explored systematically with successsive rostral penetrations, the appearance of neurons showing highly constant tactile responses was an index of the transition from F1, activated predominantly by proprioceptive stimuli, to F4. The receptive field size of the neurons was usually large, although some neurons had fields of only a few square centimetres. The receptive field locations of the F4 neurons ($n = 103$) were: lip, 16 neurons (15.5% of total); face 47 (45.6%); face, neck and chest, 11 (10.7%); chest 7 (6.8%); chest and arm, 7 (6.8%); arm, 7 (6.8%); hand, 4 (3.9%); others, 4 (3.9%). Of these fields 71% were contralateral to the recorded side, 2% were ipsilateral, and the remainder were bilateral. Note the large number of fields located on the face. These fields were found in neurons active during facial movement but also in neurons triggered by arm movements.

Most F4 neurons (85%) could be activated with visual stimuli. Strong and constant visual responses were evoked with stimuli (three-dimensional objects) moved in the space within the animal's reach (peripersonal space). Approaching stimuli were usually the most effective. Visual receptive fields were located around the tactile field, thus forming a single responsive region on the skin and in the adjacent space.

An important property of the visual neurons was that their visual field was anchored to the body and did not change position with eye movements. In other words, unlike classical visual cells, F4 neurons had receptive fields coded in terms of body coordinates. Fig. 2 illustrates this point. This neuron had its tactile receptive field on the lips and the hairy skin around them. The tactile field was almost completely contralateral to the recorded side. Visual responses were studied by moving a small piece of cotton wrapped around the tip of a metal rod supported at the other end by a vertical bar. Potentiometers connected with the joint controlling the rod movement around the bar recorded the position in space of the tip of the rod. The upper part of the figure shows the responses of the neuron to a stimulus moved towards the tactile receptive field; the lower part shows the responses to the same stimulus

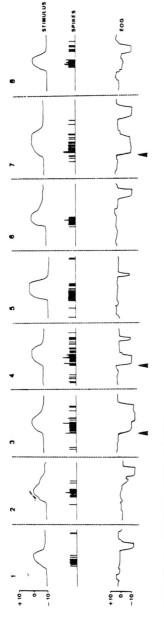

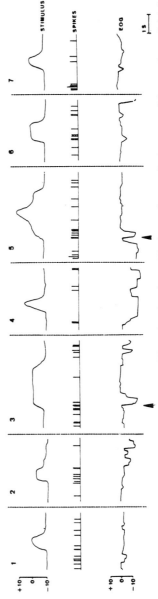

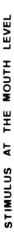

FIG. 2. Visual responses of an F4 neuron. The stimulus (a small piece of cotton) was moved from a lateral (right) position towards the animal's face along a horizontal plane. In the upper part of the figure results are shown for trials in which the stimulus was presented at mouth level, in the lower part for trials in which the stimulus was moved at eye level. For each trial the trajectory of the stimulus, action potentials (integration time 10 ms) and the horizontal electro-oculogram are shown (upper, middle and lower row respectively). On the ordinates is indicated the position of the stimulus in respect to the centre of the mouth. Negative values: positions of the stimulus on the right of the midline; positive values: position of the stimulus on the left of the midline. The arrows indicate those trials in which the stimulus triggered an ocular saccade. The unit was recorded from the left hemisphere.

moved towards the eyes. In spite of the two trajectories being only a few centimetres from each other, the unit constantly responded in the first condition, never in the second. This could not be attributed to a visual receptive field confined to the lower part of the visual field, since the response was present when the stimulus was at mouth level but absent when the stimulus was at eye level, even when the stimulus triggered a fixation saccade (trials marked by arrows). In this condition the stimulus, regardless of where it was located in space, fell on the fovea. Thus the position in relation to the head, not that in relation to the retina, was crucial for driving the neurons.

Neuronal discharge during active movements

Fifty per cent of F4 neurons fired during active movements. Arm movements were most often represented (70%), followed by face movements (25%). Among arm movements two types were very common: reaching and bringing to the mouth. 'Reaching neurons' responded to the arm being moved towards a particular, usually rather large, space sector; 'bringing-to-the-mouth neurons' fired during movements towards the mouth, independently of the initial starting point.

The receptive field location and the effective movements were organized in F4 in terms of functional relationships. Many neurons with a tactile receptive field on the face had a visual receptive field in the peripersonal upper space and were activated by reaching movements towards the upper space. Reaching neurons whose peripersonal field was around the body responded to movements towards the lower space. Similarly, there was congruence between the side where the field was located and the side towards which reaching was effective. The same functional principle was found in bringing-to-the-mouth neurons, which responded to arm movements directed to the mouth but not to the body, and had tactile and peripersonal fields around the mouth and the face. In one neuron in which the effective movement was towards the body the tactile and peripersonal field was also around the body. The organization of neurons related to facial movements was simpler, with the receptive field corresponding to the part of the face that was moved.

F5 neurons

General characteristics

It has been believed for a long time that only proximal movements are represented in area 6 (see Wiesendanger 1981). This notion, however, has not been confirmed by recent findings (Rizzolatti et al 1981a, Kurata & Tanji 1986). Our results agree with this new point of view. Of more than 200 neurons we recorded in F5 and rostral F4, only 10% were activated by

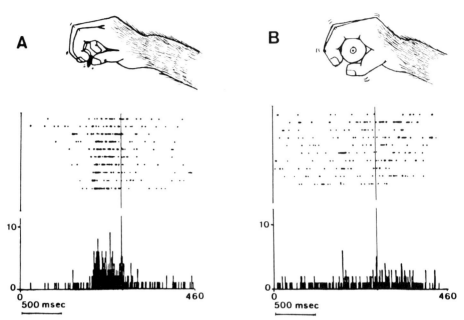

FIG. 3.   Study of a 'grasping-with-the hand' neuron. A: discharge during precision grip. B: discharge during prehension with the whole hand. The responses are aligned with the moment at which the hand touched the object (vertical bar). Each histogram is the sum of 10 trials. Bin width: 5 ms.

proximal movements or by complex movements with a possible involvement of proximal musculature. Most F5 neurons discharged during distal movements. Their properties will be described in this section.

The most interesting characteristic of the F5 neurons we recorded was that their firing correlated much better with a motor act that had a particular purpose than with any single movement made by the animal. Furthermore, movements in which the animal used the same muscles as in the effective motor acts, but for other purposes, failed to activate the neurons. Using the purposive motor act as the classification criterion we subdivided the distal neurons into four classes: 'grasping-with-the-hand neurons', 'grasping-with-the-hand-and-mouth neurons', 'holding neurons' and 'tearing neurons'.

Grasping-with-the-hand neurons

Grasping-with-the-hand neurons formed the largest class of F5 neurons (42%). Fig. 3 shows the responses of a typical neuron of this class. A strong discharge was present when the animal grasped an object with the index finger and thumb. In contrast, no movement-related discharge was observed when the animal grasped the object with the whole hand. Note that the fingers also flexed during this motor act. The neuron started to fire 500 ms before contact with the stimulus and stopped firing soon after the object had been grasped. Analysis of the temporal relations between the discharge of the neuron and the behaviour of the animal showed that the neuron started to fire before finger movements and continued to fire during hand preparation movements characterized by finger extension, as well as during the final phase of grasping, characterized by the finger flexion. Thus there was a correlation between the firing of the unit and the entire motor act, but not between the firing of the unit and the individual movements.

Most grasping neurons (85%) showed selectivity for a particular type of grasping. Some of them (40%) fired during prehension with the index finger and the thumb (precision grip), some fired during prehension with all fingers (40%), and a few (7%) discharged during grasping with the whole hand. The remaining neurons became active irrespective of how the object was picked up. These observations indicate that F5 neurons code not only the goal of a motor act but also the way in which it can be successfully accomplished.

The time relationship between the beginning of neuron discharge and the onset of movement varied from one neuron to another. In about 20% of neurons firing occurred during the last part of grasping, during finger flexion, in 50% the discharge started with finger extension and continued during finger flexion, and in 30% it started well in advance of finger movements, during arm movements. Although for these last neurons one might argue that the discharge was related to both proximal and distal movements, this does not seem likely. These neurons also showed selectively for the type of prehension, firing either during grasping of small objects (precision grip) or during grasping of large objects (other types of grasping). Since the proximal movements were identical in the two conditions, while distal movements changed, neuron activity appears to be related to distal movements.

Grasping-with-the-hand-and-mouth neurons

This class of neurons fired both when the animal grasped the objects with its hands and when it grasped them with its mouth. The discharge did not depend on synergism between hand and mouth movements, since it was present during grasping mouth movements in the absence of any hand movement and during hand grasping movements in the absence of mouth movements. It appears that these neurons code the aim of the motor act independently of the anatomical effectors used to attain it. Grasping-with-the-hand-and-mouth neurons represented about 25% of the distal neurons of inferior area 6.

Selectivity for the types of prehension described for grasping neurons was also present in this class of cells. The number of unselective neurons was higher (56%) than in grasping-with-the-hand neurons. Moreover, no neurons responding to whole-hand prehension were observed. The neurons of this class showed the same time relationships between the beginning of discharge and the onset of movement as the grasping-with-the-hand neurons.

Holding neurons

Holding neurons were less numerous than grasping neurons (10%). Unlike grasping neurons, which stopped firing when the object was grasped, holding neurons continued to discharge until the object was released. Specificity for different types of prehension was present in this class of neuron, as in the grasping classes. As far as the temporal properties are concerned, some holding neurons started to fire at the moment when the object was touched and others fired before contact.

Tearing neurons

Tearing neurons formed a tiny class of neurons (5%) which became active when the animal made movements of the fingers, hand and wrist suitable for tearing or breaking objects. In these neurons the discharge started after the hand touched the stimulus. Tearing neurons were the only F5 neurons which may code for force. However, shaping of the hand for motor acts such as tearing or breaking is not the same as shaping it for grasping. Firing of these neurons may therefore be related not to the force but to the distinctive features of the movements which require force in order to be executed.

Neuronal responses to somatosensory and visual stimuli

About 45% of distal neurons, regardless of the class they belonged to, could be activated by somatosensory stimuli. The receptive fields were located on the hands, on the mouth, or on the hands and mouth. The receptive field location corresponded to the body parts whose active movements triggered the neurons. Seventeen per cent of distal neurons responded to visual stimuli. A neuron was considered visual only if visual responses were obtained in the absence of any movement. Many visually responsive neurons were selective for the type of prehension; some were unspecific. There was a correlation between type of prehension and preferred visual stimuli. Precision-grip neurons responded only to small visual stimuli, unspecific neurons to any type of stimuli. Receptive fields were usually difficult to define.

The role of area 6 in movement

A number of proposals have been advanced about the functional role of area 6 in the control of movement. The most important of these are preparation for movement, sensory guidance of movement, control of movement sequencing.

The preparation-for-movement hypothesis has two distinct versions. The first and older one is strictly linked to the notion that area 6 controls proximal movements. According to this, the main role of area 6 is that of stabilizing the trunk and limbs in order to render possible the execution of more distal movements (see Humphrey 1979). The second version employs the term 'preparation for movement' to signify readiness to move. The empirical evidence in favour of this version is the presence in area 6 of neurons that fire in the absence of any movement when an animal that is instructed to emit a response expects a 'go' signal (Weinrich & Wise 1982). Many of these neurons (set-related neurons) show specificity for the direction of the coming movement, making it unlikely that their properties can be explained in terms of arousal. Their function is probably to facilitate spinal motor neurons and neurons linking the premotor area to the spinal cord, so allowing a fast response to the trigger stimulus.

Neither version of the preparation-for-movement hypothesis appears sufficient to explain the function of area 6 in movement control. The first version is contradicted by the finding of rich distal representation in area 6 (Rizzolatti et al 1981a, Kurata & Tanji 1986, Gentilucci et al 1987). Neurons such as those found in F5 cannot be explained by this version. The second version has limited heuristic power. As Requin (1980) convincingly argued, 'preparation is not a stage in a process, but rather a change in the functional state of a processing system'. It is not justified to consider area 6 as a 'modifier' of the excitability of area 4 and other motor centres rather than as an area which itself processes the information necessary for certain types of movement, since (a) anatomical findings show that this area has a unique role in conveying information from the parietal lobe to the motor cortex and (b) the neurons described in this paper indicate that new properties necessary for movement organization emerge in this area. Furthermore, the presence of set-related cells in many cortical areas outside area 6 points to movement preparation being a distributed function which does not specifically characterize any area (see Evarts et al 1984).

More interesting is the proposal that area 6 plays a role in sensory and especially visually guided movements (Haaxma & Kuypers 1975, Godschalk et al 1981, Rizzolatti et al 1981b). The weakness of this hypothesis has been the lack of any clear formulation on how sensory information is translated into motor commands. Some hints about this can be derived from the results presented in this paper. These show that there is a difference in the organization of proximal and distal movements. Neurons related to proximal movements respond strongly to tactile stimuli and to visual stimuli located in the peripersonal space around specific parts of the body. The visual fields are anchored to the body and do not change position with eye movements. It appears therefore that the neurons related to proximal movement encode the stimulus position in space and, as shown by their motor properties, command movements towards a specific although rather large space sector. The relationships between visual input and distal movements are more subtle. Most F5 neurons, regardless of the category they belong to, do not respond to visual stimuli but specify the motor pattern necessary to take or hold the objects. A direct relationship with visual stimuli exists, however, in about 20% of distal neurons. Furthermore, these neurons show a good correlation between the size of the stimulus effective in triggering a response and the type of motor pattern controlled by the neurons. Thus, unlike proximal neurons, distal neurons are sensitive to the size of the stimulus rather than to its location in space, and they are able to use this information to retrieve the appropriate movement.

Taken together, these findings on proximal and distal area 6 neurons are congruent with the hypothesis that this area has a functional role in sensory guidance of movements. These findings also indicate that in area 6 there is storage or a vocabulary (Rizzolatti et al 1987) of motor acts such as reaching, grasping and holding, and that this vocabulary can be addressed by visual and somatosensory stimuli. It is possible that there are other ways to retrieve the motor acts stored in area 6—for example by knowing the location or size of the object—but no data are available on this point.

The proposal that area 6 is involved in the control of movement sequencing (Fulton 1934, Deuel & Dunlop 1979) can be interpreted in several ways. The most interesting is probably that a sequence of motor acts or even an entire motor action (e.g. reach—grasp—hold—bring to the mouth) is represented in a single neuron. Our findings do not support this idea. Although it is logical to postulate that the progression from muscle contraction to movement and from movement to motor acts leads eventually to neurons which code sequences of motor acts, this type of neuron has not been observed in area 6. This high-order vocabulary, if it exists, is located in areas outside area 6.

The fascinating aspect of this idea of a vocabulary of motor acts is that it predicts that in addition to that of inferior area 6 other vocabularies should exist in the association motor areas. Some of these vocabularies may be similar in complexity to the one discussed here, but with different types of movements represented; others may be more complex. For example, one may postulate the existence of a vocubulary where eye movement and hand movements are associated, or, as already mentioned, a vocabulary where motor sequences are represented. This idea of a series of vocabularies in various cortical areas should not be difficult to test, and experiments based on it should give important information on the cortical organization of movement.

Acknowledgements

I thank R. Camarda, L. Fogassi, M. Gentilucci, G. Luppino and M. Matelli for their help in the experiments. This work was supported by NIH Grant No. 1-RO1-NS-19206-01A7 and by a CNR grant to the Unità di Parma, Gruppo Nazionale di Neuroscienze. Additional support was given by MPI.

References

Blinkov SM, Glezer II 1968 The human brain in figures and tables: a quantitative handbook. Plenum Press, New York

Deuel RK, Dunlop NL 1979 Role of the frontal polysensory cortex in guidance of limb movements. Brain Res 169:183–188

Evarts EV, Shinoda Y, Wise SP 1984 Neurophysiological approaches to higher brain functions. Wiley, New York

Fulton JF 1934 Forced grasping and groping in relation to the syndrome of the premotor area. Arch Neurol Psychiatry 31:221–235

Gentilucci M, Fogassi L, Luppino G, Matelli M, Camarda R, Rizzolatti G 1987 Somatotopic representation in inferior area 6 of the macaque monkey. Brain Behav Evol, in press

Godschalk M, Lemon RN, Nijs HGT, Kuypers HGJM 1981 Behaviour of neurons in monkey periarcuate and precentral cortex before and during visually guided arm and hand movements. Exp Brain Res 44:113–116

Haaxma R, Kuypers HGJM 1975 Intrahemispheric cortical connexions and visual guidance of hand and finger movements in the rhesus monkey. Brain 98:239–260

Humphrey DR 1979 On the cortical control of visually directed reaching: contributions by nonprecentral motor areas. In:Talbot RE, Humphrey DR (eds) Posture and movement, Raven Press, New York, p 51–112

Kurata K, Tanji J 1986 Premotor cortex neurons in macaques: activity before distal and proximal forelimb movements. J. Neurosci 6:403–411

Matelli M, Luppino G, Rizzolatti G 1985 Patterns of cytochrome oxidase activity in the frontal agranular cortex of the macaque monkey. Behav Brain Res 18: 125–137

Requin J 1980 Toward a psychobiology of preparation for action. In: Stelmach GE, Requin J (eds) Tutorials in motor behavior. Amsterdam, North-Holland, p 373–398

Rizzolatti G, Scandolara C, Matelli M, Gentilucci M 1981a Afferent properties of periarcuate neurons in macaque monkeys. I. Somato-sensory responses. Behav Brain Res 2:125–146

Rizzolatti G, Scandolara C, Matelli M, Gentilucci M 1981b Afferent properties of periarcuate neurons in macaque monkeys. II:Visual responses. Behav Brain Res 2: 147–163

Rizzolatti G, Gentilucci M, Fogassi L, Luppino G, Matelli M, Ponzoni Maggi S 1987 Neurons related to goal-directed motor acts in inferior area 6 of the macaque monkey. Exp Brain Res, in press

Von Bonin G, Bailey P 1947 The neocortex of Macaca mulatta. University of Illinois Press, Urbana

Weinrich M, Wise SP 1982 The premotor cortex of the monkey. J Neurosci 2: 1329–1345

Wiesendanger M 1981 Organization of secondary motor areas of cerebral cortex. In: Brooks VB (ed) Motor Control, part 2. American Physiological Society, Bethesda, MD (Handb Physiol Sect 1 The nervous system vol 2) p 1121–1147

Wong-Riley M 1979 Changes in the visual system of monocularly sutured or enucleated cats demonstrable with cytochrome oxidase histochemistry. Brain Res 171:11–29

DISCUSSION

Passingham: I am suspicious about the use of single-unit recording high up in the system to tell you what the area is doing. We could fit those cells to practically any theory we like. This sort of recording is essential if we are to know *how* the area does what it does but it is not a good guide as to *what* it does.

Rizzolatti: I disagree. If you were correct I should be able to assign a function to every premotor area, since, according to you, my interpretation of their function is completely arbitrary. This is not so. When we record a few millimetres medial to the spur of the arcuate sulcus, we do not understand what those neurons are doing, although they fire during the animal's movements. So our data are not so subjective as you may think. As to the lesions in area 6, my point is that there are several vocabularies in frontal and parietal lobe coding different types of movements and that among them there is a certain degree of redundancy. Thus the effect of a lesion of one of these vocabularies can be compensated by the activity of the others. The same is observed in the visual system. In the cat, for example, you can ablate area 17 and nothing dramatic happens. I don't believe that the motor system is organized according to principles radically different from those of sensory systems.

Kuypers: As I mentioned before, when this area plus the area above the arcuate sulcus plus the supplementary motor cortex are removed, Dr L. Moll and I found that the animals show a defect in the visual guidance of hand and finger movements for three months (Haaxma & Kuypers 1975).

Passingham: The defect is not there after a lateral premotor lesion.

Roland: If it is true that the premotor area is preferentially activated in visual reaching there is definitely some discrepancy between the results in monkeys and those in humans. When Laplane and co-workers ablated the SMA and the premotor cortex of a person they found lasting defects in all kinds of skilled movements—the limb became useless and it stayed like that. In human studies the premotor areas were metabolically active during visual guidance tasks, during auditory guidance tasks and during tactile guidance tasks (Roland & Friberg 1983, Roland et al 1980, Roland & Larsen 1980). It is definitely wrong to limit the functional role of the premotor cortex to visual reaching in humans.

Rizzolatti: We found that the vocabulary of inferior area 6 can be addressed by visual and somatosensory stimuli. We cannot, however, exclude other possibilities. It may even be that the vocabulary of inferior area 6 is used during internally generated actions.

Marsden: You demonstrated beautifully how that area can be addressed by a visual input, for example. I didn't detect in your recordings any signs of the vocabulary that you think the input is addressing.

Rizzolatti: The vocabulary is demonstrated by the fact that inferior area 6 neurons selectively fire during specific goal-related motor acts.

Marsden: That vocabulary sounds to me identical to the vocabulary that one can record from the motor cortex itself.

Rizzolatti: One major difference is that neurons of inferior area 6 indicate a goal regardless of whether it is achieved using the right hand, the left hand or the mouth. I don't think there is any evidence that there are neurons firing during hand and mouth movements in area 4. Furthermore, a very large number of inferior area 6 neurons are selectively activated during specific motor acts such as precision grip, finger prehension or whole-hand prehension. We have found some neurons with these properties in area 4 too, but the percentage is not very high.

Lemon: That depends heavily on what your sample is.

Rizzolatti: Yes, but goal-related neurons are found everywhere in F5.

Thach: When this area is ablated do the animals show any consistent abnormality that would indicate whether it is an intellectual deficit or a motor deficit?

Rizzolatti: It is certainly not an intellectual deficit. Deuel & Dunlop (1979) ablated the frontal premotor cortex bilaterally and the monkeys were unable to pick up their food and put it into their mouths in the normal way. In order to get the food they had to bend and take it with the mouth. This behaviour is consistent with a motor defect, not with an intellectual impairment.

Passingham: We found a visual reaching defect in monkeys with premotor lesions. We measure whether the animal puts its forefinger straight into a hole with a peanut or into neighbouring holes with no peanut. Monkeys with premotor lesions sometimes miss the correct hole or hit the divide between holes. You could argue that these are not misreaching defects but something to do with getting the hand into proper shape as it approaches the hole.

Thach: But you have just described a motor defect following ablation of a premotor area, and that is cardinally important.

Kalaska: Some of the neurons you presented, especially those that seem to have both somatomotor and visual receptive fields, are very similar to those described by Hyvarinen in parietal area 7b.

Rizzolatti: The comparison with area 7 is appropriate. Many of our observations are very similar to those of Leinonen, Hyvarinen and their colleagues (1979). F4 neurons, in particular, appear to have functional properties difficult to differentiate from those of area 7b neurons. I think this fits well with my hypothesis of a multiplicity of premotor vocabularies.

Kuypers: These two areas are strongly interconnected by corticocortical fibres (Pandya & Kuypers 1969).

Kalaska: Dr Passingham, you seem pessimistic about the value of these experiments and their potential usefulness in revealing the function of these areas. Could you suggest an experimental strategy by which single-unit experiments could yield useful data on the function of the premotor neurons?

Passingham: Single-unit recording was a great success in visual cortex and in motor cortex where we know roughly what these areas do. The method has had more troubles in areas in between. The greatest early success of single-unit recording was in parietal cortex, where it was known from lesion studies that animals with area 7 lesions misreach and where clinical studies suggested spatial functions. I only want to stress that if you have no idea of what supplementary motor cortex or some other area does, initial lesion experiments may guide you. As soon as you have some idea, unit experiments will tell you more about function. For example, psychologists have done many experiments on the functions of prefrontal cortex. Without those initial behavioural observations neither the anatomy nor the physiology could have advanced. We all talk as if we know what supplementary motor cortex does but I really don't think we do know. Lesion experiments at this point may be helpful.

Porter: You talked earlier about disabilities in animals lifting their arm to a target. Yet much of the clinical evidence seems to agree that the permanent deficit in patients in whom lesions of that midline cortex have occurred is a disorder of bimanual performance. There is some evidence that that is a permanent deficit in monkeys too. Yet no one, other than Dr Tanji, has said anything about bimanual actions.

Passingham: We have to put together what there is in common between a unimanual sequence task and doing two things together. In a bimanual sequence one hand may have to consult an instruction from the other hand. It may be as simple as that.

Kuypers: I know that Dr Passingham will support me when I emphasize that lesion studies in the postarcuate area are very difficult. If one removes the caudal bank of the arcuate sulcus and the adjoining convexity of the precentral gyrus, one always has to demonstrate first that the resulting deficit is not merely a motor defect, and this demonstration is sometimes very difficult indeed.

Marsden: Another restriction on the single-unit studies is that most of the motor paradigms examined are for very simple single movements, such as a reach. Is there any clue in either your recordings, Professor Rizzolatti, or those of Dr Tanji, that the neurons fire only when two motor programmes such as grasping and bringing to the mouth are put together, rather than firing with each individual action?

Rizzolatti: I have no evidence on that.

Tanji: I am in the process of investigating that point.

Deecke: We did experiments in which humans manually tracked a moving circle on an oscilloscope screen. The tracking was fed back to the screen as a point that always had to be kept in the circle. No learning was involved and everybody could do this successfully. Then we made an inverse paradigm in which the feedback signal was inverted between left and right and up and down. This task was very tricky to perform. At the same time we recorded the negativity over the cortex (Bereitschaftspotential). We established correlations between the increase in negativity for inverted tracking compared to normal tracking and the learning effect during the inverted tracking experiment by measuring the gradually falling error rate. The only brain regions where we found significant positive correlations were the left and right frontal convexities and the SMA. Our conclusion is that these areas may have something to do with motor learning.

Fetz: We have also been fascinated by the 'visual approach' cells in primary motor cortex. A small proportion of area 4 cells respond to approaching objects in the way you describe, Professor Rizzolatti. Some of these cells also have cutaneous receptive fields, and some are pyramidal tract neurons that also fire with active arm movement (Fetz et al 1980). What is the caudal border of the region in which you have observed these cells?

Rizzolatti: It is the border between the cytochrome oxidase areas F1 and F4. I think many people still consider F4 (FBA of von Bonin and Bailey) as part of area 4, but I think it is more correct to attribute it to area 6.

Fetz: Was it primary motor cortex?

Rizzolatti: No. We consider only F1 as primary motor cortex. Our distinction between F1 and F4 is based essentially, but not exclusively, on the organization of layer V pyramidal cells. In F1 the pyramidal cells form a continuous row of neurons with high cytochrome oxidase activity; in F4 these cells are present but organized in clusters (Matelli et al 1985). As I mentioned before, the properties of neurons in the two areas are different. However, F4 is electrically excitable; in this it is similar to F1.

Porter: But you have not tested whether the cells from which you are recording send their axons into the pyramidal tract?

Rizzolatti: That is correct.

Lemon: Some of the differences between your recordings and those obtained in other studies in the same area may be because the natural movements you are studying include the processes that are going on, such as the addressing of the programmes, and the execution of the programme itself. In our experiments (Godschalk et al 1981, 1985) most of the cells in the postarcuate area showed activity both while the animal was preparing to make a particular movement and during the execution of the movement itself, whereas cells in the caudal area 4 tended to show activity related purely to the execution of the movement. The separation of the preparation time and the execution of the movement is obviously not normal but it gives physiologists an opportunity to dissect some of these processes out. That difference still remains a very important difference between the classical motor cortex and the postarcuate area.

Rizzolatti: I am against the idea that the primary motor function of area 6 is movement preparation, if by this term is meant readiness to move. My view is that area 6 is a stage in movement control and this stage precedes that of area 4. Your finding that area 6 neurons fire before or in the absence of movement does not contradict this notion.

Lemon: I agree; but if you present the animal with a target—a purposeful movement for example—the activity you see in these areas is related to a number of different functions.

Marsden: One view is that these long-duration firing units are concerned with the preparation for a movement as well as with its execution. The alternative view is that they are a signal that continues until the movement is finished and then allows the next movement to occur. If a monkey executes a simple movement for longer than usual, do these 'preparatory' units go on firing until the movement is finished?

Rizzolatti: In our experiments we cannot rigidly separate preparation from action. My interpretation of area 6 neurons is that their activity represents the signal for a specific motor act. It is not very useful to postulate the existence of separate cortical areas for movement preparation (readiness to move) and movement execution. I prefer to think that there are various stages in motor control and that the activity of these stages eventually leads to motor action. Area 6 sends signals which, for example, command grasping and indicate how grasping has to be executed. These signals reach area 4 and various subcortical centres, the motor act is then executed, and the signal ceases.

Marsden: And when that signal ceases, it may be the trigger for doing the next thing?

Rizzolatti: Yes.

References

Deuel RK, Dunlop NI 1979 Role of frontal polysensory cortex in guidance of limb movements. Brain Res 169:183–188

Fetz EE, Finocchio DV, Baker MA, Soso MJ 1980 Sensory and motor responses of precentral cortex cells during comparable passive and active joint movements. J Neurophysiol 43:1070–1089

Godschalk M, Lemon RN, Nijs HGT, Kuypers HGJM 1981 Behaviour of neurons in monkey peri-arcuate and precentral cortex before and during visually-guided arm and hand movements. Exp Brain Res 44:113–116

Godschalk M, Lemon RN, Kuypers HGJM, van der Steen J 1985 The involvement of monkey premotor cortex neurones in preparation of visually cued arm movements. Behav Brain Res 18:137–157

Haaxma R, Kuypers HGJM 1975 Intrahemispheric cortical connections and visual guidance of hand and finger movements in the rhesus monkey. Brain 98:239–260

Laplane D, Talairach J, Meininger V et al 1977 Motor consequences of motor area ablations in man. J Neurol Sci 31:29–49

Leinonen L, Hyvarinen J, Nyman G, Linnankoski L 1979 I. Functional properties of neurons in lateral part of associative area 7 in awake monkeys. Exp Brain Res 34:299–320

Matelli M, Luppino G, Rizzolatti G 1985 Patterns of cytochrome oxidase activity in the frontal agranular cortex of the macaque monkey. Behav Brain Res 18:125–136

Pandya DN, Kuypers HGJM 1969 Cortico-cortical connections in the rhesus monkey. Brain Res 13:13–36

Roland PE, Friberg L 1983 Are cortical γ CBF increases during brain work in man due to synaptic excitation or inhibition? J Cereb Blood Flow Metab (Suppl) 3:S244–S245

Roland PE, Larsen B 1976 Focal increase of cerebral blood flow during stereognostic testing in man. Arch Neurol 33:551–558

Roland PE, Skinhoj E, Lassen NA, Larsen B 1980 Different cortical areas in man in organization of voluntary movements in extrapersonal space. J Neurophysiol 43:137–150

Motor control function of the prefrontal cortex

P.S. Goldman-Rakic

Section of Neuroanatomy, Yale University School of Medicine, 333 Cedar Street, New Haven, Connecticut 06510, USA

Abstract. The prefrontal granular cortex, with the premotor and motor areas, forms the frontal lobe. The three areas are allied by their proximity to one another and by their role in motor control. Of these three major subdivisions, the role of prefrontal cortex has been the most obscure. However, recent anatomical studies have elucidated the circuit basis for motor regulatory functions of the principal sulcus (Brodmann's area 9; Walker's area 46). In addition to well known and well worked out prominent connections with subcortical structures, e.g. the basal ganglia and deep layers of the superior colliculus, this area of prefrontal cortex is reciprocally connected to portions of the supplementary motor and premotor fields that are but one synapse removed from primary motor cortex. The principal sulcal cortex is additionally interconnected with the primary somatosensory area and the somatosensory association areas, in the frontoparietal operculum, with area PF of von Bonin and Bailey in the posterior parietal cortex, and with parts of the 'motor' thalamus. Recent behavioural and electrophysiological studies in monkeys (*Macaca mulatta*) demonstrate that the principal sulcus can influence delayed-responding, whether the response is a hand or an eye movement. The anatomical and functional evidence supports the thesis that prefrontal cortex has access to and can direct the output of several motor centres.

1987 Motor areas of the cerebral cortex. Wiley, Chichester (Ciba Foundation Symposium 132) p 187–200

The role of cerebral cortex in motor control is generally considered to involve three major 'motor' areas—primary motor cortex (Brodmann's area 4), the premotor cortex (Brodmann's area 6) and the supplementary motor cortex (medial area 6). Although motor, premotor and supplementary motor areas are involved in the highest order control over voluntary behaviour, none of them are thought of as the 'prime mover' in the chain of command. In this paper I will review recent evidence on the role that prefrontal cortex may play in the initiation, facilitation and inhibition of motor responses. Although it has been proposed that prefrontal cortex performs command functions, the necessary functional and anatomical relationships between prefrontal cortex and motor centres have proved difficult to specify precisely and are usually not provided. However, recent behavioural, anatomical and physiological

187

studies of the so-called motorically 'silent' areas of the frontal lobe indicate that such relationships exist and may provide new ways of conceptualizing the cortical and subcortical interactions underlying the regulation of voluntary motor behaviour. Although prefrontal areas are unable to directly affect the performance aspects of a single muscular contraction, they are nevertheless essential for the initiation, selection and guidance of behaviour by representational knowledge, and they might accomplish this regulation by enhancing or inhibiting responses mediated by 'lower' centres.

Nature of motor control functions of the human prefrontal cortex

Prefrontal cortical centres are widely associated with the ability to inhibit inappropriate or incorrect responses. The motor responses themselves are normal; it is their occurrence that is not. The classical example of the prefrontal type of impairment is the difficulty that patients exhibit in the Wisconsin Card Sort Test (Milner 1964, Drewe 1974). In this task, the patient is asked to sort a deck of cards which bear stimuli that vary in number, colour and shape. As each card in the stack comes up, the individual has to match it to a set of reference cards on the basis of one dimension that is arbitrarily selected by the experimenter (e.g. colour). The experimenter then tells the patient whether he or she is 'right' or 'wrong' and the patient tries to get as many correct matches as possible. After the patient achieves a specified number of consecutive correct matches, the sorting principle is shifted without warning, e.g. to shape or number, and the patients must modify their responses accordingly. Patients with right or left hemisphere prefrontal damage exhibit a strong tendency to select the dimension (i.e. perform the response) that was rewarded on the previous trial. Further, patients are impaired in the verbal regulation of their own behaviour (Milner 1964, Luria & Homskaya 1964). Although able to articulate the correct dimension on the Wisconsin Card Sort, they are nevertheless unable to guide their manual responses by verbal instruction.

The effects of prefrontal lesions do not appear to be restricted to any single motor domain. Another example of a failure to inhibit unwanted responses is illustrated in a recent study of eye movements in patients with frontal and temporal lobe damage (Guitton et al 1985). The patients with frontal lobe lesions were unable to obey the instruction to look to the visual field *opposite* to the one in which a stimulus appeared and they exhibited severe deficits in inhibiting glances to the initial cue. Moreover, corrective eye movements away from the cue and towards the opposite field were nearly always triggered by the appearance of a target in the opposite field, as if the patients had difficulty in generating an eye movement in the absence of a target stimulus.

It should be added that patients with frontal lobe lesions are not only deficient in suppressing incorrect responses but also have difficulty in generating correct responses, even when there is little or no interference from incorrect responses. Thus, patients with frontal lobe deficits are impaired in generating word lists (Milner 1964, Perrett 1974), in inventing abstract designs (Jones-Gotman & Milner 1977) and in solving problems such as the Tower of London Puzzle in which a goal has to be decomposed into subgoals and subgoals must be tackled in the correct order (Shallice 1982).

The delayed-response tests: animal model for motor disinhibition

Behaviour resembling that observed in patients with frontal lobe damage is also present in monkeys that have suffered damage to the prefrontal cortex. Such behaviour is well illustrated by the profound and selective impairments shown by such monkeys on tests of spatial delayed responses (Jacobsen 1936). In the classical version of the test, the animal is shown the location of a food morsel that is then hidden from view by an opaque screen. After a delay of several seconds, the monkey reaches to the correct location out of two or more choices. In this situation, the monkey that has been given a prefrontal lesion performs at chance levels of accuracy and makes its mistakes primarily by persevering with previously rewarded but now incorrect choices, much as patients with frontal lobe damage do in the Wisconsin Card Sort Test. Recently we have shown that the same lesions produce a marked impairment in an oculomotor delayed-response paradigm in which the animal indicates its response by saccadic eye movements rather than by manual responses (Funahashi et al 1986). Thus, monkeys with prefrontal damage, like their human counterparts, have difficulty in regulating the direction of their eye movements as well as their hands. It is relevant that both the classical and oculomotor versions of delayed response measure an animal's ability to respond to situations on the basis of stored information, rather than on the basis of 'immediate' stimulation. A crucial feature of these tests is that no information to guide the response is available to the animal at the time of response. In contrast to associative memory tasks in which environmental stimuli evoke appropriate responses, in delayed-response tasks the correct response is not an obligatory one but rather is guided by internalized knowledge based on information presented several seconds before.

It will be argued in this paper that it is only when inner models of reality are used to govern responses that prefrontal cortex is pre-eminently engaged (for review, see Goldman-Rakic 1987). Absence of this mechanism will result in heightened distractability and reliance on external cues, perseverative responding and fragmented undirected behaviour—in brief the cardinal symptoms of prefrontal lesions in humans and monkey. In humans, additionally, the symptoms of lethargy, lack of fluency and initiative are prominent symptoms of a disconnection of representational knowledge from motor control mechanisms. Viewed in this way, perseveration, distractability and ennui are

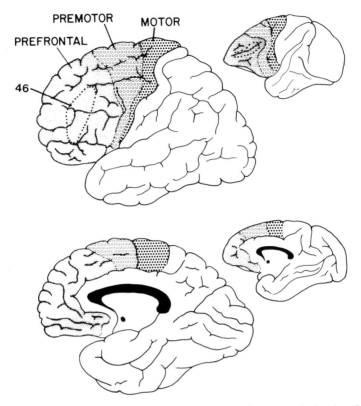

FIG. 1. Subdivisions of the frontal lobes in human and monkey, indicating the major divisions of the frontal lobe into primary motor, premotor and prefrontal zones. The prefrontal (and premotor) areas are further divisible into smaller cytoarchitectonic areas with distinctive afferent and efferent connections and functional specializations. The focus of this paper is the motor control functions of Walker's area 46 in the principal sulcus of the macaque (homologous areas in human and monkey are encircled).

consequences rather than primary causes of a more basic defect in the regulation of behaviour by representations. Indeed, these symptoms are prime examples of a cortical release phenomenon: in the absence of mechanisms for representational memory, behaviour is governed by the rules of associative or non-associative processes.

Common functional denominator

The anti-saccade test, the Wisconsin Card Sort test and delayed-response tasks are formally dissimilar to one another, yet have certain fundamental similarities. In each of these tasks, the correct response depends on stored

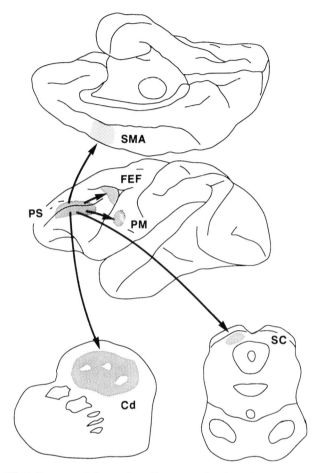

FIG. 2.   Simplified diagram of the major efferent projections from the region of the principal sulcus (PS) to motor centres, the frontal eye field (FEF), the supplementary motor (SMA) and ventral premotor cortex (PM), the caudate nucleus (Cd), and the deep layers of the superior colliculus (SC).

representations rather than on stimuli that are immediately present in the situation. In the anti-saccade test, the representation is an instruction ('look opposite') and the correct response is to look away from the target, thereby inhibiting the prepotent tendency to look at it. In the Wisconsin Card Sort Test, although the relevant features of the stimuli (colour, size, shape) are all present at the time of response, they nevertheless provide no information about the correct response—it must be provided from representational memory, in this case by a concept or category (e.g. 'colour') for guiding response choice. Although the capacity for this type of symbolic system appears to be a unique acquisition of human intelligence, undoubtedly linked to the emergence of language, it clearly must be built on a first-order representational capacity shared with other mammals.

The principal sulcus and motor control

In order to analyse the involvement of the prefrontal cortex in motor control and the possible mechanisms available to it for initiating and selecting correct responses and inhibiting incorrect responses, it is useful to consider the anatomical relationships between prefrontal centres and motor centres. However, the prefrontal cortex is not a unitary structure but is composed of several cytoarchitectonic subdivisions. The focus of this paper is on the cortex lining the principal sulcus in the macaque monkey, *Macaca mulatta* (Brodmann's area 9; Walker's area 46) (Fig. 1). The principal sulcus is particularly relevant as a model of prefrontal motor control mechanisms because damage to it is necessary and sufficient for producing profound deficits in delayed-response tasks. As will be described, the principal sulcus has strong, well organized connections with the basal ganglia, tectum and premotor cortex, putting it in an excellent anatomical position to issue and/or regulate motor commands.

Corticostriatal pathway and related feedback loops

The projections from the neocortex to the caudate nucleus and putamen form a massive system of cortical efferents, the corticostriatal system, long thought to be the major pathway by which associational and sensory cortical areas exert control over motor function (Fig. 2). The prefrontal cortex, and especially the region of the principal sulcus, projects throughout a central territory of the head, body and tail of the caudate nucleus as well as to the rostral putamen (Goldman & Nauta 1976, Selemon & Goldman-Rakic 1985). For the most part, cortical projections arising from distinctive cytoarchitectonic areas of the cortex project to separate territories within the neostriatum. For example, association cortical regions project mainly to the caudate nucleus whereas somatosensory cortex projects to the putamen. Even in areas of the caudate-putamen where two systems of cortical afferents overlap topographically, their terminals form a mosaic of interdigitated patches 500 μm in diameter (see Fig. 14 in Selemon & Goldman-Rakic 1985), suggesting a high degree of segregation in the cortical inputs to the neostriatum.

Corticostriatal fibres terminate on the medium spiny neurons of the neostriatum (e.g. Kemp & Powell 1971), which in turn project to the substantia nigra (pars reticulata) and globus pallidus. (A small complement of cortical efferents project directly to the substantia nigra as well.) If we assume that clusters of cells in the neostriatum that receive specific cortical inputs likewise have specific outputs, this could represent a 'labelled line' that extends from cortex through neostriatum to the substantia nigra or globus pallidus and continues back through the thalamus and then to cortex. Recent studies in our laboratory indeed indicate that the substantia nigra projects to portions of the ventral anterior and mediodorsal nucleus that project directly to the principal sulcus (Ilinsky et al 1985). It thus seems reasonable to suggest that the prefrontal cortex may stand at the head of a multisynaptic circuit that functions to inhibit most behaviour in order to allow the execution of single appropriate acts. Basal ganglia damage in humans disconnects this structure from the cortex and disrupts the balance of cortical influences, resulting in uncontrolled movements ranging from involuntary tremor in Parkinson's disease to ballistic thrusts in Huntington's disease, as well as slowness or confusion (or both) in motor responses and, sometimes, in thought processes.

Corticotectal pathway

Another connection from the prefrontal cortex to 'motor' structures is the corticotectal pathway (Fig. 2), long thought to arise in the frontal lobe exclusively from the frontal eye fields. Several studies have now shown that the cortical innervation of this pathway involves many parts of the cortical mantle, including the principal sulcus (Goldman & Nauta 1976, Fries 1984). These latter areas project to the intermediate and deep layers of the colliculus, the part of this premotor oculomotor centre that contains cells that discharge in relation to eye movements (e.g. Wurtz & Goldberg 1972).

The intermediate and deeper layers of the colliculus could be the points where principal sulcal innervation facilitates or inhibits head and eye movements, particularly in relation to stored information. Guitton et al (1985) have proposed that the unwanted glances generated by patients with frontal lobe deficits in their experiments result from failure of a mechanism designed to cancel the incorrect response before it has occurred. Arguments based on their experimental findings suggested that the cancellation signal might be generated elsewhere than in the frontal eye fields, though the timing of its occurrence might be governed by neurons of the prefrontal eye field. If we accept that the principal sulcus contains the mechanism for guiding specific responses on the basis of an instruction (such as 'look to the opposite locations of the target'), then it recommends itself as the structure capable of issuing the cancellation signal in the 'anti-saccade' task described above. Cancellation could occur at any or all of several levels of the neuroaxis: in the deep layers of the superior colliculus itself, in the substantia nigra or at the cortex. An interaction between the principal sulcus and frontal eye fields is likely because the two cortical areas are interconnected (e.g. Barbas & Mesulam 1985). Prefrontal eye field neurons may be involved in computing or accessing the coordinates for an intended eye movement, whereas principal sulcus neurons may be concerned more with whether to move the eyes to a particular target.

Thalamo-cortical system

An important common aspect of the corticostriatal and corticotectal projections is that they are not reciprocal, i.e. neither the caudate nor tectum project to the cortex directly. Rather they communicate with the prefrontal cortex indirectly through the thalamus. The ventral anterior and certain parts of the mediodorsal nucleus link the principal sulcus with the output from the globus pallidus and substantia nigra (Ilinsky et al 1985, Goldman-Rakic & Porrino 1985). Similarly the medial pulvinar, which may be regarded as a relay from the 'oculomotor' tectum, projects to the principal sulcus (Goldman-Rakic & Porrino 1985). In the primate, the medial pulvinar receives its most prominent subcortical input from the deep layers of the superior colliculus (Benevento & Fallon 1975, Harting et al 1980, Partlow et al 1977). Thus, unlike the thalamic input to sensory cortices, the thalamic input to prefrontal and perhaps other association areas may serve as a motor feedback mechanism rather than as a sensory relay from peripheral receptor organs. The overall organization suggests that these thalamic pathways to prefrontal cortex could participate in the putative 'corollary discharge' mechanism envisioned by Teuber (1972) as monitoring and readjusting ongoing behaviour.

Prefronto-premotor connections

For many years, the study of cortical control over movements centred around the primary motor areas or the corticostriatal circuitry. Recently, this has changed rapidly as new methods and approaches have exposed new facts concerning the organization and dynamics of the premotor areas. The study of Muakkassa & Strick (1979) was particularly helpful in showing that the somatotopically organized portions of the premotor cortex are connected with areas of similar somatotopy in motor cortex. This demonstration opened the way for analysis of prefrontal–premotor–motor pathways, and indeed recent findings show that neurons in the principal sulcus project to specific portions of the premotor cortex. For example, the principal sulcus, particularly its caudal portion, projects to the anterior supplementary motor cortex (SMA) which, in turn, projects to the upper body and head representation of the primary motor cortex (M.L. Jouandet and P.S. Goldman-Rakic, unpublished observations; Fig. 2). A portion of the same area of the principal sulcus that projects to the anterior SMA receives afferents from the specific area of the posterior parietal cortex (von Bonin and Bailey's PF) that serves as a relay for somaesthetic information (Cavada & Goldman-Rakic 1985, 1986). Further, neurons in this region project to the area of premotor cortex that projects to the mouth area of the primary motor cortex (Fig. 2A; Matelli et al 1986) as well as to the orofacial representation of the primary somatosensory area and the somatosensory association areas in the frontoparietal operculum

(Preuss & Goldman-Rakic 1985). Thus, neurons in the caudal portion of the principal sulcus are, via either SMA or ventral premotor cortex, only one synapse removed from the primary motor cortex. Inasmuch as the SMA has been implicated in motor programming, the principal sulcus is in a position to modulate (trigger or cancel) the 'release' of 'SMA' programmes to the motor cortex. Since the SMA is a major target of the pallido-thalamo-cortical feedback loop (Ilinsky et al 1985, Schell & Strick 1984), it is also possible that the prefronto-SMA projections could interact with and influence thalamic activation of the SMA.

Summary

Neurons lying in the caudal principal sulcus contribute to many cortical and subcortical pathways that influence motor output. While probably not able independently to specify the parameters of motor action, the principal sulcal cortex nevertheless may regulate motor output by initiating, facilitating and cancelling commands to structures directly involved in the programming, computational and performance aspects of specific motor acts. The cortical circuitry indicates that the control of eye movements may be exerted primarily through efferent connections with the frontal eye fields, substantia nigra and superior colliculus, while influences on upper body, head and/or arm movements may be issued via the somatotopically organized SMA and premotor relays, globus pallidus and other brainstem/pontine centres. In contrast to both the SMA and the frontal eye fields, the principal sulcus alone has access to the spatial map represented in posterior parietal cortex and is not tied to any single output modality, i.e. any single muscle group. This gives it the potential to regulate the responses of any part of the upper body, head, mouth and eyes so as to react or not when environmental contingencies arise.

References

Barbas H, Mesulam M-M 1985 Cortical afferent input to the principalis region of the rhesus monkey. Neuroscience 15:619-637
Benevento LA, Fallon JH 1975 The ascending projections of the superior colliculus in the rhesus monkey (*Macaca mulatta*). Brain Res 160:339–362
Cavada C, Goldman-Rakic PS 1985 Parieto-prefrontal connections in the monkey: Topographic distribution within the prefrontal cortex of sectors connected with the lateral and medial posterior parietal cortex. Soc Neurosci Abstr 11:323
Cavada C, Goldman-Rakic PS 1986 Subdivisions of area 7 in the rhesus monkey exhibit selective patterns of connectivity with limbic, visual and somatosensory cortical areas. Soc Neurosci Abstr 12:262
Drewe EA 1974 The effect of type and area of brain lesion on Wisconsin card sorting test performance. Cortex 10:159–170
Fries W 1984 Cortical projections to the superior colliculus in the macaque monkey: a retrograde study using horseradish peroxidase. J Comp Neurol 230:55–76
Funahashi S, Bruce CJ, Goldman-Rakic PS 1986 Perimetry of spatial memory repre-

sentation in primate prefrontal cortex: evidence for a mnemonic hemianopia. Soc Neurosci Abstr 12:554

Goldman-Rakic PS Circuitry of primate prefrontal cortex and regulation of behavior by representational memory. In: Plum F (ed) The nervous system. Higher functions of the brain. American Physiological Society, Bethesda, MD (Handb Physiol sect 1: The nervous system, vol. 5) p 373–417

Goldman PS, Nauta WJH 1976 Autoradiographic demonstration of a projection from prefrontal association cortex to the superior colliculus in the rhesus monkey. Brain Res 116:145–149

Goldman-Rakic PS, Porrino LJ 1985 The primate mediodorsal (MD) nucleus and its projections to the frontal lobe. J Comp Neurol 242:535–560

Guitton D, Buchtel HA, Douglas RM 1985 Frontal lobe lesions in man cause difficulties in suppressing reflexive glances and in generating goal-directed saccades. Exp Brain Res 58:455–472

Harting JK, Huerta MF, Frankfurter AJ, Strominger NL, Royce GJ 1980 Ascending pathways from the monkey superior colliculus: an autoradiographic analysis. J Comp Neurol 192:853–882

Ilinsky IA, Jouandet ML, Goldman-Rakic PS 1985 Organization of the nigrothalamocortical system in the rhesus monkey. J Comp Neurol 236:315–330

Jacobsen CF 1936 Studies of cerebral function in primates. Comp Psychol Monogr 13:1–68

Jones-Gotman M, Milner B 1977 Design fluency: the invention of nonsense drawings after focal lesions. Neuropsychologia 15:653–674

Kemp JM, Powell TPS 1971 The site of termination of afferent fibers in the caudate nucleus. Philos Trans R Soc Lond B Biol Sci 262:413–427

Luria AR, Homskaya ED 1964 Disturbances in the regulative role of speech with frontal lobe lesions. In: Warren JM, Akert K (eds) The frontal granular cortex and behavior. McGraw-Hill, New York, p 353-371

Milner B 1964 Some effects of frontal lobectomy in man. In: Warren JM, Akert K (eds) The frontal granular cortex and behavior. McGraw Hill, New York, p 313–334

Matelli M, Carmarda R, Glickstein M, Rizzolatti G 1986 Afferent and efferent projections of the inferior area 6 in the macaque monkey. J Comp Neurol 251:281–298

Muakkassa KF, Strick PL 1979 Frontal lobe inputs to primate motor cortex: Evidence for four somatopically organized 'premotor' areas. Brain Res 177:176–182

Partlow GD, Colonier M, Szabo J 1977 Thalamic projections of the superior colliculus in the rhesus monkey. Light and electron microscopic study. J Comp Neurol 171:285–318

Perret E 1974 The left frontal lobe of man and the suppression of habitual responses in verbal categorical behaviour. Neuropsychologia 12:323–330

Preuss T, Goldman-Rakic PS 1985 Somatosensory representation in primate prefrontal cortex: connections of the principal sulcus with S-I, S-II and adjacent areas of the frontoparietal operculum. Soc Neurosci Abstr 11:677

Schell GR, Strick PL 1984 Origin of thalamic input to the arcuate premotor and supplementary motor areas. J Neurosci 4:539–560

Selemon LD, Goldman-Rakic PS 1985 Common cortical and subcortical target areas of the dorsolateral prefrontal and posterior parietal cortices in the rhesus monkey. Soc Neurosci Abstr 11:323

Shallice T 1982 Specific impairments in planning. Philos Trans R Soc Lond B Biol Sci 298:199–209

Teuber H-L 1972 Unity and diversity of frontal lobe functions. Acta Neurobiol Exp (Warsaw) 32:615–656

Wurtz RH, Goldberg ME 1972 Activity of superior colliculus in behaving monkey. III. Cells discharging before eye movements. J Neurophysiol 35:575

DISCUSSION

Kuypers: You showed several corticocortical connections which we have not been able to see with the old degeneration technique. However, to my surprise, you did not show some of the connections that the degeneration technique revealed. For example, from the anterior part of area 7 you showed no projections to the posterior bank of the arcuate sulcus and the adjoining precentral areas, from where a pronounced projection to the rostral bank of central sulcus arises.

Goldman-Rakic: There are some projections to the posterior bank of the arcuate sulcus, in accord with previous studies. Our results with wheat germ agglutinin-horseradish peroxidase agree with our autoradiographic studies and with other transport studies.

Kuypers: It is surprising that you don't get a more extensive fibre distribution after some of the injections.

Goldman-Rakic: These are small injections. If the injection were larger there would be a larger terminal field. Both the premotor and prefrontal cortex receive projections from the posterior parietal cortex. I think the differences between our results are a question of a large lesion versus a restricted injection.

Deecke: There is a very nice point-to-point connection between parietal association areas and prefrontal areas. The parietal association area is the classical area where apraxia occurs in patients, but apraxia, unlike aphasia, never lasts for ever. The explanation for this recovery may be by way of the connections you showed. Apraxia also occurs with disconnection syndromes and there is callosal apraxia not only with lesions of the central and posterior corpus callosum but also with anterior callosal lesions. These clinical syndromes can be nicely explained by your findings.

Goldman-Rakic: One point about prefrontal cortex is that it is only one synapse removed from the primary motor cortex. Further, in its relationship to the motor cortex, the prefrontal cortex may express the 'wishes' of the entire network of associational areas with which it is reciprocally connected.

Strick: While we may disagree about minor issues, I think we have both observed that the parietal lobe has substantial projections to the premotor areas. Projections to the premotor areas from the prefrontal cortex are meagre by comparison. Thus, if one wants to view the prefrontal cortex in classical terms as one of the steps in a chain of commands through premotor areas to the primary motor cortex, this view is not supported by the density of anatomical connections between these cortical areas. One might want to examine an alternative route, namely that the prefrontal cortex may gain access to the motor system at the cortical level via its dense connections with the parietal lobe.

Goldman-Rakic: I think we have the answer to that. I would agree with you that in the monkey the parietal cortex has more intense projections to the premotor area. Regarding cortical versus subcortical access to the motor centres, I have the following speculation. Monkeys are much more dominated by the external world than humans are; that is, they don't walk around like miniature human beings with internal concepts and plans for action. There are two sources of information that finally come into the premotor area or into the motor cortex. One is via corticocortical connections (via both prefrontal and parietal cortex) and the other is by the descending subcortical projections, the parallel pathways, which we both know so well. Perhaps in monkeys the subcortical—that is, basal ganglia—route to the premotor cortex is more developed than are the corticocortical projections to the same area. I would say the monkey has less corticocortical influence than humans but this is not exactly testable. In humans the corticocortical connections are probably more prominent than in the monkey. We might say there is dual control or a ratio of control.

As to the density of projections, how can we say that these prefronto-premotor projections are not enough to have some influence on motor output? They project into the premotor cortex and everybody here agrees that the premotor cortex projects to the motor cortex (Muakkassa & Strick 1979). All I am saying is that these cells are of value to the animal when it is behaving in the absence of external stimuli.

Marsden: The corticocortical projection from your area 47 into the premotor cortex and supplementary motor area is not very dense. Your findings suggest that this is not very strong in the monkey, so you are making a special case by saying it may be much stronger in the human being. The alternative route to get information from that prefrontal area into the premotor and supplementary motor area via the basal ganglia may not work if there is true parallel processing through the basal ganglia. Corticostriatal projections from prefrontal areas may not go back into the premotor area and supplementary motor area; they may go back to the region of the principal sulcus.

Goldman-Rakic: The degree of parallelism is not fully known and is under investigation. However, should basal ganglia-to-cortex (via thalamus) pathways turn out to be strictly parallel loops (and I doubt this), the motor command operations of the principal sulcus would have to rely on the prefronto-premotor pathways that I described, even though their density is not impressive.

Thach: I was just wondering how a physiologist might attack the question of demonstrating a memory loop. It is some years since Lorente de Nó (Fulton's Textbook of Physiology, 17th edn) talked about the possibility of a reverberating loop. N. Tsukahara (unpublished) was interested in the possibility of demonstrating a loop between the cerebellar nuclei and the pons. He tried various strategies, such as introducing a train of pulses into the putative loop with the recording microelectrode and seeing whether the pulses came back round again to the microelectrode. 'Set' and 'memory' discharge can be seen as a continuous firing in cells long after the stimulus has gone. How is that maintained? The most plausible possibility is that it is a loop function of some kind. Could one do stimulations with the recording electrode and see whether that introduces periodicities in the subsequent discharge, such as to support a loop function? Or could one give a large shock and see if the discharge is erased?

Goldman-Rakic: We are planning such experiments.

Passingham: I was bothered by your speculation that in human brains things might be organized differently from the way they are organized in monkey brains. With development of language, corticocortical routes to the motor apparatus may be more prominent in human than in monkey brains.

Goldman-Rakic: The connections from the prefrontal cortex to the premotor areas exist. Their existence should not be denied just because they are not the densest projections seen. Perhaps there is a correspondence between the density of a given connection and the nature of motor control. When ideas guide behaviour, prefrontal control may predominate; when stimuli guide behaviour, other areas may predominate. I see the differences between monkey and human as qualitative in this respect.

Calne: Your critics say that if a pathway is large and anatomically obvious it is important. But I don't think there is much clinical evidence to support that view. The corpus callosum, for example, is a huge projection but we can manage quite well without it. The pituitary, one of the smallest components of the brain, is one of the most important. The nigrostriatal pathway is very small, yet the effect is devastating when it dies. Why is a big pathway thought to be more important than a small pathway?

Goldman-Rakic: Obviously my presentation evoked some kind of response. That is not unexpected because there is very strong resistance in science dating to the 18th century, and in our culture in general, to looking for the area of the brain that might have a bit more control than any other area. It has always been difficult to study the prefrontal cortex; it has always aroused controversy and it has always been something that people resist tremendously.

The facts are very clear in this case. There are parallel distributed pathways linking the association areas. Our double-label paradigm shows that subdivisions of parietal and prefrontal areas are interconnected in topographically segregated circuits and that the parieto-prefrontal connection follows a 'feedforward' pattern (Seleman & Goldman-Rakic 1985). The prefrontal and parietal areas are also interconnected with more than 12 other association areas. These parallel distributed circuits are the knowledge base on which higher cortical function is elaborated. Prefrontal cortex is pre-eminent in motor control only when motor action is based on internal cues, i.e. representations or ideas. Under all other circumstances it is dispensable!

Reference

Muakkassa KF, Strick PL 1979 Frontal lobe inputs to primate motor cortex: evidence for four somatotopically organized 'premotor' areas. Brain Res 177:176–182

Seleman LD, Goldman-Rakic PS 1985 Common cortical and subcortical target areas of the dorsolateral prefrontal and posterior parietal cortices in the rhesus monkey. Soc Neurosci Abstr 11:323

Cerebellar inputs to motor cortex

W.T. Thach

Departments of Anatomy & Neurobiology, Neurology and Neurological Surgery and The McDonnell Center for Higher Brain Function, Washington University School of Medicine, Box 8108, 660 South Euclid Avenue, St Louis, MO 63110, USA

Abstract. The macaque cerebellar nuclei all project topically onto a common thalamic field that is somatotopically organized in its projection to motor cortex. The complete overlap (except at the cellular level) of dentate and interpositus (and possibly fastigius and vestibular nuclei) projection onto the somatotopic thalamic field implies a complete body representation within each cerebellar nucleus, rather than a preferential representation of trunk in fastigius, proximal limb in interpositus and digits in dentate, as is sometimes supposed. Dentate receives from association cortex and generates the earliest signals, which assist motor cortex in initiating goal-directed movements. Interpositus receives the spinocerebellar projection and provides a fast input to motor cortex from the periphery, perhaps used in transcortical 'reflex' responses and in the control of oscillation. Fastigius and vestibular nuclei provide an opportunity for labyrinthine control of motor cortex activities—even for the digits. What is unique about cerebellar input to motor cortex? Recent work has emphasized two aspects: switching of a cerebellar signal on or off through Purkinje cell inhibition, and adjusting the magnitude of the signal to optimize motor performance.

1987 Motor areas of the cerebral cortex. Wiley, Chichester (Ciba Foundation Symposium 132) p 201–220

A common thalamic route of all cerebellar nuclei to motor cortex

Until recently, the outputs of the basal ganglia and the cerebellum were believed to merge and fall on a common thalamic field en route to motor cortex. Modern pathway tracing methods have shown this to be incorrect: basal ganglia project separately to the ventral anterior nucleus (VA), the ventral lateral nucleus, medial division (VL_m), the ventral lateral nucleus, oral division (VL_o), and the centre median nucleus (cf. Asanuma et al 1983b). The cerebellum projects to a thalamic field composed of the ventrolateral nucleus, caudal division (VL_c), the ventrolateral nucleus, pars postrema (VL_{ps}), the ventral posterolateral nucleus, oral division (VPL_o), the nucleus X (Olszewski), and the central lateral nucleus (CL) (Asanuma et al 1983a, b). The basal ganglia thalamus has been shown to project to medial area 6 (supplementary motor area: SMA), and only thereby to motor cortex (cf. Asanuma, 1983b). The cerebellar thalamus has two parts, one projecting directly and somatotopically to motor cortex (VL_o, VL_{ps}, VPL_o, and X), the other projecting more diffusely to wider regions of cerebral cortex (CL) (Asanuma et al 1983b).

Another misconception was that the cerebellar contribution to motor cortex came exclusively from the lateral 'dentate' nucleus, the interposed and fastigial nuclei being supposed to influence only brainstem and spinal mechanisms. Yet modern methods have shown that all cerebellar nuclei—dentate, interpositus, fastigius and even the vestibular complex (the deepest of the deep cerebellar nuclei)—merge and fall onto the common thalamic field (Asanuma et al 1983b, c). This has been shown most clearly for dentate and interpositus: the outputs arrive in contralateral thalamus topically organized and in register, the interpositus projection being only slightly less prominent than that from dentate.

A complete somatic representation within each cerebellar nucleus

Since cerebellar thalamus projects topically onto motor cortex, and since motor cortex is somatotopically organized, a somatotopic map may be inferred for cerebellar thalamus, with head medial and tail lateral, trunk dorsal and extremities ventral (Strick 1976). Since dentate and interpositus project topically to this contralateral thalamic field, a somatotopic organization may also be inferred for both cerebellar nuclei, with head caudal, tail rostral, trunk lateral and extremities medial (Asanuma et al 1983c). In the lateral two cerebellar nuclei, this somatotopic organization has been confirmed in the rostrocaudal dimension independently by three different methods: (1) electrical stimulation of monkey cerebral cortex and peripheral somatosensory receptors while recording in the nuclei (cf. Allen & Tsukahara 1974), (2) recording of single-unit activity within the nuclei in relation to isolated limb and head movements made by trained monkeys (cf. Brooks & Thach 1981), and (3) positron emission tomography (PET) of local increases in cerebellar blood flow in humans as they move their limbs and eyes (Fox et al 1985).

The fastigial and vestibular nuclei project bilaterally to the common thalamic field and although they have been less well studied than dentate and interpositus they appear also to project with topographic order. The few injected sites in fastigius permit one to infer that at least the rostrocaudal body mapping is as in dentate and interpositus (Asanuma et al 1983c), and the vestibular nuclei are known to be somatotopically organized to the extent of representation of eye and head movement in the medial and body movement in the lateral nuclei. Both fastigial (Asanuma et al 1983c, Fig. 16, 17) and vestibular (Asanuma et al 1983b, Fig. 17) nuclei project onto the *entire* thalamic field, suggesting that they, like dentate and interpositus, exert control over all parts of the body.

What cortical motor areas are influenced by the cerebellum?

Since the output of the main cerebellar thalamic target—VL_c, VL_{ps}, VPL_o and

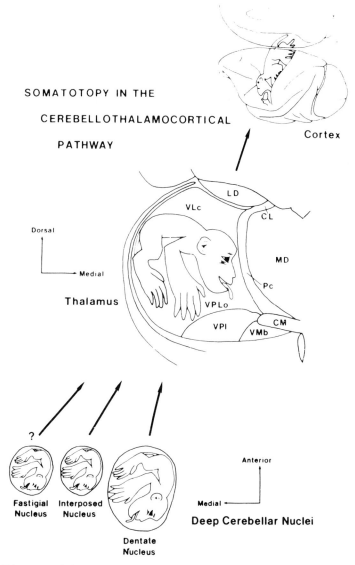

FIG. 1. Diagram of the somatotopic organization of each of the deep cerebellar nuclei and their projection via thalamus to motor cortex (from Asanuma et al 1983c).

X—goes exclusively to motor cortex (Strick 1976), the output of the cerebellum would appear to be chiefly directed to motor cortex. An exception would be the relatively smaller cerebellar projection to CL, which could influence the wider extent of cortex to which CL is known to project (cf. Asanuma et al 1983b). Whether this projection is somatotopically organized, whether it

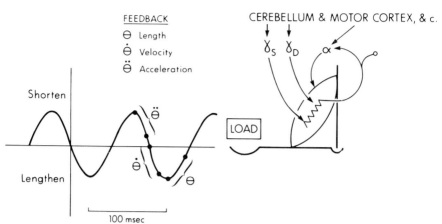

FIG. 2.   Diagram of the hypothetical action of segmental stretch reflexes on mechanical tremor. The mechanical tremor results from the underdamped mass-spring properties of the limb, set in motion by any of a variety of perturbations. Stretch reflex receptors (only the primary is shown; the argument applies to the secondary also) are controlled by gamma static and gamma dynamic motorneurons, to render the overall sensitivity closer to length (θ) or velocity ($\dot{\theta}$) or acceleration ($\ddot{\theta}$) of stretch. If receptors are maximally sensitive to length of stretch, θ, their action is maximal at peak stretch which, because of the loop time delay, causes muscle contraction during the passive shortening phase, thereby augmenting the mechanical tremor. If receptors are more sensitive to velocity of stretch, $\dot{\theta}$, the contraction is earlier in the stretch cycle and actively limits the passive stretch, thereby damping the mechanical tremor. If receptors are more sensitive to acceleration, $\ddot{\theta}$, or higher time derivatives of stretch, the contraction is earlier still, providing even more effective damping of the mechanical tremor.

represents all four nuclei equally, and whether it represents all parts of each nucleus are not yet known. This projection could, conceivably, form a basis for cerebellar influences on the supplementary motor area, premotor area, periarcuate area, prefrontal cortex and sensory and associational areas as well, though again the strength and topographic organization would not appear to be comparable to that of VL_c, VL_{ps}, VLP_o and X to motor cortex. Schell & Strick (1983) raise the question of whether the cerebellar nuclei form a strong and topographically organized projection to the periarcuate area (area 6) anterior to motor cortex (area 4), in which they believe there is a complete body representation independent of that in motor cortex. In their scheme, the periarcuate cortex receives a projection from the thalamic X nucleus, to which project the caudal portions of the cerebellar nuclei. Since Schell & Strick (1983) posit a complete body representation in periarcuate cortex (yet to be shown), they require a complete body representation also in X (separate from that in VL_c, VL_{ps}, VLP_o, and at least lateral X), and in caudal cerebellar nuclei (separate from that in the bulk of the nuclei anterior). The pathway tracing study of Asanuma et al (1983b, c) interpreted the

KNOWN CIRCUITRY

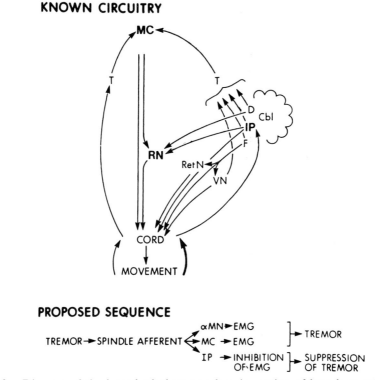

PROPOSED SEQUENCE

FIG. 3.   Diagram of the hypothetical tremor-damping action of long loop reflexes using circuits described by Asanuma et al (1983a, b, c, d). D, dentate; IP, interposed; F, fastigial; VN, vestibular; RetN, reticular; RN, red; and T, cerebellothalamic nuclei. MC, motor cortex. Model based on data from Schieber & Thach (1985) and Elble et al (1984).

caudal cerebellar nuclei and thalamic X as representing the head only, since the topographic progression was continuous from the cerebellar nuclei caudorostral mapping onto the thalamic mediolateral dimension, and since previous studies had suggested that at least a portion of X projected to the head area of the motor cortex. The interpretation hinges on how much X projects to periarcuate as distinct from motor cortex, and how fully the body is represented within periarcuate as distinct from motor cortex. If one looks simply at the cerebellar nuclear somatic representation, none of the three different independent mapping methods have yet indicated more than one map within each nucleus. Instead, these methods have independently indicated a single representation, with head caudal and tail rostral (Asanuma et al 1983c). Thus, the interpretation of Asanuma et al would be that, while cerebellar outflow may to some extent influence any part of wide regions of motor cortex via thalamic CL, the strongest and most somatotopically organized output is to motor cortex.

Dentate helps initiate activity in motor cortex in voluntary movement

Knowing that the output of the lateral cerebellum projects to thalamus and thence to motor cortex we measured the timing of dentate discharge in relation to that of motor cortex and the onset of trained flexion and extension of the wrist (Thach 1975). Microelectrode penetrations were made on alternative days into dentate and motor cortex in each of three rhesus monkeys as they performed wrist movements in response to a light signal. The timing distributions covered about 300 ms and overlapped considerably, and the median dentate change preceded that of motor cortex by 33, 12 and 15 ms respectively in each of the three monkeys. This timing difference, with dentate preceding motor cortex, was confirmed in a later study in two monkeys in which all recordings were made first in motor cortex (one monkey) or in dentate (the second monkey) (Thach 1978).

Does the overlapping but slightly earlier discharge in dentate cause changes in motor cortex? Meyer-Lohmann et al (1977) trained cebus monkeys to flex and extend the elbow in response to a light signal and they recorded in the motor cortex, with and without inactivation of the lateral cerebellum by a previously implanted cooling probe. Like Evarts (1974) and others they found that on the average most motor cortex neurons changed their discharge before movement onset. With the lateral cerebellum (dentate) inactivated, not only was movement onset delayed by 50–150 ms, but change in the motor cortex neurons was delayed by an equivalent amount. These results confirmed the interpretation that, while dentate is not necessary for activation of motor cortex, it is necessary for maintaining the shortest reaction time. Thus, dentate helps to initiate activity of motor cortex in arbitrarily triggered volitional goal-directed movements.

Strick used the Tanji–Evarts paradigm (Tanji & Evarts 1976) to study dentate and interpositus discharge in relation to prior intention and triggered initiation of movement (Strick 1983). In this task, the first cue (red or green light) 'instructs' the monkey in which direction to move (flex or extend); after a random delay, a second cue (perturbation by a manipulandum that stretches flexor or extensor muscles) serves as the 'go' signal. The direction of the instruction cue and the direction of the go cue were pseudorandomly dissociated across trials. Strick found that the first change in interpositus neurons was determined by which muscle was stretched by the go cue, with the stimulus presumably carried over the rapidly conducting spinocerebellar pathways. By contrast, the first changes in the dentate, though timed to the go cue and following it by a scant 30–50 ms, had their direction (increase or decrease firing) determined by the instruction cue (flex or extend). Though the time of dentate change was not compared with that of motor cortex in these studies, from previous work it seemed likely to precede at least the later components of motor cortex discharge and therefore possibly to be a site of sensorimotor transformation of a sensory stimulus to a motor command.

Interpositus controls an early component of transcortical reflexes and oscillation

In light-triggered reaction-time movements, interpositus lagged behind dentate by 26 ms and motor cortex by 10 ms (median changes; Thach 1978). The late timing implies that interpositus could not have initiated these movements but must rather have played a role in the 'ongoing control' of movement in progress. By contrast, in movements triggered by perturbation of the limb to be moved, interpositus changes preceded the median dentate changes by 24 ms, and a second component of motor cortex change by 10 ms (Thach 1978). As interpositus has now been shown to project to motor cortex via thalamus, interpositus may help to cause some of the earlier changes in motor cortex in the transcortical reflex. This would also fit with the observation that the sign of change in interpositus (increase or decrease) is determined by the sign of the stimulus (stretch or slack of agonist to be used) and that the transcortical reflex works fastest when the muscle to be contracted is stretched by the go signal (Evarts & Tanji 1976). Does interpositus initiate the *first* changes in motor cortex? The only pertinent timing studies suggest a biphasic response in motor cortex to limb perturbation, with interpositus preceding only the second (by 10 ms), and following the first by about 5 ms (Thach 1978). Since it is known that a direct non-lemniscal spinothalamic input to thalamus (VL_c, VL_{ps}, VPL_o, X) overlaps the cerebellar input, this has been suggested as potentially the fastest path to motor cortex (Asanuma et al 1983b). What is now needed is an experiment on localized inactivation of interpositus, with recording from motor cortex during the transcortical reflex. The prediction would be that interpositus inactivation would abolish the second motor cortex response but not the first. The relatively late timing of dentate after hand perturbation (Thach 1978, Strick 1983), and its coding for direction of intended move (and which muscle is to be contracted) rather than for which muscle is stretched, suggests it can play only a tertiary or later temporal role in the transcortical stretch reflex.

A second major role for interpositus is its control of oscillation. In slow tracking movements, interpositus discharged in striking relation to a monkey's own physiological tremor (Schieber & Thach 1985, Elble et al 1984). The tremor modulation was superimposed on an apparent 'carrier' discharge pattern that uniformly increased during all slow movements, relatively independently of movement direction, velocity ($10–30°/s$) and load. Since this discharge was mirrored in the discharge of Ia spindle afferents, which was also very different from the EMG pattern of the parent muscle, we argued (Schieber & Thach 1985) that the cerebellum dissociated the activity of γ motor neurons from that of α motor neurons and made the γ neurons

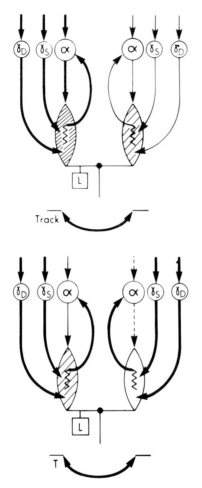

FIG. 4.   Diagram of the relative activities of antagonist wrist muscles and their α
skeletomotor and γ fusimotor motorneuron and primary spindle afferent innervation
while flexing and extending under torque load in the naive (top) and the adapted
(bottom) state. Muscle activity is graded from highest (dense cross-hatch) through
intermediate (coarse cross-hatch) to nil (no cross-hatch). Neural activity is graded
from highest (heavy line) to intermediate (fine line) to nil (dashed line). Track, wrist
excursion in flexion and extension. Top: in the naive state, there is coactivation of α
and γ motorneurons, and spindle afferent firing is less in the passive muscle than in the
active. Bottom: in the adapted state, the activities of α and γ motorneurons have been
dissociated, resulting in a high maintained firing frequency of the primary spindle
afferents in the unloaded silent muscle as well as in the loaded active muscle. The
heightened maintained discharge of all primary afferents from both muscles is proposed to increase the sensitivity of tremor detection and correction at segmental and
higher levels. Model based on data from Schieber & Thach (1985).

fire, so rendering the muscle spindles maximally sensitive to tremor, regardless of whether the parent muscle was active or relaxed, lengthening or
shortening.

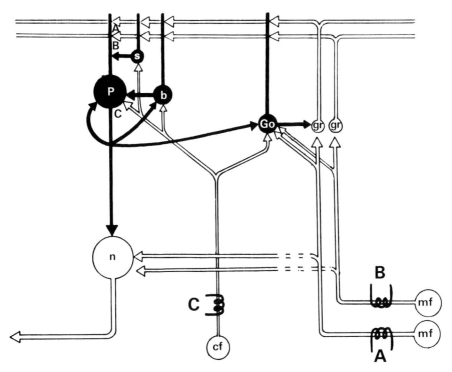

FIG. 5. Diagram of the basic cerebellar circuit and its proposed actions in switching cerebellar output on or off and in modifying the input/output gain. n, nuclear cell; P, Purkinje cell; s, stellate cell; b, basket cell; Go, Golgi cell; gr, granule cell and its axon (parallel fibre); mf, mossy fibre; cf, climbing fibre. White cells are excitatory, black are inhibitory. A, B, and C are stimulating electrodes placed on climbing fibres (C) and two different sets of mossy fibres (A and B). Stimulus A and stimulus B represent two different conditions which may switch off the nuclear cell output by the inhibition from increased Purkinje cell discharge. If the mossy fibre stimulus A is repeatedly coupled in time with the climbing fibre stimulus C, the Purkinje cell – parallel fibre A synapse becomes progressively weakened, while the B synapse remains unaltered in its ability to excite the Purkinje cell. A decreased excitation of the Purkinje cell results in disinhibition = increased excitation of the nuclear cell.

Why was tremor monitored? We argued that the information is used to control the natural tendency of the limbs to oscillate. The tendency arises from at least three factors: (1) the underdamped mass-spring characteristics of muscle and soft tissues, (2) the spring characteristics of length-sensitive stretch reflexes, and (3) the feedback delay of the stretch reflex. Thus, a length-sensitive stretch reflex is maximally activated when the muscle is at peak stretch during the mechanical oscillation at the joint. The reflex contraction, because of the delay, occurs only after the shortening phase of the oscillation has begun; this therefore adds to the oscillation. The argument runs (Thach et al 1986, 1987) that to minimize oscillation the aggregate stretch reflex sensitivity is shifted away from length sensitivity and more towards velocity sensitivity or even acceleration sensitivity. The stretch reflex is then activated earlier in the stretching phase of the tremor cycle and the contraction occurs before stretching is complete, thereby serving to limit the amplitude of the oscillation. This therefore serves an obvious damping function. The mechanism could involve any or all of the following: a shift in sensitivity from length to velocity of Ia and II receptors (but cf. Matthews 1981), an increase in bias or gain of Ia receptor activity over II receptor activity, or a change in sensitivity of a transcerebellar long loop (Elble et al 1984). The postulate that interpositus actively minimizes unwanted oscillation in the course of movements is supported by our observation that local temporary inactivation of interpositus with muscimol injections immediately produces a tremor much larger in amplitude (and slower in frequency) then physiological tremor (J.W. Mink & W.T. Thach, unpublished observations). Similar inactivation of dentate produces only the delay in movement onset, but no tremor.

In addition to minimizing unwanted oscillation, the cerebellum helps to produce wanted oscillation. The ability to make rapid alternating movements is one of the standard neurological tests for cerebellar damage. We believe that this activity may also be localized to interpositus, and that the mechanism is a shift of stretch reflex sensitivity (again through gamma motor neurons or transcerebellar reflexes, or both) away from acceleration or velocity sensitivity and towards length sensitivity, increasing the spring and decreasing the viscous damping components. The evidence for this idea is twofold: (1) local muscimol inactivation of interpositus in rhesus monkeys makes attempted rapid alternating movements slow and irregular (dentate inactivation does not have this effect: J.W. Mink & W.T. Thach, unpublished observations) and (2) interpositus neurons discharge at peak modulation in relation to rapid alternating movements (Thach 1968). Control of wanted oscillation may be a unique feature among the various inputs to motor cortex; globus pallidus neurons discharge conspicuously little in relation to rapid alternating movement (Mink & Thach 1987). The fact that interpositus neurons *do* so modulate indicates that the mechanism is not simply an increase in length sensitivity of segmental stretch reflexes via a tonic cerebellar signal descending to excite gamma static neurons, but rather to some extent is a transcerebellar loop operation.

Fastigius and vestibular nuclei modulate alpha motor neurons

The fastigial nucleus, like interpositus and dentate, projects to the whole body map in the thalamus. It must therefore, like its neighbours, serve a unique function for the whole body, rather than a like function for only part of the body. What might the function be for fastigius? It is possible that fastigius shares with the vestibular nuclei the extension of vestibular control of the whole body, even at the motor cortex level. The fastigial nucleus receives information from the spinocerebellar paths and from the vestibular system, and is thus part of both the spinocerebellum and the vestibulocerebellum. Observations of truncal ataxia with midline cerebellar lesions have led clinicians (Victor et al 1959) to assume that the sole concern of the midline cerebellar nuclei is the truncal musculature. This cannot be fully correct, since the fastigial nuclei projecting to the cerebellar thalamus project as extensively to the digital representation area as to the truncal. The projection may therefore play a role in the automatic gravity and deceleration-induced motions of the whole body, including those splaying movements of the distal digits that are so obvious in cats and monkeys (Goldberger & Growdon 1973).

A second role may be the matching of muscle properties at motor cortex and α motor neuron levels of synergist muscles on both sides of the body. Fastigial neurons in cat and monkey make monosynaptic contacts with neck α motor neurons (Asanuma et al 1983d, Wilson et al 1978). These are exclusively contralateral, seemingly forming an exception to the rule that the cerebellum controls only the ipsilateral body. Vilis and Hore have implicated fastigius in the compensation for disparate length of bilateral yoke-pair extraocular muscles, and in correction of the otherwise resulting strabismus (Vilis et al 1983, Snow et al 1985). The contralateral projection to neck muscle motor neurons may adjust the synergic actions of these muscles to match those of their ipsilateral muscle partners in head–neck movements. This would be consistent with the bilateral fastigial projection to thalamus.

The vestibular nuclei have long been known to contact spinal α and oculomotor neurons. The cerebellum controls the vestibular nuclei in dual synergic movements of head and eyes (the vestibular ocular reflex: VOR) and their gain adjustment, in the cancellation of the VOR to permit head and eye movement in the same direction (or with eyes fixed in head), and in the production of smooth-pursuit eye movement. These mechanisms have been implicated in bodily movements as well, and they provide clues to what makes the cerebellar control unique.

Motor adaptation, mode switching and motor programmes: what makes the cerebellum unique?

Ablation of the cerebellum has been shown to prevent adaptations of the vestibulo-ocular reflex (Ito et al 1974, Robinson 1975), pulse-step matching for saccades (Optican & Robinson 1980), strabismus compensation (Vilis et al 1983, Snow et al 1985), conditioned eye-blink (McCormick & Thompson 1984, Yeo et al 1984), functional stretch reflexes (Nashner & Grimm 1978), and startle-response habituation (Leaton & Supple 1986). Stimulation of the mossy fibre–parallel fibre system in conjunction with the climbing fibre system of the inferior olive specifically weakens the input of that mossy fibre–

parallel–fibre subset to the Purkinje cell (Ito et al 1982; but see Llinas et al 1975). The Purkinje cell therefore appears to exert less inhibition on the nuclear cell, and the mainline throughput may be increased even though the mossy fibre input is the same. Recording from Purkinje cells during adaptation of stretch reflexes (Gilbert & Thach 1977) and the VOR (Watanabe 1984) shows increased climbing fibre activity during the adaptation, and a progressively weakened response to the mossy fibre–parallel fibre input. As the adaptation is made, the climbing fibre activity returns to baseline and the Purkinje cell response to the mossy fibre parallel input remains weakened. These observations fit the Albus version (Albus 1971) of the cerebellar adaptive control theories in which the mossy fibre input–nuclear cell output relation is transformed because an alteration at the level of the Purkinje cell produces appropriate behaviour.

Purkinje cell modulation has been shown to increase when the head is turned and the VOR is cancelled (fixing the eyes in the head), and to decrease when the head is turned and the VOR operates (fixing the eyes on an extrapersonal target) (Lisberger & Fuchs 1978). Ablation of the cerebellum prevents VOR cancellation (cf. Leigh & Zee 1983). This has supported the idea that VOR cancellation is accomplished by increased Purkinje cell inhibition affecting the appropriate vestibular nuclear cells (Lisberger & Fuchs 1974). When the thumb and forefinger are used for pinching, wrist flexors and extensors co-contract. During a pinch the majority of Purkinje cells (62%) decrease their activity while the majority of interposed nuclear cells (91%) increase their activity (Frysinger et al 1984, Wetts et al 1987). This suggested a mechanism in which Purkinje cell inhibition turns off and allows nuclear cell excitation to increase and activate both synergist muscle pairs. In flexion and extension of the wrist during moves and holds, both Purkinje cells and nuclear cells alternated between higher and lower firing levels. The suggestion was made (Frysinger et al 1984) that the Purkinje cells increased inhibitory discharge and thereby relaxed the antagonist muscle when reciprocal agonist–antagonist was wanted. The problem with this interpretation is that ablation of cerebellar cortex does not result in forced co-contraction, which this interpretation implies should occur. A general increase in interposed cell activity (bidirectional increased discharge) has also been seen in slow tracking flexion–extension movements, in which the *antagonist muscle* relaxes but the *antagonist γ loop* is co-active with that of the agonist (Schieber & Thach 1985). This and the previous experiment have been interpreted as suggesting that the interposed cell activity influences the γ loop but not the α motor neuron, and that in both pinching and smooth pursuit-tracking the agonist and antagonist γ loops are both turned 'on'. A possible purpose of this effect would be to increase stretch reflex sensitivity to assist the control of muscle length in pinching and the control of length and stability in tracking. Certainly, cerebellar nuclear ablation is known to suppress and stimulation to increase gamma motor neuronal activity, and spinocerebellar cortical ablation is known to increase stretch reflex sensitivity (cf. Dow & Moruzzi 1958, Gilman et al 1981). Thus, in both the VOR and stretch reflexes a role of the Purkinje cell may be to inhibit and disinhibit the operation of the VOR and the stretch reflexes.

It is not known whether the cerebellum contains more than reflex gain control in the way of motor programmes, such as multi-joint and body part combinations or movement sequences. Eye-in-head and head-in-world signals balanced to equally excite Purkinje cells conceivably provide a mechanism for gaze control (eye-on-world) across two moving members (Lisberger 1982). It has been suggested that a similar arrangement could in principle control fingertip trajectory (in world) across multiple moving proximal and distal limb joints (Lisberger 1982, p 513). It is not yet clear from recording and ablation studies whether fingertip trajectory is the sum of the cerebellar controls at each proximal joint or of some coordinating control across all joints.

As to motor sequences, no mechanism within the cerebellum is known to be capable of sustaining an activity for longer than 300 ms once the input is off. The Marr model (Marr 1969) of a chain of movements each fully triggered by context-recognition of the preceding movement appears unlikely, because cerebellar outflow does not seem strong enough to fully generate any one movement in the sequence. Cerebellar stimulation does not lead to persistent movements or postures, and after acute total cerebellar ablation motor sequences can still be performed, albeit imperfectly. This implies that motor sequences are generated by structures other than the cerebellum.

References

Albus JS 1971 A theory of cerebellar function. Math Biosci 10:25–61

Allen GI, Tsukahara N 1974 Cerebrocerebellar communication systems. Physiol Rev 54:957–1006

Asanuma C, Thach WT, Jones EG 1983a Cytoarchitectonic delineation of the ventral lateral thalamic region in the monkey. Brain Res Rev 5:219–235

Asanuma C, Thach WT, Jones EG 1983b Distribution of cerebellar terminations and their relation to other afferent terminations in the ventral thalamic region of the monkey. Brain Res Rev 5:237–265

Asanuma C, Thach WT, Jones EG 1983c Anatomical evidence for segregated focal grouping of efferent cells and their terminal ramifications in the cerebellothalamic pathway of the monkey. Brain Res Rev 5:267–297

Asanuma C, Thach WT, Jones EG 1983d Brain stem and spinal projections of the deep cerebellar nuclei, with observations on the brain stem projections of the dorsal column nuclei. Brain Res Rev 5:299–322

Brooks VB, Thach WT 1981 Cerebellar control of posture and movement. In: Brooks VB (ed) Motor control, part 2. American Physiological Society, Bethesda, Maryland (Handb Physiol sect 1 The nervous system vol 2) p 877–946

Dow RS, Moruzzi G 1958 The physiology and pathology of the cerebellum. Minnesota Press, Minneapolis

Elble RJ, Schieber MH, Thach WT 1984 Activity of muscle spindles, motor cortex and cerebellar nuclei during action tremor. Brain Res 323:330–334

Evarts EV 1974 Precentral and postcentral cortical activity in association with visually triggered movement. J Neurophysiol 37:373–381

Evarts EV, Tanji J 1976 Reflexes and intended responses in motor cortex pyramidal tract neurons of monkey. J Neurophysiol 39:1069–1080

Fox PT, Raichle ME, Thach WT 1985 Functional mapping of the human cerebellum with positron emission tomography. Proc Natl Acad Sci USA 82:7462–7466

Frysinger RC, Bourbonnais D, Kalaska JF, Smith AM 1984 Cerebellar cortical activity during antagonist cocontraction and reciprocal inhibition of forearm muscles. J Neurophysiol 51:32–49

Gilbert PFC, Thach WT 1977 Purkinje cell activity during motor learning. Brain Res 128:309–328

Gilman S, Bloedel JR, Lechtenberg R 1981 Disorders of the cerebellum. Davis, Philadelphia

Goldberger ME, Growdon JH 1973 Pattern of recovery following cerebellar deep nuclear lesions in monkeys. Exp Neurol 39:307–322

Ito M, Shiida T, Yagi N, Yamamoto M 1974 The cerebellar modification of rabbit's horizontal vestibulo-ocular reflex in stimulation. Proc Jpn Acad 50:85–89

Ito M, Sakurai M, Tongroach P 1982 Climbing induced depression of both mossy fiber responsiveness and glutamate sensitivity of cerebellar Purkinje cells. J Physiol (Lond) 324:113–134

Leaton RN, Supple WF Jr 1986 Cerebellar vermis: essential for long term habituation of the acoustic startle response. Science (Wash DC) 232:513–515

Leigh RJ, Zee DS 1983 The neurology of eye movements. Davis, Philadelphia

Lisberger SG 1982 The signal processing and function of the flocculus during smooth eye movement in the monkey. In: Palay SL, Chan-Palay V (eds) The cerebellum: new vistas. Exp Brain Res Suppl 6:501–511, 513

Lisberger SG, Fuchs AF 1974 Responses of flocculus Purkinje cells to adequate vestibular stimulation in the alert monkey: fixation vs. compensatory eye movements. Brain Res 69:347–353

Llinas R, Walton K, Hillman DE, Sotelo C 1975 Inferior olive: its role in motor learning. Science (Wash DC) 190:1230–1231

MacKay WA, Murphy JT 1979 Cerebellar modulation of reflex gain. Prog Neurobiol 13:361–417

Marr D 1969 A theory of cerebellar cortex. J Physiol (Lond) 202:437–470

Matthews PBC 1981 Muscle spindles, their messages and their fusimotor supply. In: Brooks VB (ed), Motor control, pt 1. American Physiological Society, Bethesda, Maryland (Handb Physiol sect 1 The nervous system vol 2) p 189–228

McCormick DA, Thompson RF 1984 Cerebellum: essential involvement in the classically conditioned eyelid response. Science (Wash DC) 223:296–299

Meyer-Lohmann J, Hore J, Brooks VB 1977 Cerebellar participation in generation of prompt arm movements. J Neurophysiol 40:1038–1050

Mink JW, Thach WT 1987 Preferential relation of pallidal neurons to ballistic movements. Brain Res, in press

Nashner LM, Grimm RJ 1978 Analysis of multiloop dyscontrols in standing cerebellar patients. Prog Clin Neurophysiol 4:300–319

Optican LM, Robinson DA 1980 Cerebellar-dependent adaptive control of primate saccadic system. J Neurophysiol 44:1058–1980

Robinson DA 1976 Adaptive gain control of the vestibuloocular reflex by the cerebellum. J Neurophysiol 39:954–969

Schell GR, Strick PL 1983 The origin of thalamic inputs to the arcuate premotor and supplementary motor area. J Neurosci 4:539–560

Schieber MH, Thach WT 1985 Trained slow tracking. II. Bidirectional discharge patterns of cerebellar nuclear, motor cortex, and spindle afferent neurons. J Neurophysiol 55:1228–1270

Snow R, Hore J, Vilis T 1985 Adaptation of saccadic and vestibulo-ocular systems after extraocular muscle tenectomy. Invest Ophthalmol Vis Sci 26:928–931

Strick PL 1976 Anatomical analysis of ventrolateral thalamic input to the primate motor cortex. J Neurophysiol 39:1020–1031

Strick PL 1983 The influence of motor preparation on the response of cerebellar neurons to limb displacements. J Neurosci 3:2007–2020

Tanji J, Evarts EV 1976 Anticipatory activity of motor cortex in relation to direction of an intended movement. J Neurophysiol 39:1062–1068

Thach WT 1968 Discharge of Purkinje and cerebellar nuclear neurons during rapidly alternating arm movements in the monkey. J Neurophysiol 31:785–797

Thach WT 1975 Timing of activity in the cerebellar dentate nucleus and cerebral motor cortex during prompt volitional movement. Brain Res 169:168–172

Thach WT 1978 Correlation of neural discharge with pattern and force of muscular activity, joint position, and direction of intended next movement in motor cortex and cerebellum. J Neurophysiol 41:654–676

Thach WT, Schieber MH, Mink JW, Kane SA, Horne MK 1986 Cerebellar relation to muscle spindles in hand tracking. Prog Brain Res 64:217–224

Thach WT, Schieber MH, Horne MK, Kane SA, Mink JW 1987 Selective adaptation of stretch reflexes and its behavioral effect in monkey and man. Glickstein M, Stein J (eds) Cerebellar learning. Oxford University Press, in press

Victor M, Adams RD, Mancall EL 1959 A restricted form of cerebellar cortical degeneration occurring in alcoholic patients. Arch Neurol 1:579–688

Vilis T, Snow R, Hore J 1983 Cerebellar saccadic dysmetria is not equal in the two eyes. Exp Brain Res 51:343–350

Watanabe E 1984 Neuronal events correlated with long-term adaptation to the horizontal vestibulo-ocular reflex in the primate flocculus. Brain Res 297:169–174

Wetts R, Kalaska JF, Smith AM 1987 Cerebellar nuclear cell activity during antagonist cocontraction and reciprocal inhibition of forearm muscles. J Neurophysiol, in press

Wilson VJ, Uchino Y, Maunz RA, Susswein A, Fukushima K 1978 Properties and connections of cat fastigiospinal neurons. Exp Brain Res 32:1–17

Yeo CH, Hardiman MJ, Glickstein M 1984 Discrete lesions of the cerebellar cortex abolish classically conditioned nictitating membrane response of the rabbit. Behav Brain Res 13:261–266

DISCUSSION

Roland: These are all extracellular recordings, but to prove the Marr–Albus–Ito hypothesis you have to do intracellular recordings to show that you can modulate the parallel fibre–Purkinje cell synaptic efficiency by training the animal.

Thach: At present, stability is not good enough to permit intracellular recording in the Purkinje cells of awake animals. The experiment has been done in the decerebrate paralysed cat (Ito et al 1982). But, as in any research of

this sort, a number of different approaches are required. Extracellular recording is particularly useful because you can look at the interaction of the two
inputs on the Purkinje cell for relatively long periods of time during which the
behaviour is adapting. This is a unique advantage offered by the Purkinje cell,
first shown by Granit & Phillips (1956, 1957), who demonstrated the two types
of spike response in the Purkinje cell.

Armstrong: Did you find a relationship between interpositus neuronal discharge rates and the velocity of the movements?

Thach: Not in the range of velocities examined, which were relatively slow
velocities (10° to 30°/s). There were some very slight changes that were not
systematic, which was unexpected.

Armstrong: Presumably they were unexpected because of the Burton &
Onoda (1977, 1978) findings, where in cats making a voluntary elbow flexion
the discharge rate varied in parallel with the velocity of the movement.

Thach: Yes.

Armstrong: It is perhaps in line with your findings that Stephen Edgley and I
(in preparation) have recorded interpositus discharges in cats walking at two
different speeds with the same gait pattern, and during locomotion at 0.5 m/s or
0.9 m/s there is virtually no difference in the pattern of interpositus discharge,
either in the phasing of the discharges or in the peak frequencies. Occasional
cells show substantial changes in peak frequency but most alter very little so
that, on average, the changes are not impressive—of the order of an increase of
6% for a near-doubling of walking speed.

Porter: Does that disagree with your recordings which showed the responsiveness of interpositus neurons to physiological tremor? The neurons were
locked into that tremor in a way that suggested a direct input from muscle
spindle receptors, also sensitive to those small perturbations.

Thach: We do not at present know whether the interpositus and spindle
afferent neurons were responding to the displacement (length) or velocity or
some higher time-derivative of stretch in the tremor. In any case, the sensitivity
appears to be narrowed to the small range occupied by the tremor.

Porter: That has also been shown for dorsospinal cerebellar tract neurons
(Rymer 1972).

Freund: You showed that oscillatory input may come from the muscle
spindles. On the other hand you have an additional input with an intrinsic
oscillator from the inferior olive. Could you comment on their possible inter-
relationship?

Thach: The oscillatory signals that we record from the spindle afferents and
the interpositus neurons seem to be peripherally initiated: we can influence
both of them with the application of a tuning fork to the arm. Despite the
proposition by Llinas (1970) that there is an average driving frequency of 10/s
across inferior olive neurons, we do not see a 10/s periodicity in interpositus
discharge if there is no peripheral tremor. We are now using Fourier analysis to

further look for this. The oscillations that we see are more consistent with a mass-spring stretch reflex oscillation than with a central oscillator.

Freund: This implies that these frequencies are different for different parts of the body representation, because the resonant frequencies are different.

Thach: We have only looked at this in the hand. We know that we can change the oscillation frequency by mass loadings, which slow the frequency, and by adding external springs, which increases the frequency. This would be consistent with the idea of a peripheral oscillator.

Porter: How much of the influence of the cerebellum, for example in switching between α activation and the dynamic or static fusimotor activation of reflexes, is exerted via the cerebral cortex, and how much of it may be due to an activity directed through other descending pathways into the spinal cord?

Thach: Although we have monitored some of the output at the level of the motor cortex, we have not independently measured output by separate routes. When the animals had tremor in the interpositus discharge, we also observed it in the discharge of motor cortex neurons. It could be transmitted from the periphery through the interpositus to the motor cortex, but there are other possible routes.

Porter: Concerning the pathways from detectors of a disturbance in movement, either muscle stretch receptors or other peripheral afferents, could the pathway come through the interpositus to the part of the thalamus that projects onto area 4?

Thach: It may. The questions are how effective is it and does it account solely for the initial changes in the cortical stretch reflex? There may be other contributing routes with similar short latencies, although the one through interpositus is very short.

Marsden: The leading edge of the long latency stretch reflex in humans in the first five or ten milliseconds seems to be proprioceptively driven, after which there is a peripheral cutaneous component. This does not fit exactly with your description of the early spinothalamic input directly into the motor cortex followed by an interpositus loop, which may then feed into the motor cortex.

You raise the question of the extent to which the cerebellum controls spinal inhibition and whether co-contraction is a feature of cerebellar deficit. Hallett, Berardelli and I (unpublished observations) have analysed ballistic movement in cerebellar disease; co-contraction is the commonest abnormality, quite apart from variability of the size and duration of the initial agonist pulse.

Thach: This agrees with Smith & Bourbonnais's (1981) original interpretation that the cerebellum controls antagonist inhibition.

Shinoda: Which part of the cerebral cortex do you think is responsible for conveying information to the dentate nucleus?

Thach: Brodal (1982) looked to the cerebropontine projection and the pontocerebellar projection. Originally, the electroanatomical studies of Robert Dow (1942) suggested that input came mainly from parietal and frontal association cortex to lateral cerebellum via this pontine route. Brodal questioned this, saying that the main input to the lateral cerebellum was from motor cortex, somatosensory cortex and possibly anterior area 6. That agreed with results from Allen and colleagues, summarized by Allen & Tsukahara (1974), in animals where electrical stimulations were given to cerebral cortex and recordings made in the dentate nucleus. They found that it is very difficult to get transmission from frontal and parietal association cortex to dentate. Brodal has now shown that there are inputs from association cortex but they are not as numerous. Yet M. Glickstein's injections with horseradish peroxidase into the pontocerebellar projection nuclei show retrograde transport to cerebral cortex association areas, including the visual cortex. At present we have no clear idea of the correct interpretation of these different results.

Rizzolatti: According to the maps of Snider (1950) there is one homunculus in the anterior lobe of the cerebellum and one in the posterior lobe. You have described three motor maps organized mediolaterally, but only one rostrocaudally. What happened to Snider's two homunculi? Is there a convergence from homologous points represented rostrally and caudally in the cortex to the deep cerebellar nuclei?

Thach: Snider & Stowell (1944) and Snider & Eldred (1952) mapped a homunculus in the anterior lobe and simplex, and one in the paramedian lobules. Snider drew a midline figure with extremities pointing laterally. Subsequent studies of the responses of cortical neurons to peripheral inputs have shown a complicated microsomatotopy across the cortex (Bower et al 1981). Whatever is in cortex must converge on the nuclei. It remains to be seen to what degree the cortical and the nuclear body maps are in register.

Armstrong: In barbiturate-anaesthetized cats Robertson et al (1982) showed good climbing fibre representation of distal parts of the body even in the vermis. However, Gert Andersson and I (Andersson & Armstrong 1987 and in preparation) looked in the lateral vermis (b zone) in unanaesthetized cats and found very little representation of the distal parts of the limbs. Most Purkinje cells had complex spike (and simple spike) receptive fields related to axial or proximal parts of the body such as the neck, the spinal column, the shoulder girdle or the region around the hip. We cannot at present reconcile the two sets of findings.

Kalaska: Dr Thach, you propose that the dentate nucleus assists in the initiation of movement, but how is it doing this?

Thach: I do not think it is an exclusive input; it has to be accompanied by others, which may be quantitatively more important. Our animals with a dentate injection of muscimol continue to do the task with only the very slightest delay and no tremor. That means that something else must also be driving motor cortex, phasically or tonically; the dentate helps but does only a fraction of the whole job. That fraction may become critical as the performance requirement becomes more stringent, such as playing a musical instrument.

Kalaska: Then what is the information content of the signals that the dentate provides? In 1978 you described that in a three-step task against different directions of load and so on, three possible types of cell signal (pattern and force of muscle activity, joint position, or direction of intended next movement) were equally represented in the dentate, suggesting that there was no one predominant signal or type of information coming from the dentate.

Thach: In that study we found cells related to the held position, the pattern of muscle activity used to hold, and the anticipated direction of the next move. These were the only variables that were dissociated in the task, and we found cells relating to each variable in equal proportions. More sophisticated task designs may reveal more complicated cell–behaviour correlations.

Lemon: The influence of some of these connections between the dentate and the motor cortex might not be evident from a single trial. The changes may be subtle and occur only in subsequent trials; therefore, when looking at the average activity of a motor cortex neuron over a large number of trials, you will not detect the expected modulation of the motor cortex output, particularly if it is influenced by processes occurring in the lateral parts of the cerebellum.

Secondly, there is the possibility that the cerebellum plays a part in the control of sensory feedback to the motor cortex. Although people have been able to record responses of motor cortex neurons to peripheral stimuli, there is little evidence for these responses in the thalamus. This might be because people have not looked in precisely the right area, but I consider this unlikely.

Deecke: Dentate cooling increases the reaction time but in the parallel pathway, via the basal ganglia, cooling shortens the reaction time (Trouche et al 1984, Amato et al 1978).

Thach: Horak & Anderson (1984) have done ablations and detect no change in reaction time but a prolongation of movement time. In patients with Parkinson's disease the reaction time is not prolonged but movement time is (Evarts et al 1981).

References

Allen GI, Tsukuhara N 1974 Cerebrocerebellar communication systems. Physiol Rev 54:957–1006

Amato G, Trouche E, Beaubaton D, Grangetto A 1978 The role of internal pallidal segment on the initiation of a goal directed movement. Neurosci Lett 9:159–163

Andersson G, Armstrong DM 1987 Complex spikes in Purkinje cells in the lateral vermis (b zone) of the cat cerebellum during locomotion. J Physiol (Lond) 385:107–134

Bower JM, Beermann DH, Gibson JM, Shambes GM, Welker W 1981 Principles of organization of a cerebro-cerebellar circuit. Micromapping the projections from cerebral (SI) to cerebellar (granule cell layer) tactile areas of rats. Brain Behav Evol 18:1–18

Brodal P 1982 The cerebropontocerebellar pathway: salient features of its organization. Exp Brain Res Suppl 6:108–133

Burton JE, Onoda N 1977 Interpositus neuron discharge in relation to voluntary movement. Brain Res 121:167–172

Burton JE, Onoda N 1978 Dependence of the activity of interpositus and red nucleus neurons on sensory input data generated by movement. Brain Res 152:41–64

Dow RS 1942 Cerebellar action potentials in response to stimulation of the cerebral cortex in monkeys and cats. J Neurophysiol 5:121–136

Evarts EV, Teravainen H, Calne DB 1981 Reaction time in Parkinson's disease. Brain 104:167–186

Granit R, Phillips CG 1956 Excitatory and inhibitory processes acting upon individual Purkinje cells of the cerebellum of cats. J Physiol (Lond) 133:520–547

Granit R, Phillips CG 1957 Effects on Purkinje cells on surface stimulation of the cerebellum. J Physiol (Lond) 135:73–92

Horak FB, Anderson ME 1984 Influence of globus pallidus on arm movements in monkeys. I. Effects of kainic acid-induced lesions. J Neurophysiol 52:290–304

Ito M, Sakurai M, Tongroach P 1982 Climbing induced depression of both mossy fiber responsiveness and glutamate sensitivity of Purkinje cells. J Physiol (Lond) 324:113–134

Llinas R 1970 Neuronal operations in cerebellar transactions. In: Schmitt FO (ed) The neurosciences: second study program. Rockefeller University Press, New York, p 409–426

Robertson LT, Laxer KD, Rushmer DS 1982 Organization of climbing fiber input from mechanoreceptors to lobule V vermal cortex of the cat. Exp Brain Res 46:281–291

Rymer WZ 1972 A comparison between muscle spindle receptors and dorsal spinocerebellar tract cells. PhD Thesis, Monash University

Smith AM, Bourbonnais D 1981 Neuronal activity in cerebellar cortex related to the control of prehensile force. J Neurophysiol 45:286–303

Snider RS 1950 Interrelation of cerebellum and brain stem. Res Publ Assoc Res Nerv Ment Dis 30:267–281

Snider RS, Eldred E 1952 Cerebro-cerebellar relationships in the monkey. J Neurophysiol 15:27–40

Snider RS, Stowell 1944 Receiving areas of the tactile, auditory, and visual systems in the cerebellum. J Neurophysiol 7:331–357

Trouche E, Beaubaton D, Amato G, Viallet F, Legallet E 1984 Changes in reaction time after pallidal or nigral lesion in the monkey. Adv Neurol 40:29

General discussion 3

Shinoda: I would like to make two comments on the cerebello-thalamo-cortical pathway. Dr Jones showed us earlier that dentate terminals and interpositus terminals interdigitate anatomically within the same thalamic area. But this does not necessarily indicate that the two systems are physiologically separate. In fact, our electrophysiological study has shown that a large proportion of ventrolateral (VL) projection neurons receive convergent inputs from both nuclei (Shinoda et al 1985b). This finding has been confirmed more recently by L. Rispal-Padel (personal communication).

Briefly, to examine inputs to different corticofugal neurons from the dentate and the interpositus nuclei, we recorded intracellular potentials in areas 4 and 6 in anaesthetized cats. Such an experiment is shown in Fig. 1. Stimulation of the interpositus (INP) (Fig. 1C) and the dentate nucleus (DN) (Fig. 1D) produced large excitatory postsynaptic potentials (EPSPs) in a fast pyramidal tract neuron (PTN). These EPSPs are disynaptic from each nucleus, since EPSPs are evoked monosynaptically from the VL in the same cell (Fig. 1B), and they are mediated via the VL of the thalamus (Fig. 1E–L). In this series of experiments, the majority of fast and slow PTNs in areas 4 and 6 receive convergent inputs from both INP and DN (Shinoda et al 1985a); other corticofugal neurons such as corticorubral and corticopontine neurons also receive convergent inputs (Futami et al 1986). The site of convergence of the two inputs was determined by analysing the interaction of INP- and DN-evoked EPSPs. Fig. 1M–P shows an experiment investigating whether the inputs converge at the level of the cortex or at the level of the VL. Simultaneous stimulation of the INP and the DN at weak stimulus intensities evoked EPSPs (Fig. 1O) larger than the algebraic sum (Fig. 1P) of individual EPSPs evoked separately from the INP (Fig. 1M) and the DN (Fig. 1N), indicating that there is spatial facilitation at the last-order relay neurons in the pathway. It was concluded that at least some of the convergence of the dentate and the interpositus inputs occurs at the level of the thalamus.

To confirm this finding more directly, we recorded intracellular potentials from thalamocortical neurons in the VL and examined the effects of stimulating both nuclei. Fig. 1Q–S shows a typical example of inputs from the cerebellar nuclei to a thalamocortical neuron. Unitary EPSPs of different shapes were evoked at threshold by stimulation of two sites in the INP (Fig. 1S 1,2) and another two sites in the DN (Fig. 1S 3,4). Judging from the positions of the stimulating electrodes and the low stimulus intensities, we concluded that this thalamocortical neuron received convergent inputs from both the INP and the DN (Shinoda et al 1985b). The distribution of inputs from the INP and the DN

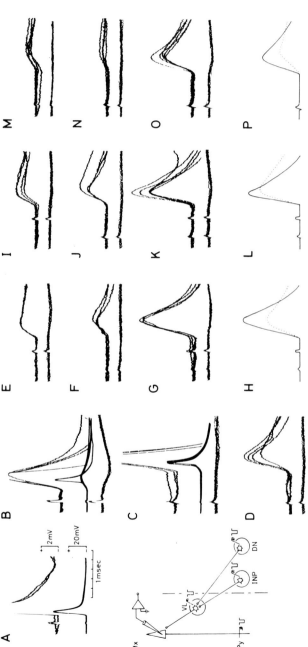

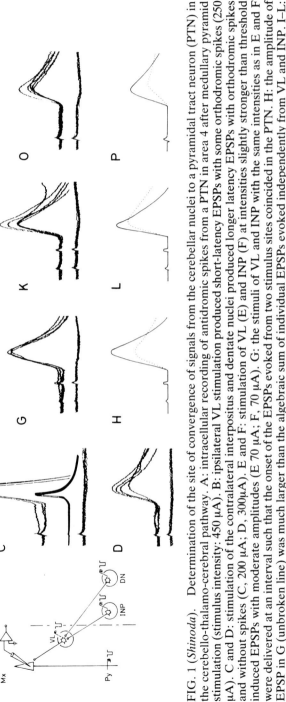

FIG. 1 (*Shinoda*). Determination of the site of convergence of signals from the cerebellar nuclei to a pyramidal tract neuron (PTN) in the cerebello-thalamo-cerebral pathway. A: intracellular recording of antidromic spikes from a PTN in area 4 after medullary pyramid stimulation (stimulus intensity: 450 μA). B: ipsilateral VL stimulation produced short-latency EPSPs with some orthodromic spikes (250 μA). C and D: stimulation of the contralateral interpositus and dentate nuclei produced longer latency EPSPs with orthodromic spikes and without spikes (C, 200 μA; D, 300μA). E and F: stimulation of VL (E) and INP (F) at intensities slightly stronger than threshold induced EPSPs with moderate amplitudes (E 70 μA; F, 70 μA). G: the stimuli of VL and INP with the same intensities as in E and F were delivered at an interval such that the onset of the EPSPs evoked from two stimulus sites coincided in the PTN. H: the amplitude of EPSP in G (unbroken line) was much larger than the algebraic sum of individual EPSPs evoked independently from VL and INP. I–L: similar to E–H, but VL and DN were stimulated (I, 70 μA; J, 250 μA). M–P: spatial facilitation of the interpositus and the dentate inputs. Stimulation of INP (M) and DN (N) at just above threshold produced small EPSPs in the same neuron (M, 60 μA; N, 200 μA).

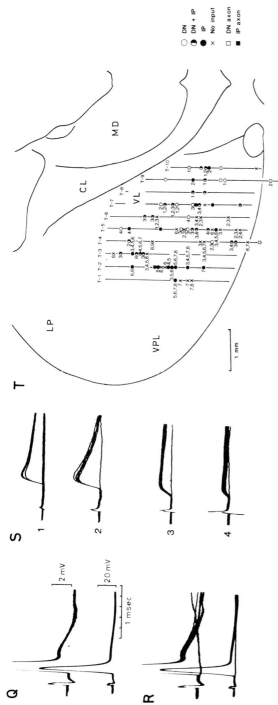

Simultaneous stimulation of INP and DN at the same intensities as in M and N induced large EPSPs in O. P: the amplitude in O (solid line) was much larger than the algebraic sum of the EPSPs in M and N (dotted line). The lower trace in records B–O is an extracellular field potential taken after withdrawal. The experimental set-up and the presumed neural connections are shown schematically, above left. (From Fig. 7 in Shinoda et al 1985a.) O–T: convergence of interpositus and dentate inputs to a single thalamocortical neuron in VL. Intracellular recording of antidromic spikes from a thalamocortical neuron in VL activated antidromically from the motor cortex at suprathreshold (Q) and at threshold (R). S: monosynaptic EPSPs evoked in an all-or-none manner by stimulating the interpositus (S1,2) and the dentate (S3,4) nuclei at juxta-threshold intensities with 110, 75, 70 and 80 μA respectively. These EPSPs had different shapes and time courses. Upward deflection indicates positivity in this figure. T: thalamic distribution of thalamocortical neurons receiving inputs from the interpositus and the dentate nuclei. Seventy-three cells and three axons were penetrated intracellularly, using a single micropipette throughout the experiment. Mapping was done systematically at 300 μm intervals lateromedially at the same frontal plane of the thalamus 10.0 mm anterior to the ear bar position. The electrode was advanced dorsoventrally in one direction and was not pulled back until the ventral margin of the thalamus was reached. Circles: neurons receiving inputs as indicated. Crosses: neurons in which PSPs could not be evoked from either nucleus. Numbers in T indicate stimulating sites placed at 1 mm intervals from which neurons were antidromically activated. (From Figs. 1 and 7 in Shinoda et al 1985b.)

onto single thalamocortical neurons is shown in Fig. 1T. In this example, 73 TC neurons were recorded in the same frontal plane of the VL in the same cat, using the same microelectrode. Twenty-one of 50 neurons receiving cerebellar inputs (42%) received convergent inputs from both the DN and the INP. Some cells in the medial portion of the VL received mainly from the DN, some in the lateral portion of the VL mainly from the INP. The thalamic projection areas of the DN and the INP are wide and there is considerable overlap between the dentate and the interpositus projection areas in the VL. And in this overlapping area a considerable number of thalamocortical neurons receive convergent inputs from both the DN and the INP.

So far I have discussed convergence of inputs. This kind of convergence of inputs onto single cells from different sources has been extensively analysed in various parts of the mammalian central nervous system, using electrophysiological techniques. However, the divergent properties of single neurons to various targets have been less thoroughly examined, mainly for technical reasons. The morphology of axon branches of single efferent cerebellar nucleus neurons and thalamocortical neurons has not been described, since it is difficult to trace the total trajectory of long axons in a Golgi preparation. I would like to describe our recent data on divergent properties of single neurons in the cerebello-thalamo-cerebral pathway.

Axonal branching patterns of physiologically identified cerebellar nucleus neurons were investigated in the cat, using intra-axonal horseradish peroxidase (HRP) injection and three-dimensional reconstruction from serial sections (Shinoda et al 1987). Penetrated axons were identified as axons originating from dentate or interpositus neurons by their direct spike responses to stimulation of individual nuclei. Axons of dentate and interpositus neurons project to the VL of the thalamus and, on their way, several axon collaterals are given off from stem axons to the red nucleus. Some of them also send their descending axons to the nucleus reticularis tegmenti pontis. In this way, single cerebellar nucleus neurons have very wide divergent projections to different nuclei. Axon terminals of interpositus neurons are very extensive and terminate as a sagittal sheet of arborizations in the caudal portion of the red nucleus. The approximate dimension of this sheet of arborizations is 1 to 2 mm retrocaudally, 200 to 500 μm mediolaterally, and 500 to 800 μm dorsoventrally. This distribution of terminals suggests some organization of rubrospinal neurons; an output functional unit seems to be organized in a rostrocaudally elongated vertical plate. Axon terminals make apparent contact with cell bodies and proximal dendrites of rubrospinal neurons very densely. These structures seem to be functional correlates of large unitary EPSPs observed in rubrospinal neurons after stimulation of the INP. The axons from the DN, after passing through the caudal portion of the red nucleus, enter its rostral portion and give off axon collaterals there. These collaterals are very thin and axon terminals are usually very sparse. So far, we cannot find any cerebellar nucleus neurons specifically projecting to the red nucleus without further projecting to the VL. After the entrance into the VL, axons branch successively and spread widely in a delta-like fashion. Synaptic boutons are clustered within about 200 μm and more than 10 such clusters arise from a single stem axon. These clusters must innervate the rod-like structures of thalamocortical neurons reported by Dr Jones.

To analyse the branching patterns of thalamic neurons in the motor cortex, intracellular recordings were made from thalamocortical neurons in the VL which received inputs from the INP and the DN. About 40% of them were antidromically activated from three or more sites in the motor cortex separated from each other by 1.5–2 mm, indicating that single thalamocortical neurons project to multiple zones in the motor cortex (Shinoda et al 1985b). This electrophysiological finding of multiple projection was further investigated morphologically by intra-axonal injection of HRP in physiologically identified thalamocortical neurons. Single thalamocortical axons ascend through the white matter and divide repeatedly into numerous branches, forming clusters of terminals in the motor cortex. These clusters have an extension of 0.3–1.5 mm and are separated by a terminal-free gap. Individual thalamocortical axons have two to eight such clusters and project to a wide area in the motor cortex. In a thalamocortical axon (Fig. 2) terminals are distributed over a distance of 5.0 mm rostrocaudally and 4.8 mm mediolaterally in the 'forelimb area' of the motor cortex. At least five clusters are identified in this axon, although four of them overlap in the lateral view. Terminal boutons are located most extensively in layer III. This very wide and multiple distribution of a single thalamocortical axon suggests that a single such neuron might innervate multiple 'motor efferent columns' defined by intracortical microstimulation. But, given multiple representation of a single muscle in the motor cortex, it is also possible that a single thalamocortical axon might control the excitability of a single muscle. Moreover, this anatomical divergence does not necessarily imply functional divergence. In spite of a wide morphological divergence, functionally this system may have a focusing effect on its target. If that is so, the dynamic filtering mechanism will be needed. Earlier Ted Jones showed us beautiful slides of GABAergic neurons in the motor cortex. Those inhibitory neurons must be very important for such functional focusing.

Jones: Those are some of the most spectacular filled axons I have ever seen. Is this really divergence, because the distribution of axons in the cortex is very focal? A single axon forms multiple foci; this seems to be equally focused, though on multiple patches. This is comparable to the Y-type axon in the visual cortex which forms multiple patches, each focused on individual ocular dominance columns. So it may be inappropriate to use the term 'divergence' here, because each of the patches may have some common function.

Shinoda: All the thalamocortical neurons I showed had fast axonal conduction velocities. We have filled with HRP the very thin axons which might correspond to X-type cells in the lateral geniculate body, but those cells also

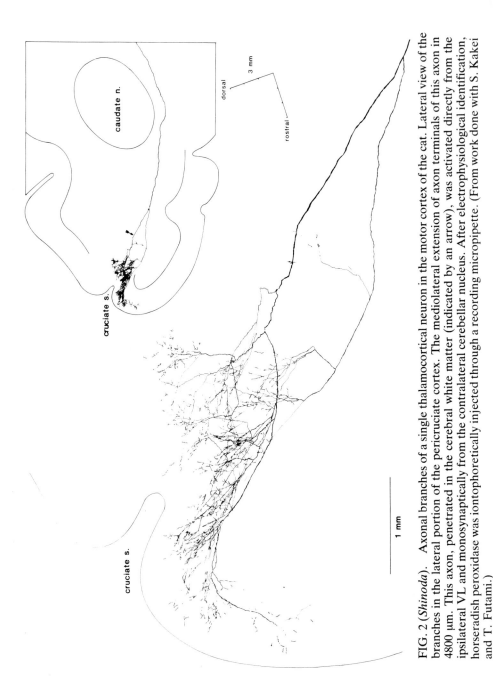

FIG. 2 (*Shinoda*). Axonal branches of a single thalamocortical neuron in the motor cortex of the cat. Lateral view of the branches in the lateral portion of the pericruciate cortex. The mediolateral extension of axon terminals of this axon in 4800 μm. This axon, penetrated in the cerebral white matter (indicated by an arrow), was activated directly from the ipsilateral VL and monosynaptically from the contralateral cerebellar nucleus. After electrophysiological identification, horseradish peroxidase was iontophoretically injected through a recording micropipette. (From work done with S. Kakei and T. Futami.)

have multiple projection sites and so far we have not found any neurons with narrow projection areas.

I used the term divergence in a morphological sense, to show that an axon tends in different directions from a common point to separate sites. I agree with you that those clusters of terminals arising from a single thalamocortical axon might govern cell colonies with a common function, although it is hard to believe that all colonies have common functional features in every respect.

Porter: There is not necessarily any reason why the term 'divergence' should not be used. An axon can diverge its influence and link several systems, whether they be in the cortex or elsewhere.

Jones: The implication of divergence is spreading and perhaps combining, but here I see no evidence for that spreading.

Thach: Divergence does not necessarily mean diffuseness.

Goldman-Rakic: We have made small injections in the mediodorsal nucleus of monkeys, although not single-axon injections, and have examined the terminal fields in prefrontal cortex by light microscopy. We find for many of our injection sites that the terminal territories correspond in some ways to the extent of branching of one of your labelled cells; that is, it seems as though half of a gyrus or a part of a sulcus receives its input from a particular subnucleus of the thalamus. Might the projections of many cells together form an overlapping field in a particular cytoarchitectonic area?

Shinoda: I have not done that kind of experiment. From my work with single-axon injections, there seems to be a slight tendency for axon terminals of single thalamocortical axons to spread widely in a rostrocaudal direction rather than in a mediolateral direction.

Strick: In the cat, we examined the pattern of degeneration in the cortex which resulted from small lesions in either VL or the ventrobasal complex (Strick 1973). After small lesions in VL, degeneration was found in a remarkably large region of the primary motor cortex. In contrast, small lesions in the ventrobasal complex caused a very focal cluster of degeneration in the primary somatosensory cortex. We argued that these different patterns of degeneration reflected different patterns of thalamocortical arbors for VL and ventrobasal complex neurons. We thought that the VL arbor would be extensively branched, spreading horizontally over considerable distances, and that the arbors of ventrobasal complex neurons would be spatially more compact. These suggestions appear to be supported by the Golgi studies of Professor Jones and the intracellular injections of thalamic afferents by Dr Shinoda and others.

Jones: One should not attribute homogeneity to the nuclei of the thalamus. There is good evidence from a number of sites that you can have different populations of cells in the same nucleus, which have radically different axonal distributions in the cortex, both in terms of layers and degree of focused terminations.

Dr Shinoda, I was interested in your data from the VL which showed convergence on some single cells of inputs from the interpositus and dentate nuclei, but also a significant population of cells receiving only from the interpositus or the dentate nucleus. Is there evidence for distinct populations?

Shinoda: I have no such evidence. We found that many cells have convergent inputs from both nuclei but others have input either from the dentate or from the interpositus nucleus. However, in this kind of experiment it is hard to conclude that those cells really receive input from only one nucleus, because we have to use weak stimuli in order to avoid inadvertent current spread to the other nucleus, so that only a portion of each nucleus is stimulated. Therefore, the number of VL cells receiving convergent inputs must be underestimated. So far we have found no correlation between the branching pattern of VL neurons and the mode of cerebellar input to those neurons.

Xi: Your results did not show that the postcruciate area and hindlimb areas of the motor cortex, which correspond to the forelimb in the cat, received projections from neurons in the ventrolateral nucleus. As we know, there is also a representation of forelimb and hindlimb muscles in ventrolateral nucleus. Why does the postcruciate area not receive inputs from ventrolateral nucleus in the thalamus?

Shinoda: I showed only VL neurons projecting to the 'forelimb area'. There are other VL neurons that project to the postcruciate gyrus of the motor cortex, the so-called hindlimb area. Common branching patterns are observed in VL neurons terminating in the forelimb area, in the hindlimb area and also in the trunk area of the motor cortex.

Lemon: I was impressed by the size of some of these EPSPs. We should remember that when we stimulate in the motor cortex, by recruiting groups of fibres such as those described by Dr Shinoda, we probably activate cells over quite large areas of the cerebral cortex.

Georgopoulos: Can one produce a delayed response defect by disconnecting the principalis and the parietal area?

Goldman-Rakic: Lesions of parietal cortex do not produce obvious delayed response loss but they do produce some kinds of spatial deficit, such as spatial neglect.

Georgopoulos: What about undercutting the principalis?

Goldman-Rakic: That has not been done. I would say that studies involving parietal cortex lesions need to be repeated with either a disconnection or a total lesion paradigm, because the posterior parietal cortex has at least four different subdivisions. It might be necessary to ensure that all subdivisions are removed to obtain a delayed response deficit. In addition, an important consideration in all neuropsychological studies is the control of behaviour. Since the animals can do the task in a number of ways, it is essential to prove that they perform the task by memory, not by using other subtle cues.

Georgopoulos: Some lesions of other areas, for example of the caudate nucleus, have produced a delayed response defect.

Goldman-Rakic: Lesions of the caudate nucleus (Goldman & Rosvolds

1972) and also of the mediodorsal nucleus (Isseroff et al 1982) do produce delayed response deficits, so the subcortical projections may be disconnected more easily.

Georgopoulos: That suggests that all the circuits would be necessary for correct performance in delayed response tasks.

Goldman-Rakic: We interpret many of the cognitive deficits associated with basal ganglia damage as some kind of disconnection from the prefrontal cortex. The mediodorsal nucleus is instructive. It was known for a long time that a small lesion in this nucleus was insufficient to produce a delayed response deficit. We now know from anatomical tracing that the anteriomedial group, the mediodorsal nucleus and the medial pulvinar all project to the prefrontal cortex, and if all these nuclei are damaged, a delayed response deficit results (Isseroff et al 1982), but if you spare some of them you do not necessarily get the deficit. There is strong support from the behavioural literature for a circuit basis underlying just this kind of cognition, namely knowledge of where things are in space.

Xi: By using extracellular unit recording techniques many different response patterns of neurons can be recorded in one cortical area. The problem is that most of these neurons have not been identified physiologically. It seems to me that the different response patterns we recorded are due to responses of different kinds of neurons. There are many kinds of neurons in the cortex and I think it is important to identify the type of neuron from which you record, whether they are pyramidal tract neurons, corticocortical neurons or neurons projecting to other neuronal structures.

Porter: Dr Tanji showed that at least some of the cells he had been recording from in the supplementary motor area projected axons into the motor cortex. While that does not prove that they are only one synapse removed from corticomotoneuronal projections, it does mean they are linked by their output into another area of cortex whose function is at least partially determined.

Deecke: Can you identify neurons by more aspects than just distinguishing between pyramidal tract and non-pyramidal tract neurons?

Porter: Kitai and other workers (Kitai & Deniau 1981) have attempted to isolate from areas of the cortex those cells which can be activated by stimulation of the putamen or other parts of the input system of the basal ganglia. There are still questions about the cells which project axons into the thalamus. One of the big challenges is to understand how the cerebral cortex may control its own inputs by actions on the thalamus. I am not aware that anyone has convincingly demonstrated that behaviour of cells in any area of the cortex, including the visual cortex, can be attributed to an output from that area to the appropriate nuclear region of the thalamus.

References

Futami T, Kano M, Sento S, Shinoda Y 1986 Synaptic organization of the cerebello-thalamo-cerebral pathway in the cat. III. Cerebellar input to corticofugal neurons destined for different subcortical nuclei in areas 4 and 6. Neurosci Res 3:321–344

Goldman PS, Rosvold HE 1972 The effects of selective caudate lesions in infant and juvenile rhesus monkeys. Brain Res 43:53–66

Isseroff A, Galkin T, Rosvold HE, Goldman-Rakic PS 1982 Spatial memory impairments following damage to the mediodorsal nucleus of the thalamus in rhesus monkeys. Brain Res 232:97–113

Kitai ST, Deniau JM 1981 Cortical inputs to the subthalamus: intracellular analysis. Brain Res 214:411–415

Shinoda Y, Kano M, Futami T 1985a Synaptic organization of the cerebello-thalamo-cerebral pathway in the cat. I. Projection of individual cerebellar nuclei to single pyramidal tract neurons in areas 4 and 6. Neurosci Res 2:133–156

Shinoda Y, Futami T, Kano M 1985b Synaptic organization of the cerebello-thalamo-cerebral pathway in the cat. II. Input-output organization of single thalamocortical neurons in the ventrolateral thalamus. Neurosci Res 2:157–180

Shinoda Y, Futami T, Mitoma H, Yokota J 1987 Morphology of single neurons in the cerebello-rubro-spinal system. Behav Brain Res, in press

Bereitschaftspotential as an indicator of movement preparation in supplementary motor area and motor cortex

L. Deecke

Neurologische Universitätsklinik, Lazarettgasse 14, A-1097 Vienna, Austria

Abstract. Topographical studies in humans of the Bereitschaftspotential (BP, or readiness potential, as averaged from the electroencephalogram) and the Bereitschaftsmagnetfeld (BM, or readiness magnetic field, as averaged from the magnetoencephalogram) revealed a widespread distribution of motor preparation over both hemispheres even before unilateral movement. This indicates the existence of several generators responsible for the BP, including generators in the ipsilateral hemisphere, which is in agreement with measurements of regional cerebral blood flow or regional cerebral energy metabolism. Nevertheless, two principal generators seem to prevail: (1) An early generator, starting its activity 1s or more before the motor act, with its maximum at the vertex. For this and other reasons, early BP generation probably stems from cortical tissue representing or including the supplementary motor area (SMA). (2) A later generator, starting its activity about 0.5s before the onset of movement and biased towards the contralateral hemisphere (contralateral preponderance of negativity, CPN). For unilateral finger movements the CPN succeeds the BP's initial bilateral symmetry in the later preparation period. Thus, this lateralized BP component probably stems from the primary motor area, MI (area 4, hand representation).

While regional cerebral blood flow or regional cerebral energy metabolism show that the SMA is active *in conjunction* with motor acts, these data do not permit the conclusion that SMA activity *precedes* motor acts. This can only be shown by the Bereitschaftspotential, which proves that SMA activity occurs before the onset of movement and, what is more, before the onset of MI activity. This important order of events (first SMA, then MI activation) has been elucidated by our BP studies. It gives the SMA an important functional role: the initiation of voluntary movement. The recording of movement-related potentials associated with manual hand-tracking and motor learning points to the SMA and frontal cortex having an important role in these functions.

1987 Motor areas of the cerebral cortex. Wiley, Chichester (Ciba Foundation Symposium 132) p 231–250

For the human brain it makes a great difference whether we make movements in response to stimuli from the outer world—*re-actions*—or whether we

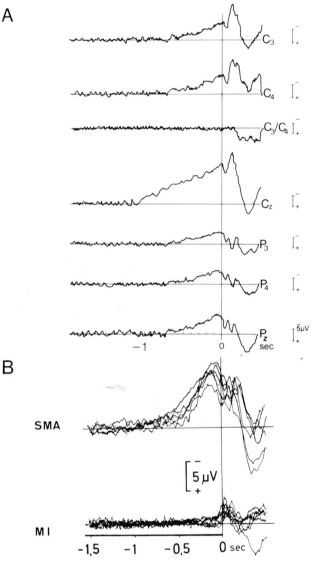

FIG. 1. (A) Bereitschaftspotential (BP) before bilateral flexion of the index fingers (n = 128) in an individual who was left-handed, except for handwriting. Note early BP onset (1.2s before first EMG activity, 0) in C_z (roughly overlying SMA) compared to C_3 (left MI) and C_4 (right MI), where BP starts only 0.7s before EMG onset, indicating that SMA is 'upstream' of MI in the temporal chain. (From Kristeva & Deecke 1980.)

(B) Superimposed recordings of the BP of six experiments on different days in a right-handed subject flexing the right index finger. Off-time of the BP (reversal to positivity, 'relaxation', pre-motion positivity, PMP) 90 ms before the first EMG activity (0) over SMA (upper trace). Bipolar left versus right precentral recordings, showing additional negativity over left precentral cortex (MI; motor potential, MP) 60 ms before first EMG activity (lower trace). The difference of 30 ms between BP off-time in SMA and MP onset in MI allows motor commands to be conveyed via cortico-cerebello-cortical or cortico-basal ganglia-cortical loops. (From Kornhuber & Deecke 1985.)

perform purely volitional 'endogenous' movements, which are really voluntary in nature and deserve the term *actions*. In the latter case the brain itself has to trigger the movement. Consequently, there must be a structure in the brain by which we can initiate our voluntary, purely endogenous movements. While diencephalic and limbic structures are probably also involved in volition (on which it is difficult to obtain information), the earliest sign of brain activity to be recorded by non-invasive means in humans is slowly increasing cortical negativity over the frontocentral midline, which probably reflects or contains activity from the supplementary motor area (SMA).

Bereitschaftspotential of SMA origin

The slowly increasing cortical negativity before voluntary, purely endogenous, movement has been termed the Bereitschaftspotential (BP) or readiness potential (Kornhuber & Deecke 1965, Deecke et al 1969, 1976). Depending on the complexity of the action the BP starts as early as 1–2s or more before the onset of movement. Initially it is bilaterally symmetrical, with its earliest onset over the frontocentral midline and—in healthy subjects—its maximum amplitude at this position. An example is given in Fig. 1A from Kristeva & Deecke (1980). Before bilateral flexion of the index fingers the BP clearly starts at the midline (C_z) as early as 1.2s before onset of movement but it does not start in the precentral (C_3, C_4) or parietal (P_3, P_4) lateral brain regions until about 0.7s before the onset of movement. Thus, there must be an early BP generator in frontocentral midline structures, probably including the SMA. This early strong BP onset in SMA is particularly pronounced for the bilateral finger movements in Fig. 1A, and we believe that SMA is especially important for bilateral movement coordination.

The emphasis above on distinguishing two principal generators does not mean that the SMA and, later, the primary motor cortex (MI, see below) are the only generators responsible for the BP. Rather, such preparatory activity before volitional movements shows a widespread distribution over both hemispheres even before unilateral movement, a concept that is supported by recordings of the Bereitschaftsmagnetfeld (BM) or readiness magnetic field (Deecke et al 1982) and by regional cerebral metabolic activity (Roland 1987, this volume).

With these reservations I return to BP topographies which, like the one in Fig. 1A, suggest that the two principal generators SMA and MI prevail. Not only does the onset time (Fig. 1A) suggest that SMA precedes MI but the off-time also favours this idea. Fig. IB indicates that negativity of the midline source (SMA) stops before the onset of movement (upper trace of Fig. 1B), a phenomenon discovered long ago as pre-motion positivity (PMP) (Deecke et al 1969). The PMP has a mean onset time, which at the same time is the off-time or resolution of the BP, of 90 ms before the electromyographic onset

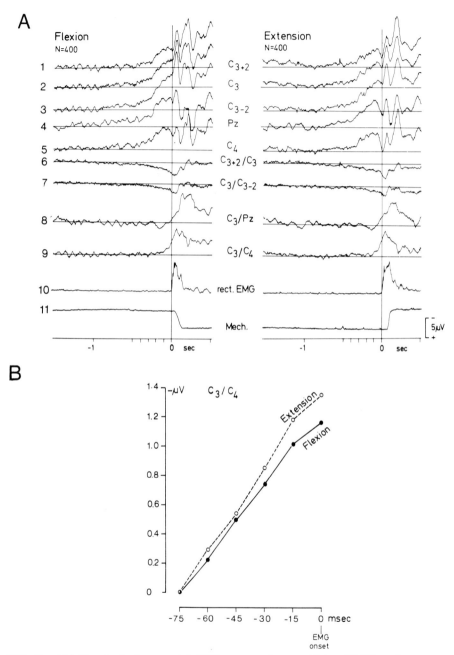

FIG. 2. (A) Bereitschaftspotential (BP), pre-motion positivity (PMP) and motor potential (MP) when the right index finger is flexed or extended in a typical right-handed subject. There is no difference in the BP (traces 1–5), but note the larger MP for extension than for flexion in trace 9.

(B) When the contralateral extra negativity in the bipolar C_3/C_4 derivation is measured in steps of 15 ms from −75 ms to 0, a significantly larger (P <0.05, two-tailed) MP is found for extension than for flexion, in agreement with the findings of Fetz & Cheney (1979) in the monkey. (From Deecke el al 1980.)

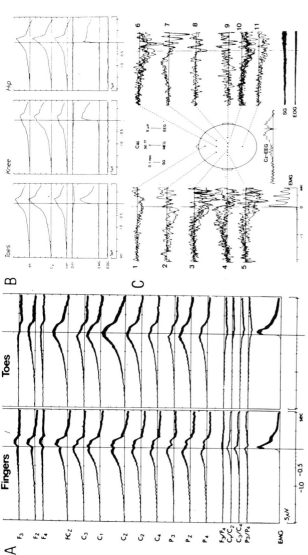

FIG. 3. (A) Grand averages over 30 subjects, with double standard error (thickness of the lines), of the Bereitschaftspotential before flexion of the right fingers and right toes. BP is twice as large for fingers as for toes in C_z due to lateralized MI generator for fingers. However, BP is twice as large for toes as for fingers in C_z due to accumulation of negativity from both generators SMA and MI in C_z for toe movements. In the four bipolar derivations there is contralateral preponderance of negativity (CPN) for fingers (upward) but ipsilateral preponderance (IPN) for toes (downward), due to different dipole orientation of active cortical tissue. (From Boschert et al 1983.)

(B) Mapping the motor homunculus by non-invasive voluntary movement physiology. When the IPN of the Bereitschaftspotential in the bipolar contralateral precentral derivation is compared to the ipsilateral precentral derivation (Diff.), an IPN for toes is seen, and a smaller one for the knee, but there is no IPN for hip movements. Grand averages over 10 subjects. (From Boschert & Deecke 1986.)

(C) Magnetoencephalographic (MEG) mapping of movement-related cortical fields during sophisticated right-finger tapping task, which the individual performs accurately (see rectified EMG average at lower left). There are two reversals of the Bereitschaftsmagnetfeld (BM), or readiness magnetic field: an early one between trace 7 (field lines coming out of the head, upward deflection) and traces 10/11 (BM field lines going into the head, downward deflection), indicating a current dipole between the two, with its negative pole pointing to the right (SMA generator). The second reversal involves the late BM component and is seen in trace 4 (MI generator). Each of the superimposed recordings represents the average of 40 artifact-free trials. (From Deecke et al 1985.)

of movement (Deecke et al 1976). As shown in the lower trace of Fig. 1B, additional negativity in the contralateral motor cortex (measured in the bipolar contralateral versus ipsilateral precentral derivation) starts about 60 ms before the electromyographic onset of finger movement; this is called the motor potential (MP, Deecke et al 1969). The difference of 30 ms in onset times between PMP and MP allows not only for direct transfer from SMA to MI but also for conveyance of motor command activity via subcortical loops such as the cortico-cerebello-cortical or the cortico-basal ganglia-cortical loop. Pre-movement activity of both subcortical sites has been established in animal experiments (cf. Thach 1987, this volume, and DeLong & Strick 1974).

The MP is believed to reflect the activation of the motor cortex while it is generating the pyramidal tract (PT) volley immediately before the onset of EMG activity. If this is so, the MP should share certain characteristics of motor cortex activity, e.g. differences between extension and flexion movements of the fingers. In a study with H. Eisinger and H.H. Kornhuber, extensions and flexions of the forefinger in the same experiment in a randomized order were compared (Deecke et al 1980). A typical example in one individual is shown in Fig. 2A. As seen in traces 1–5, early preparation for extension and for flexion is similar: there is no difference in the readiness potential, BP. Traces 9–11 show the last three events of the final motor pathway in their temporal order: trace 9 shows the discharge of the motor cortex (MP, larger for extension than for flexion), trace 10 gives the rectified electrical activity of the agonist muscle, and trace 11 displays the physical course of the finger movement itself (mechanogram, position signal).

Fig. 2B gives the average MP over the total of 30 right-handed people tested, showing a larger MP for extension than for flexion. This finding is in good agreement with the results of Fetz & Cheney (1979), who found that extensor-related motor cortex cells in the monkey have a higher discharge rate per unit of force ('motor gain') than have flexor-related motor cortex cells.

The study of voluntary movements of the toes can also contribute some evidence on the SMA origin of the early BP. As shown in a large group of subjects ($n = 32$), a comparison of toe and finger movements in the same experiment revealed characteristic differences in BP topography (Fig. 3A, Boschert et al 1983): over the contralateral precentral hand area (C_3), the BP preceding finger movement is twice as large as the BP preceding toe movement. Over the central midline (C_z, vertex) the BP preceding toe movement is twice as large as that preceding finger movement. A plausible explanation for this difference in topography can be found in the two principal BP generators under discussion. In finger movement, these generators are dissociated: SMA is on the mesial cortical surface of the midline and MI over the convexity, i.e. the hand area of the motor cortex. In toe movement, the generators are juxtaposed on the mesial cortical surface of the midline, summing to an extra large BP at the vertex.

Bereitschaftspotential of MI origin

We have seen that the BP is bilaterally symmetrical in the first half of the preparation period, even for unilateral voluntary finger movements, and that this is due to the SMA generator. Indeed, both SMAs seem to be active during early preparation for voluntary movement. In the second half of the period before such movement, the BP before unilateral movements becomes asymmetrical. This asymmetrical component of the BP is probably due to preparatory activity of MI. Support for this view again comes from comparative investigation of unilateral finger movements and toe movements (Boschert et al 1983). Interestingly, unilateral finger movements showed a contralateral preponderance of negativity (CPN) in the second half of the preparation period, whereas toe movements revealed an ipsilateral preponderance of negativity (IPN). This is seen in the bipolar leads of Fig. 3A:F_3/F_4,C_1/C_2,C_3/C_4 and P_3/P_4. For finger movement the bipolar contralateral versus ipsilateral derivations show an upward deflection (CPN); for toe movement they show a downward deflection (IPN).

IPN means that for movements of the right toes there is more negativity over the right hemisphere than over the left (cf. Fig. 3A, toes). As there is usually a cross-over relationship between the hemispheres and the sides of the body, this ipsilateral preponderance seems paradoxical (Brunia 1980). However, it can be explained by the spatial configuration of the respective generator dipoles. For finger movement, the generator tissue is on the convexity of the contralateral hemisphere (area 4, hand respresentation of the precentral gyrus), with the cortical surface being negative and the depth positive. The respective vector or dipole is oriented perpendicularly to the skull with its negative pole pointing out of the head. Thus, it points in the 'right' direction, namely towards the contralateral hemisphere, and causes the known plausible topography of the finger movement-related BP with its asymmetrical component shifted contralaterally. For toe movements, the active generator tissue (cf. Penfield's homunculus) is on the mesial cortical surface between the hemispheres, the relevant dipole being perpendicular to the falx and pointing in the 'wrong' direction, namely towards the ipsilateral hemisphere. Consequently, this orientation causes the asymmetrical component of the BP to shift ipsilaterally in surface maps.

If this explanation were true, movements of leg muscles, whose motor cortex cells are in the transition zone of the precentral gyrus between the convexity and the mesial surface ('mantle edge'), should show no BP asymmetry at all. Fig. 3B shows the results of a study with J. Boschert in which movements of the toes, knee and hip were compared (Boschert & Deecke

1986). As seen in the bipolar contralateral versus ipsilateral precentral leads ('Diff.' in Fig. 3B), there is an IPN (downward deflection) for toe movements, a lesser one for knee movements but no IPN (an absolutely isoelectric course) for hip movements. Thus, the generator tissue for hip movements must be right at the mantle edge, while creating a dipole standing upright in the sagittal direction, which fits the somatotopic organization of the primary motor cortex as mapped by Penfield & Rasmussen (1950) through electrical stimulation. This is confirmed here by physiological non-invasive means, i.e. voluntary-movement-related potentials.

The readiness magnetic field (Bereitschaftsmagnetfeld, BM) also confirms the view that there are two separate principal generators in voluntary finger movement. Fig. 3C shows the results of a study carried out with J. Boschert, P. Brickett and H. Weinberg at the Brain and Behaviour Laboratory, Simon Fraser University, Vancouver (Deecke et al 1985). This new method using the SQUID (superconducting quantum interference device) makes it possible to detect the minute magnetic field changes in the human brain that occur in relation to electrical cortical activity. Basically, the magnetoencephalogram (MEG) contains the same elements as the electroencephalogram (EEG). The evoked fields and movement-related fields can be extracted from the MEG by averaging the records. Recording the magnetoencephalographic fields, however, provides a unique opportunity for obtaining far better localization than will ever be possible in recordings of EEG potentials. In fact, by mapping the field lines on the skull surface, one can establish the maximum position of field lines coming out of the head at one position and the maximum of field lines going into the head at another position. Once such a reversal is demonstrated, the electrical current dipole lies in the middle of the connecting line between the two maxima at a 90° angle to the line.

In a first series of experiments, we were able to show that the Bereitschaftspotential of the EEG has an analogous phenomenon in the MEG, the Bereitschaftsmagnetfeld, and that it has—for finger movement—a reversal around the hand representation of the rolandic area (Deecke et al 1982). In a second set of experiments, we investigated movements of the right foot: the BM maximum with field lines going into the head was found in the left parietal region, while the BM maximum with field lines coming out of the head was found in the right frontal region (Deecke et al 1983). This pointed to an electrical current dipole in the midline, which—following the 90° rule—is obliquely oriented, with its negative pole pointing in a right posterior direction. This finding, which was confirmed by Hari et al (1983), agrees with the anatomical orientation of area 4 foot representation which is situated partly on the mesial cortical surface and partly in the anterior wall of the central sulcus, thus creating a resultant dipole with its negative pole pointing in an oblique ipsilateral-posterior direction.

The SMA, being juxtaposed to area 4 foot representation on the mesial cortical surface, should cause a BM topography similar to the MI foot area. Indeed, for a right-finger-tapping task thought to need strong SMA activation (Fig. 3C), a BM going into the head (downward) was found at the vertex and at a mid-occipital position (traces 10 and 11), and a BM coming out of the head (upward) was found in the right frontal region (trace 7), indicating a current dipole midway between the two. As seen in Fig. 3C, it is the early part of the BM which reverses between traces 10/11 and 7, another indication that the SMA generator leads in time. This becomes obvious when it is compared to the second reversal in Fig. 3C, occurring later in time in trace 4. In fact, the four recordings of this trace start homonymously at 1.5s in an upward direction. Later on, at 0.7s, they diverge. Two of the superimposed traces go up and the other two go down. This reversal around the hand area of the rolandic region thus describes the second—MI—generator. Trace 7, which picks up the field lines of the SMA generator coming out of the head, tells us that SMA shows activity in the early preparatory period but not in the late one (note downward deflection of trace 7 at about 0.7 s before the onset of movement). In conclusion, the MEG recordings using the SQUID technique support our distinction between two principal generators, SMA and MI, before a voluntary sequential finger movement, the SMA generator being upstream of MI in the temporal chain.

Bereitschaftspotential with tracking

We are now in a position to consider the movement-related cortical potentials accompanying more complex movements than those discussed above. In a study with W. Lang, M. Lang, B. Heise and H.H. Kornhuber, tracking movements of the right hand under voluntary starting conditions were investigated (Deecke et al 1984). As seen in the inset of Fig. 4, the individuals fixated on a point straight ahead of them and held a ballpoint pen in the right hand. As soon as he or she pressed the pen onto the paper, a contact in the pen was closed and started a visual (V) or a tactile (T) stimulus to move. V was a light spot on a television screen in the subject's left visual field, which moved for 1s in a random direction and for 1s in a second random direction, then quickly returned to the starting position. T was a skin indentation in the subject's left palm produced by a suspended plastic stylus driven by a modified X–Y-plotter which, like the light spot, moved in two random directions, then returned to the starting position. The subjects had to track the stimulus as soon as it moved, using the pen in the right hand. After the stimulus returned to the starting position, the individuals lifted the pen and this caused the paper to be advanced by a few centimetres. The subjects were told that the paper drawings would be compared with the original stimulus patterns, that we would give marks on both the promptness and the accuracy of performance, and that this would influence the monetary reward for the experiments.

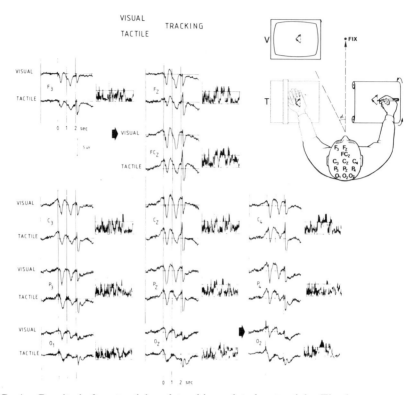

FIG. 4. Bereitschaftspotential and tracking-related potentials. The inset at upper right shows the experimental paradigm (and see text). Hearing was masked by white noise via earphones. The main part of the figure displays the grand averages over 16 individuals of cortical potentials for visual and tactile tracking in 12 different recording locations, F_3 to 0_2 (indicated on the head in the inset). The graphs to the right of each pair of visual and tactile averages are plots of paired-difference Wilcoxon tests over time calculated for each of the 1024 data points per recording and per person, testing differences between visual and tactile tracking potentials for significance (black areas extending beyond the horizontal line of the 2-tailed 0.05 level, without Bonferroni's correction). In FC_z/SMA (bold arrow at upper left), black areas indicate significantly larger positive potentials (relaxation positivity, RXP) for visual than for tactile tracking. In C_4 the black areas of the graph indicate significantly larger negative directed attention potentials (DAP) for tactile than for visual tracking, due to activity of the somatosensory projection and association areas contralateral to the tactile stimuli. The reverse is true for 0_2 (bold arrow at lower right), where the black area of significance indicates a larger DAP for visual than for tactile tracking. For further details see text. (Experiment with Lang, Lang, Heise & Kornhuber.)

Visual and tactile stimuli were investigated in separate runs of $n = 128$ each. Thus, the subjects were in a certain set during the experiment, treating sensory information in the right hemisphere and elaborating motor actions in the left hemisphere. The monetary reward motivated them strongly in this paradigm where temporal events were predictable (start to move, s 0; change in direction, s 1, and return to starting position, s 2 on the abscissae of the main part of Fig. 4) but spatial events (randomized directions) were unpredictable.

The main part of Fig. 4 shows the summed averages for 16 subjects of movement-related potentials in the 12 scalp recordings as viewed from above, negative up. Before the voluntary self-initiated start of pressing the pen onto the paper (which triggered the first stimulus trajectory at s 0 on the abscissae), a BP is seen in almost all recordings, even occipitally. Before the change in direction (s 1 on the abscissae) and before the return to the starting position (s 2), typical expectancy waves or contingent negative variation (CNV)-like negativities are generated in anticipation of these events.

A striking feature of the cortical potentials accompanying this paradigm are the sharp positive 'notches' in the wave form that seem to separate each component of this multisequential task, as if they were related to operant changes in the motor performance. These positive 'operant change potentials' (OCP) or 'relaxation positivities' (RXP), if surface negativity is taken as cortical activity (for which there are good reasons), are particularly pronounced over the frontocentral midline (FC_z and C_z) and are larger in the visual experiment than they are in the tactile one.

If we consider FC_z (which overlies SMA) in the visual task (bold arrow), we get the impression that SMA activity is 'switched on' (negativity) and 'off' (positivity) while the tracking task is conducted. If we now look at the activity in the right occipital cortex receiving the visual stimuli (O_2, second bold arrow), we realize that the visual projection and association areas switch on and off at different times than in the SMA: whereas SMA switches off shortly (90 ms) before the pen is pressed down (PMP, cf. Fig. 1B) and considerably (300 ms) before the change in direction, the right visual cortex at O_2 switches off (or 'relaxes') only later (about 200 ms after these events). Obviously, negativity (= activity) is maintained until the direction of the trajectory has been analysed, which is essential for tracking. In fact considering the change in direction (at s 1) SMA 'relaxes' as much as 0.5 s earlier than O_2 can afford to relax. O_2 still has to pay attention to the relevant stimulus while SMA has already done its (motivational) job in initiating or timing the motor consequences of the task. When the sides are compared (O_2 versus O_1) it is clear O_2 generates both a larger BP before the onset (at s 0) and a larger expectancy wave before the change in direction (at s 1) than O_1. This is remarkable since at least for the expectancy wave or CNV such a notion about asymmetry has never been produced in experimental paradigms. The term 'directed attention potential' (DAP) has been coined (Deecke et al 1984) for this significant additional negativity contralateral to the relevant stimulus.

Our interpretation of these observations is that with this particular paradigm we can regard the human cerebrum as consisting of a rostral *motivational brain* (frontocentral midline, SMA) and a posterior *attentional brain* (sensory projection and association cortex contralateral to the stimuli) which behave differently in time. One can also say that SMA becomes active early in the preparatory period and when it has fulfilled its motivational task it can relax and delegate the execution of the task (tracking) to other cortical areas that are expert in conducting such sensory controlled tracking tasks (O_2 region for visual or C_4 for tactile tracking, cf. legend to Fig. 4).

Bereitschaftspotential with motor learning

In continuation of the tracking experiment, we did another study which involved motor learning (Lang et al 1983). The experimental set-up (Fig. 5A) was similar to that in Fig. 4, with the following exceptions: (1) the moving target stimulus was now a circle, and the position of the pen held in the subject's right hand was coupled back to the TV screen as a light point, thus providing continuous visual feedback. It was the subject's task to keep the light-spot within the circle. (2) Instead of two trajectories, the circle moved in three different random directions, the duration of each trajectory being 1.5 s instead of 1.0 s. (3) A learning task was included by multiplying the feedback signal by -1 (inverted or mirror tracking: IT).

The results are shown for the SMA electrode only (FC_z). Fig. 5B gives the grand averages across 14 subjects. In the upper trace (no-tracking: NT) the subjects initiated the stimulus programme by leading the stylus onto the plate but did not track it. We see only a BP before this voluntary act, with no negativity while the stimulus is moving. This absolute absence of tracking negativity in NT compared to T (normal tracking with $+1$ feedback) was statistically significant at the 1% level. In the lower trace of Fig. 5B the learning experiment of IT (inverted tracking, using -1 feedback) is shown. Due to the difficulty of the learning task, another increase in tracking negativity occurs for IT compared to T, the difference being significant at the 1% level during the first trajectory, then at the 5% level.

The difference between target circle and feedback point (average of horizontal and vertical components) was measured as error. In Fig. 5C, learning in motor performance is described as the percentage reduction in error (i.e. mean tracking error $\bar{E}$ in the first third minus $\bar{E}$ in the last third of 96 trials related to the mean error). This difference is labelled dE% on the ordinates and is correlated with the mean enhancement of cortical negativity (dN, abscissae) when the T and IT tasks are compared for each of the 14 subjects during the first 1.5 s of tracking. Significant correlations were found only for the three recordings shown (F_3, F_4 and FC_z/SMA), giving highly significant correlation coefficients, from $r = 0.7$ (SMA) to $r = 0.82$ (left frontal, P<0.01 to P<0.001). When the coefficients of determination, d ($= r^2$), are plotted as areas of circles over the 12 recording positions, as in Fig. 5C, the main result of the study becomes obvious: significant positive correlations (open circles)

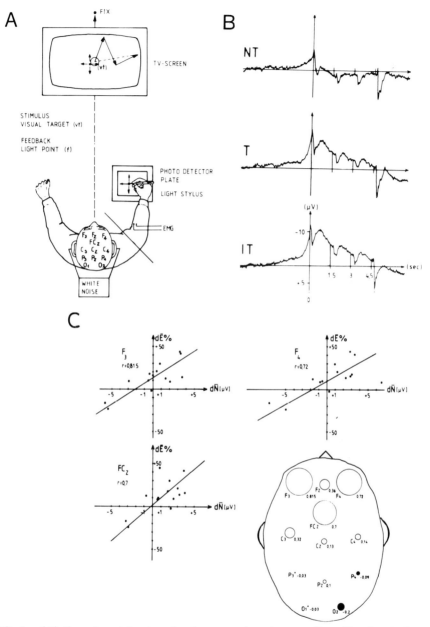

FIG. 5. (A) Experimental set-up for the motor learning paradigm (for description see text).

(B) Bereitschaftspotential and tracking-related potentials for no-tracking (NT), tracking (T) and inverted tracking (IT) tasks. For description see text.

(C) Correlations between the relative reduction of error (dĒ%) during the learning experiment of IT (ordinates) and the increase in negativity during the first trajectory in IT compared to T (dN̄, abscissae) for each of 14 individuals. There are good learners and bad learners among these individuals; good learners show a large increase in negativity between IT and T, whereas bad learners show equal or less negativity in IT compared to T. (B and C from Lang et al 1983.)

are seen only over the frontal cortex, in particular over the frontolateral convexity of both hemispheres and the frontomedial SMA region. We believe that this is essential electrophysiological evidence in humans for the importance of the frontal cortex in learning.

In a recent study with W. Lang, I Podreka and others (so far unpublished), the motor learning experiment for horizontal inverted tracking (-1 feedback only in the horizontal plane) was investigated using the regional cerebral blood flow method. Regional cerebral blood flow was measured using the single photon emission computer tomogram (SPECT) at our Neurological University Clinic in Vienna and a new technetium-bound compound (hexamethylpropylene amine oxime) which is trapped in the cell, thus enabling time resolution down to 3 min. The results using 16 subjects show significant differences in brain activity between T and IT only in frontal cortex (SMA and middle frontal gyrus of both sides) similar to the electrical findings shown in Fig. 5C. In the regional cerebral blood flow study, the maximum increase in cortical activity due to learning was found in the *right* middle frontal gyrus, which may be related to the spatial task of tracking and its feedback addressing the right hemisphere. The results will be published when the same subjects have been studied with the Bereitschaftspotential method as well.

References

Boschert J, Deecke L 1986 Cerebral potentials preceding voluntary toe, knee and hip movements and their vectors in human precentral gyrus. Brain Res 376:175–179
Boschert J, Hink RF, Deecke L 1983 Finger movement versus toe movement-related potentials: Further evidence for supplementary motor area (SMA) participation prior to voluntary action. Exp Brain Res 55:73–80
Brunia CHM 1980 What is wrong with legs in motor preparation? In: Kornhuber HH, Deecke L (eds) Motivation, motor and sensory processes of the brain: electrical potentials, behaviour and clinical use. Amsterdam, Elsevier (Prog Brain Res vol 54) p 232–236
Deecke L, Scheid P, Kornhuber HH 1969 Distribution of readiness potential, pre-motion positivity, and motor potential of the human cerebral cortex preceding voluntary finger movements. Exp Brain Res 7:158–168
Deecke L, Grözinger B, Kornhuber HH 1976 Voluntary finger movement in man: Cerebral potentials and theory. Biol Cybern 23:99–119
Deecke L, Eisinger H, Kornhuber HH 1980 Comparison of Bereitschaftspotential, pre-motion positivity and motor potential preceding voluntary flexion and extension movements in man. In: Kornhuber HH, Deecke L (eds) Motivation, motor and sensory processes of the brain: electrical potentials, behaviour and clinical use. Amsterdam, Elsevier (Prog Brain Res vol 54) p 171–176
Deecke L, Weinberg H, Brickett P 1982 Magnetic fields of the human brain accompanying voluntary movement. Bereitschaftsmagnetfeld. Exp Brain Res 48:144–148
Deecke L, Boschert J, Weinberg H, Brickett P 1983 Magnetic fields of the human brain (Bereitschaftsmagnetfeld) preceding voluntary foot and toe movements. Exp Brain Res 52:81–86

Deecke L, Heise B, Kornhuber HH, Lang M, Lang W 1984 Brain potentials associated with voluntary manual tracking: Bereitschaftspotential, conditioned premotion positivity, directed attention potential, and relaxation potential. Anticipatory activity of the limbic and frontal cortex. Ann NY Acad Sci 425:450–464

Deecke L, Boschert J, Brickett P, Weinberg H 1985 Magnetoencephalographic evidence for possible supplementary motor area participation in human voluntary movement. In: Weinberg H et al (eds) Biomagnetism: applications and theory. Pergamon Press, New York, p 369–372

DeLong MR, Strick P 1984 Relation of basal ganglia, cerebellum, and motor cortex units to ramp and ballistic movements. Brain Res 71:327–355m

Fetz EE, Cheney PD 1979 Muscle fields and response properties of primate corticomotoneuronal cells. In: Granit R, Pompeiano O (eds) Reflex control of posture and movement. Elsevier, Amsterdam (Prog Brain Res vol 50) p 137–146

Hari R, Antervo A, Katila T, Poutanen T, Seppanen N, Tuomisto T, Varpula T 1983 Cerebral magnetic fields associated with voluntary limb movements. Nuovo Cimento 2D:484–494

Kornhuber HH, Deecke L 1965 Hirnpotentialänderungen bei Willkürbewegungen und passiven Bewegungen des Menschen: Bereitschaftspotential und reafferente Potentiale. Pflügers Arch 284:1–17

Kornhuber HH, Deecke L 1985 The starting function of the SMA. Behav Brain Sci 8:591–592

Kristeva R, Deecke L 1980 Cerebral potentials preceding right and left unilateral and bilateral finger movements in sinistrals. In: Kornhuber HH, Deecke L (eds) Motivation, motor and sensory processes of the brain: Electrical potentials, behaviour and clinical use. Amsterdam, Elsevier (Prog Brain Res vol 54) p 748–754

Lang W, Lang M, Kornhuber A, Deecke L, Kornhuber HH 1983 Human cerebral potentials and visuomotor learning. Pflügers Arch 399:342–344

Penfield W, Rasmussen T 1950 The cerebral cortex of man. Macmillan, New York

Roland PE 1987 Metabolic mapping of sensorimotor integration in the human brain. This volume, p 251–268

Thach WT 1987 Cerebellar inputs to motor cortex. This volume, p 201–220

DISCUSSION

Wiesendanger: You propose that the SMA is the main source generating the readiness potentials. How confident are you about the uniqueness or special role played by the SMA? To what extent might other regions of the cortex also be implicated? You suggest that in animal studies one should use self-paced movements. Sasaki and his colleague (Gemba & Sasaki 1984) have in fact done this and they found similar pre-movement potentials in the monkey. The distribution was wide and those in the premotor cortex had a higher amplitude than those in the SMA, which were disappointingly small in the monkey.

Deecke: We pointed out that pre-movement preparation is widespread, with both hemipheres involved. With right-sided finger movements, for example, the ipsilateral precentral region and maybe other regions are also active, so we have to imagine several generators. However, if I restrict the number of principal generators to two, I think that the SMA (or roughly the fronto-central midline) in humans is one of them. The people working on regional cerebral blood flow agree. Our method does not prove that this activity is restricted to the SMA but certainly the fronto-central midline is active before voluntary movement.

If you do animal experiments I would suggest that you should not ignore field potentials, even if you are recording from single units. It would be easy to measure the surface field potentials at the same time. The two need to be put together in the same animal but this hasn't been done yet. Field potentials might allow you to see the area being switched on and off.

Goldman-Rakic: You seemed to indicate that during the inverted tracking task the individual was learning the task and that this explained why the right frontal or prefrontal areas were involved. Rather than new learning engaging the prefrontal cortex, maybe the inverted tracking test brings in the necessity of regulating behaviour by representation. I think your task is not a straightforward visually guided response but has some element of representational guidance of behaviour. That would be consistent with what I presented earlier, as we are also studying the spatial system in the non-human primate. Have you looked at this in subjects after they have learnt the task? I suspect you would see the same as we see in animals.

Deecke: I thought these findings were nicely confirmed by yours. The sensory association area which is also necessary for tracking does not show the learning effect—that is, the significant correlation between the reduction in error and the increase in negativity. The learning effect was seen only in frontal areas. The evidence presented makes us think that this area has something to do with learning, but it is not the only learning centre in the brain. It is part of a memory loop, which may also include the hippocampus. However, I think activity of the frontal convexity is a necessary prerequisite for learning. We are in the process of studying people who have learnt the inverted tracking test.

Goldman-Rakic: I think that prefrontal cortex may still be needed to regulate behaviour after the task has been learnt. In the overtrained person you may see the same engagement of this area.

Kuypers: With magnetoencephalography one can localize activity to a much greater extent than with electroencephalography. Can you really pinpoint activity to the medial aspect of the hemisphere and, in particular, exclude the activity of the cingulate gyrus as being the real source?

Deecke: We cannot distinguish whether the cingulate gyrus or the medial cortical surface above the cingulate sulcus is the active area, or whether both of these are active. We just find the potential over the fronto-central midline. In theory, magnetoencephalography will be able to pinpoint the activity precisely, when combined with EEG. At present only one channel at a time is used for recording the magnetic field. This is a bit tricky methodologically because you never know whether the brain is in the same set from one experiment to the next. We will have to wait for multichannel recordings.

This method has also been used to map the representation of tones in the human auditory cortex, in Heschl's gyrus. With high pitch the generator was different from that with low pitch and one was able to localize the tones of different pitch in a three-dimensional manner.

Porter: The method still has the disadvantage of needing to average a number of repetitions over a period of time.

Marsden: What sort of spatial resolution will multichannel magnetoencephalograms achieve?

Deecke: It will be in the range of millimetres.

Wu: You showed that the readiness potential in the midline started much earlier than the readiness potential presumably generated by the motor cortex. However, in animal experiments the difference in onset times of unit activities in SMA and the motor area, in relation to a task movement, is not conspicuous. Also the onset time of midline readiness potential is much earlier than that of the unit activity in SMA. How do you explain these discrepancies?

Deecke: I think that the readiness potential is a summation of the synaptic events, i.e. the sum of EPSPs. What we investigate is a synaptic drive or facilitation involving these areas. This paradigm shows, in an anticipatory foreperiod, which cortical areas will be active in a certain task and which will not. You should not take our onset times literally and try to correlate them with the single units. We are not recording the spike activity but the synaptic/postsynaptic activity of the apical dendrites in superficial cortical layers.

Wu: You mean it takes some time to build up to the threshold of spike activity?

Deecke: Yes.

Lemon: Those EPSPs have to come eventually from spike-generating neurons. People who have looked at self-paced movements in the main structures upstream of area 4 have not found cells generating action potentials that fire at those sorts of times ahead of movement.

Deecke: This synaptic drive can come from other areas, for instance from the SMA, the basal ganglia, the cerebellum or elsewhere. The spike activity may be low at this time but synaptic drive is already there. Other people's work on animals shows that the spike as such is not propagated enough to be measurable in the scalp EEG.

Lemon: Yes, but the synaptic drive should be detectable.

Deecke: The EPSPs are propagated very widely and I think that glia cells help in propagation.

Marsden: The question of whether one is looking at neuronal discharge within the cortex itself, with synaptic activity driving the neuronal discharge, is crucial. My understanding is that discharges from large pyramidal tract neurons produce a negative field potential deep within layer V which is reflected as positivity of the cortical surface. Elger et al's (1981) work with intracortical penicillin injection to produce local discharge in different cortical layers supports that conclusion. Your surface EEG recordings show exactly the opposite to what one would expect from a deep discharge of corticomotoneurons. That is confirmed to some extent by examination of surface potentials in patients with cortical myoclonus, where deep cortical discharges generate muscle twitches and positivity on the surface, not negativity. I support your interpretation that this is synaptic activity within the cortex, not the output of neurons in layer V. Therefore you have to look at the input to SMA and lateral premotor areas, such as that from the basal ganglia, to decipher what generates the negative Bereitschaftspotential.

Deecke: I underline this vigorously. We can see negativity only in superficial cortical layers, not in deeper structures.

Marsden: You are talking about 1s before movement occurs, but people examining single units in deep structures have not looked at this so early.

Deecke: Other components, for instance the P300 component, are positive in the EEG. Magnetoencephalography shows that this component stems from the hippocampus. So a structure as deep as the hippocampus—the P300 probably being negative there—gives positive components at the scalp surface. C.C. Wood et al (personal communication) have shown in epileptic patients, in whom intracerebral electrical recordings were made using a probe penetrating the temporal lobe from lateral posterior to medial anterior (roughly parallel to the sylvian fissure), that the P300 was positive on approaching the hippocampus, negative in the hippocampus itself and positive on leaving the hippocampus.

Fetz: One of the advantages of the magnetic recording seems to be its capacity to pick up sources at subcortical as well as cortical levels. What is the relative contribution of subcortical and cortical sources in your records?

Deecke: Other people, including the group at the Burden Neurological Institute in Bristol (McCallum et al 1976), have made recordings from electrodes in patients with 'fractionated lobotomy'. When they recorded from the surface both the readiness potential and the contingent negative variation were negative. In the white matter both were positive and in the thalamus they were negative again. Therefore, the barrage of negativities may come from deeper structures.

Tanji: We have done some work on self-paced versus visually triggered movement in monkeys. The animal had to push keys in two modes. In one mode it pushed a key in response to a visual cue and then released it. The full cycle took 2.2 to 3.5s. In the self-paced mode there was no visual cue and the animal had to wait for at least 5s before pressing the key to get the reward. In both these modes we observed movement-related changes in both SMA and premotor cortex. Long-lasting changes (400 ms to more than 1s), however, are more often seen in the SMA cells. So there were some differences between the activity of SMA and that of premotor cortex.

Deecke: That the SMA shows sustained firing during holding periods would be in line with our belief that it has a timing function.

Tanji: I think you are correct about the cell activity. We also tried to record the slowly developing field potentials. We put a surface electrode on top of the SMA but strangely we did not get clear activity changes from that electrode. We think that the direction of the electrical dipole in the SMA is not properly oriented for surface recording in the monkey. I am not sure what happens in humans.

Thach: Is this kind of gradual build-up not present in motor cortex? In other movement experiments you have recorded both in SMA and in motor cortex. Would you predict a difference in this case?

Tanji: We did see long-lasting activity in the motor cortex but the frequency of occurrence is less than in area 6. We observed more of that activity in the SMA.

Calne: Professor Deecke, have you studied the influence of the nature of the task on the build-up of the preparation potential? For example, how does the potential differ when there is a very sensitive delicate movement as opposed to a situation where maximal force has to be applied?

Deecke: We tried to relate force to the amplitude of the readiness potential. This holds to a certain degree for a small amplitude.

Calne: Is that so, even if the precision is much greater for the weak force?

Deecke: We did experiments with complex movements in which the amplitude was increased. It is not force alone but also effort or engagement in the motor task which builds up high amplitudes. When someone makes a careless movement without attention or engagement the potential is low in amplitude. If the individual really engages in the movement the potential is high. When we investigated bilateral simultaneous movement in right-handed subjects we expected to find an effect of handedness because when we compare right-sided movement with left-sided we get a larger readiness potential on the dominant hemisphere for the preferred hand. But with this bilateral movement the minor hemisphere showed the larger potential. Our explanation is that the non-preferred hand had difficulty in keeping up with the preferred hand, so the effort needed was greater.

Porter: The regional cerebral blood flow studies by Per Roland and his colleagues (1980) indicated that there was considerable difference in cerebral blood flow in the supplementary motor area, depending on the complexity of the task.

Deecke: The complexity has two effects, as seen in the writing experiments; it increases the amplitude and the onset time. Preparation starts earlier with complex tasks. Furthermore, it is our impression that the maximum Bereitschaftspotential over the midline was more anterior for writing and drawing than for simple movements.

References

Elger CE, Speckmann EJ, Prohaska O, Caspers H 1981 Pattern of intracortical potential distribution during focal interictal epileptiform discharges (FIED) and its relation to spinal field potentials in the rat. Electroencephalogr Clin Neurophysiol 51:393–402

Gemba H, Sasaki K 1984 Distribution of potentials preceding visually initiated and self-paced hand movements in various cortical areas of the monkey. Brain Res 306:207–214

McCallum WC, Papakostopoulos D, Griffith HB 1976 Distribution of CNV and other slow potential changes in human brainstem structures. In: McCallum WC, Knott JR (eds) The responsive brain. John Wright & Sons, Bristol, p 205–210

Roland PE, Larsen B, Lassen NA, Skinhoj E 1980 Supplementary and other cortical areas in organization of voluntary movements in man. J Neurophysiol 43:118–136

Metabolic mapping of sensorimotor integration in the human brain

P.E. Roland

Department of Clinical Neurophysiology, Karolinska Hospital, S10401, Solna, Sweden

Abstract. Studies of regional cerebral flow and regional cerebral oxidative metabolism have revealed that humans have three major cortical motor areas: the premotor, supplementary motor and primary motor areas. The premotor area participates in organizing non-routine voluntary movements, especially those carried out contingent to or dependent on sensory information. The supplementary motor area participates in the planning of all motor subroutines. The primary motor area is the executive locus for voluntary movements. Subcortically the caudate nucleus, putamen, globus pallidus, parasagittal cerebellum and ventral thalamus are the main structures which increase their metabolism during voluntary movements of the upper limbs. All these cortical and subcortical structures except the primary motor area are bilaterally activated even during strictly unilateral movements of the upper limbs. However, recent studies of oxidative metabolism show that the caudate nucleus, putamen and lateral cerebellum also participate in cognitive functions and non-motor learning. Before any specific brain work is executed, voluntary movements included, the brain tunes and prepares cortical fields measuring a few square centimetres in the areas that are supposed to participate in information transmission. The superior prefrontal cortex has a special role in this recruitment of cortical fields. Depending on the information needed to execute the voluntary movements, cortical fields are activated in the anterior parietal lobe and the dysgranular frontal cortex.

1987 Motor areas of the cerebral cortex. Wiley, Chichester (Ciba Foundation Symposium 132) p 251–268

In this short paper I shall try to describe and analyse the patterns of cerebral metabolic activation that accompany voluntary motor activity in humans. In particular I will try to analyse the metabolic patterns that emerge when sensory information is used for programming voluntary movements. These patterns emerged in experiments in which normal individuals were asked or (sometimes) trained to perform different types of voluntary motor activities while their regional metabolism was measured in all parts of the brain. In this way these human studies are fundamentally different from studies of reinforcement in animals. Yet there seems to be general agreement between human studies and other primate studies on the structures which change activity during the planning and execution of voluntary movements (Kennedy et al 1980, and Georgopoulos, Tanji, Thach and Passingham in this volume).

The techniques of single photon tomography and intracarotid injection of single photon tracers allow one to measure regional blood flow in the cortex, and positron emission tomography allows one to measure the regional metabolism of the whole brain. As in other types of behavioural neurophysiology, regional cerebral blood flow (rCBF) and metabolic activity during motor activity has to be compared with the rCBF or metabolic activity during a control state, rest (Roland & Larsen 1976), in which the subject does not move, has no detailed plans for moving, and no intention of moving. Unlike autoradiographic studies, in these studies one can measure the changes in metabolism associated with the production of voluntary behaviour in the same individual.

In the normal brain rCBF is adjusted to local metabolic demands. That is, a change in regional cerebral oxygen consumption is followed by a proportional change in rCBF (Roland et al 1987). Because the brain uses glucose almost exclusively as an energy source, changes in the regional cerebral metabolic rate of glucose are also linearly correlated with changes in regional cerebral oxygen consumption. Measurements of regional cerebral oxygen and glucose consumption and of rCBF thus provide quantitative measures of local neuronal and glial metabolism. In the normal cerebral neocortex an increase in local metabolism presumably indicates a net local increase in average excitation (Roland & Friberg 1983). Increases in metabolism after physiological brain work occur predominantly in the neuropil and predominantly where the density of active synapses is greatest (Mata et al 1980, Hand et al 1978). If a cortical field shows an increase in metabolism this could therefore be due to increased excitation by afferent synapses or to increased excitation of intrinsic synapses.

Cortical field activation

One of the main findings from metabolic mapping studies is that cortical neurons always seem to be activated in a large ensemble that covers a cortical area of 3–9 cm^2. This is the cortical field activation hypothesis (Roland 1985a) which applies to physiological activation of the motor areas (Roland & Larsen 1976, Larsen et al 1978, 1979, Orgogozo & Larsen 1979) as well as to other neocortical areas (Roland 1985a, 1985b) (see also Figs. 3,4,5). Within such a field the estimated number of neurons ranges from 3×10^6 to 9×10^6 and the number of synapses from 2.6×10^{11} to 7.8×10^{11} (Cragg 1967, Huttenlocher 1979). Presumably only a few of these synapses are active during physiological brain work, but this would still leave a few million neurons participating in information transformation in each field.

In the primary motor area (MI) and the primary somatosensory area (SI) fields are activated in a somatotopical fashion (Roland & Larsen 1976,

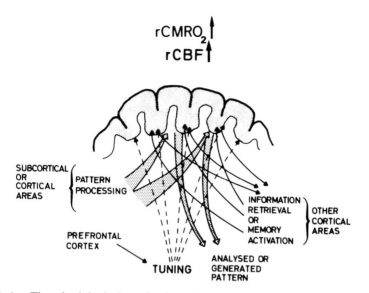

FIG. 1. The physiological mechanisms that can increase the metabolism and the regional cerebral blood flow (rCBF) of a cortical field. The metabolism can increase because the neurons constituting the field are transforming information. The information transformation or pattern processing is assumed to be spread over the entire field. Direction of attention towards the field results in a tuning of its neurons. When the field is recruited for retrieval of its memory content the metabolism also increases over the entire field. rCMRO$_2$, regional cerebral oxygen consumption. (Modified slightly from Roland 1984c.)

Orgogozo & Larsen 1979). In the non-primary sensory areas and the non-primary motor areas as well as in the rest of the homotypical cortex fields are activated in a non-somatotopical fashion (Roland & Larsen 1976, Orgogozo & Larsen 1979, Roland & Friberg 1985). Studies of the effects of circumscribed brain lesions in humans have shown that, with the exception of the primary motor and primary sensory areas, damage to part of a cortical area is not associated with any measurable loss of information; only a total or a nearly total lesion of a cortical area gives rise to loss of information (Roland 1987). The information representation and information processing that take place in a cortical field are therefore almost uniformly spread within the field. When a cortical field participates in specific brain work it thus displays a kind of distributed information processing (Roland 1985a, 1987). Macroscopically the size, shape and location of a participating cortical field is unaltered even when the content of the information to be retrieved or processed in the field is changed (Roland & Friberg 1985). From autoradiographic studies in monkeys one can estimate that each metabolically active field presumably consists of multiple metabolically active bands, which in turn consist of multiple metabolically active columns (Juliano et al 1981, 1983, Goldman-Rakic et al 1983).

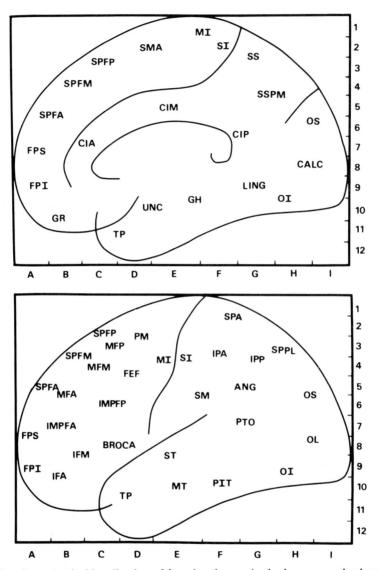

FIG. 2.   Stereotactical localization of functional areas in the human cerebral cortex.
Some areas, such as ST, PTO and IMPFA, probably consist of functionally different
subareas. As the number of metabolic experiments increases, the number of functional subdivisions can also be expected to increase. FP, frontal pole; SPF, superior
prefrontal; IMPF, intermediate prefrontal; MF, mid-frontal; CI, cingular; SMA,
supplementary motor area; PM, premotor area; SS, supplementary sensory; SSP,
superior parietal posterior; SPA, superior parietal anterior; IP, intraparietal; LING,
lingualis; GH, gyrus hippocampalis; UNC, uncinate gyrus; SM, supramarginal; ANG,
angular; PTO, parieto-temporo-occipital; O, occipital; T, temporal; F, frontal.

The active fields in monkeys are smaller than the human fields.

A cortical field may increase its metabolism because it is participating in information transformation (Roland & Larsen 1976, Roland et al 1977, 1980a, 1980b, 1985) because its memory content is being retrieved (Roland & Friberg 1985, Roland et al 1987), and because it is being tuned—that is, prepared for treatment of later-arriving information (Roland 1981). This is illustrated in Fig. 1.

In the human cerebral cortex transformation of information takes place simultaneously in several cortical *fields*. Planning and execution of voluntary movements is no exception. The experiments of Georgopoulos and collaborators (see Georgopoulos, this volume) on the population coding of vectors for the direction of voluntary movements are excellent demonstrations of the distributed information processing that takes place in the motor fields.

Studies of the location of metabolically active fields during various test procedures have revealed that the cerebral neocortex is composed of at least 32 functionally different areas plus at least five different insular regions in each hemisphere (Fig. 2). Few of these areas are consistently active during the planning and execution of voluntary movements. That is, the non-motor areas are not consistently active when the task performed by the brain does not include movement or the disposition to move.

The anatomical structures participating in the planning and execution of voluntary movements

Metabolic measurements of the cerebral cortex during motor tasks and non-motor tasks have revealed that humans have three major motor areas: MI, the supplementary motor area (SMA) and the premotor area (PM). The SMA and PM are not always active during voluntary movements but they have so far never been active in non-motor tasks.

MI is activated whenever voluntary movements are executed (Olesen 1971, Risberg & Ingvar 1973, Roland & Larsen 1976, Mazziotta & Phelps 1984) but not when subjects have no voluntary motor activity (Roland & Larsen 1976, Roland & Friberg 1985). Since an increase in metabolism in a cortical area means that the synapses increase their metabolism, other areas or structures must increase excitation in MI, or MI must increase its intrinsic activity, or both must happen, whenever voluntary movements are executed. Since MI is always metabolically active when voluntary movements are executed it has been called the executive locus for voluntary movements (Roland et al 1980b). Very often MI is coactivated with SMA.

SMA and PM can be activated without there being any voluntary motor activity (Roland & Larsen 1976, Roland et al 1977, 1980a). However, SMA and PM should be considered motor areas since active fields appear in these

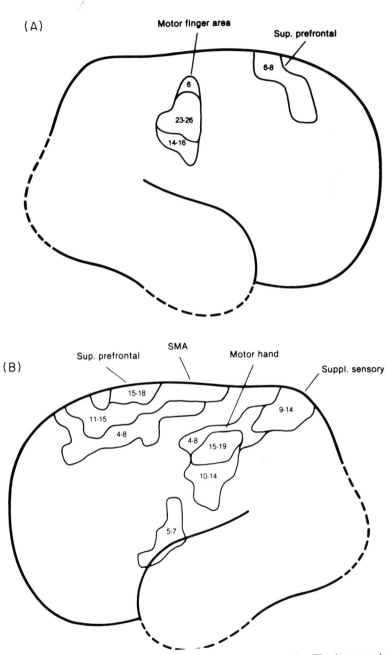

FIG. 3. Examples of cortical field activation in motor tasks. The increase in regional cerebral blood flow in each field is shown in ml 100 g^{-1} min^{-1}. (A) This person repetitively flexed the left index finger (right hemisphere). (B) This person did the motor sequence test with the right hand. In this test the thumb has to touch the index finger twice, the middle finger once, the ring finger three times and the little finger twice, all in quick succession (Roland et al 1977) (left hemisphere).

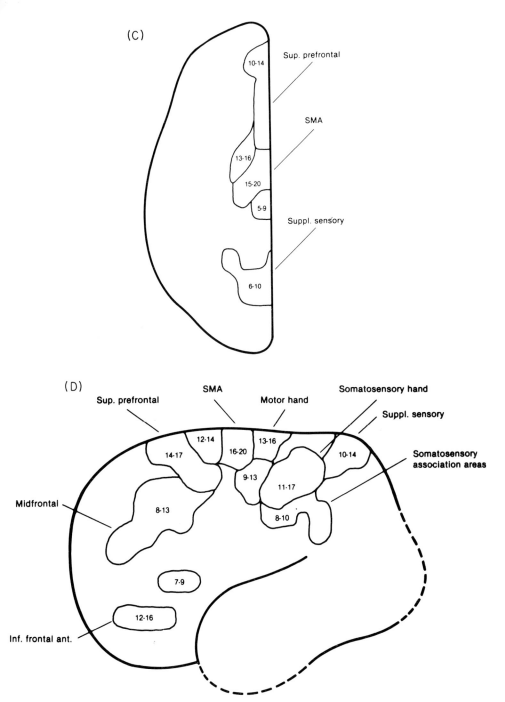

(C) Purely internal programming of the motor sequence test without any movements (vertex view, left hemisphere). (D) Discrimination of the shape of ellipsoids with the right hand (left hemisphere).

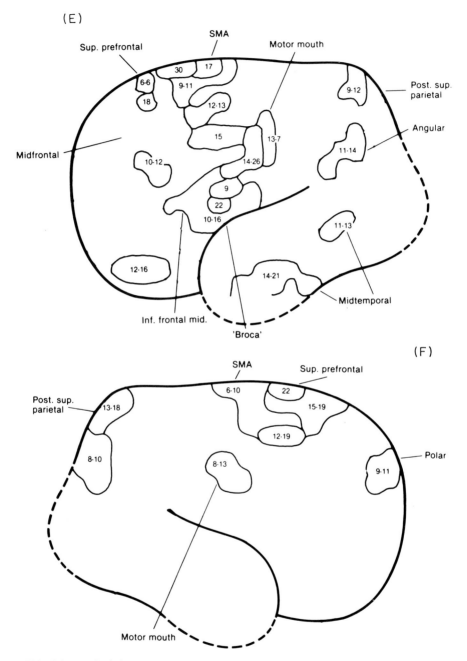

FIG. 3 (contd.). (E) Fluent descriptive speech in which the individual described every piece of furniture in his living-room (left hemisphere). (F) Same procedure as previous individual (right hemisphere). (From Roland 1985a, with permission from Raven Press.)

areas under conditions that include the disposition to move. SMA has not been coactivated in any fixed pattern with other cortical areas (Roland 1984a, 1985b). SMA is activated during the planning and execution of voluntary motor activity that consists of complicated movement sequences (Fig. 3) (Roland et al 1980a). Well-learnt sequences of movements for which no sensory information is necessary, including speech, activate SMA but not PM (Roland et al 1977, 1980a, 1982, 1985, Larsen et al 1978, 1979, Fox et al 1985a). SMA is programming motor subroutines. Simple non-deterministic movements and more complex sequences that are conditioned in response to sensory signals will activate SMA (Fox et al 1985a). In contrast to MI, SMA is always bilaterally activated (Roland et al 1977, Fox et al 1985a). In front of SMA is another area which is activated during eye movements (Melamed & Larsen 1979, Roland et al 1981, Fox et al 1985a).

PM participates in non-routine voluntary movements, in particular those performed under sensory guidance (auditory, visual, somatosensory) (Roland & Larsen 1976, Ingvar & Philipson 1977, Roland et al 1980b) (see also Fig. 5, and Passingham, Georgopoulos and Tanji in this volume). Pure motor subroutines, such as very routine tasks not dependent on sensory information and speech, do not activate PM (Larsen et al 1978, Roland et al 1980a). So far SMA has been activated in most instances where the PM has been activated (Roland 1985b). However, metabolic increases in PM and SMA have not been correlated (Roland 1985b). The PM does not appear in any fixed coactivation pattern with other cortical areas. As mentioned above, metabolic increase in SMA or PM mean (1) that the area is tuned, (2) that it participates in information transformation in motor control or (3) that its memory content is being retrieved. The metabolic increase does not tell us which of these possibilities applies in a given situation.

Subcortically the caudate nucleus, putamen and globus pallidus are bilaterally metabolically active during unilateral limb movements (Fig. 4) (Roland et al 1982, Mazziotta & Phelps 1984). Although the basal ganglia participate in voluntary motor activity they are by no means exclusively motor structures. Thinking, without any motor elements, also increases metabolism bilaterally in the basal ganglia (Roland et al 1987). Presumably different sectors of the basal ganglia are devoted to motor control and cognitive processing (Dauth et al 1985). The ventral thalamus has also been bilaterally metabolically active during voluntary movements (Figs. 3 and 5) (Roland et al 1982, Mazziotta & Phelps 1984).

The cerebellum is activated in motor tasks but, like the basal ganglia and thalamus, it cannot be considered exclusively a motor structure. The parasagittal part is bilaterally activated during unilateral finger movements (Plate I) (Fox et al 1985b). The parasagittal and lateral parts of lobus posterius are bilaterally activated during tactile learning (Plate I). The lateral part of lobus posterius is also activated during thinking (Roland et al 1987).

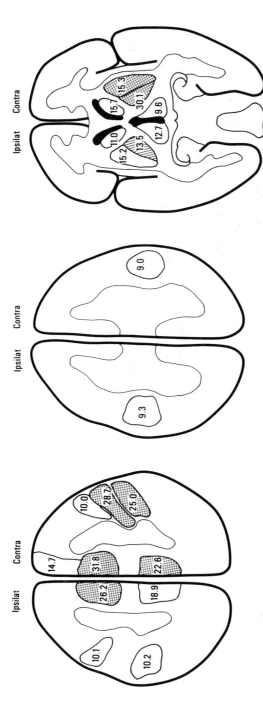

FIG. 4.   Mean percentage increase in regional cerebral blood flow and mean extensions of the increases while the motor sequence test (see text) was performed with one hand by 10 normal volunteers. Three sections of the brain are shown with a separation of 17.5 mm. Cross-hatched areas $P<0.001$, hatched areas $P<0.01$, other areas $P<0.05$ (t test, Dunnet's corrections). (From Roland et al 1982, by permission of the American Physiological Society.)

The cerebellum, basal ganglia and thalamus may therefore consist of sections devoted to motor control and sections devoted to non-motor functions.

Sensorimotor integration

Posterior to the cortical motor zones there are other cortical areas which are frequently coactivated with PM, SMA and MI during sensorimotor tasks. These are the primary somatosensory area (SI) and the somatosensory association areas (SII), the supplementary sensory area (SS), the anterior part of lobulus parietalis superior (SPA) and the parietal operculum-retroinsular cortex (RI-PO).

Tactile discrimination of the shapes of previously unknown objects elicits an array of manipulatory movements which are controlled by PM, SMA and MI (Plate I) (Roland & Larsen 1976, Roland 1985c). During tactile explorations of unknown objects these areas are coactivated with SI, SS, SPA and SII (Roland 1985c) (Plate I). The manipulatory movements are highly differentiated independent scanning movements of one, two or three fingers, interchanged with rolling and rotation of the unknown object. It can be demonstrated that the scanning movements are so well planned that the maximum information about the unknown object is extracted in each scanning movement (Roland & Mortensen 1987). Unilateral damage to the motor areas PM, SMA and MI, and to SI, severely impair these exploratory movements (Roland 1987). However, subtotal and total selective damage to any one of the areas SS, RI-PO and in particular SII also impairs the scanning movements and the rolling and rotation (Roland 1987). The sensory information which is provided by these areas, especially SII, is thus indispensable for programming tactile exploration.

How the human brain integrates sensory information and motor control is shown in Plate I. Here regional cerebral oxygen consumption is measured during a tactile recognition task. The individual first has to learn 10 complicated objects, each consisting of several geometrical shapes. The information content of each object is known exactly. After three learning sessions the 10 objects are mixed with other similar but previously unknown objects. Unknown and known objects are then presented with a probability of 0.5 in a randomized schedule. The probability of success in this task is, as in our previous sensory tasks, 0.75. Each person has 3s in which to manipulate each object presented. During this time the person has to determine whether he has a known or an unknown object in his hands. If he thinks he has a known object, he quickly raises his thumb. All the objects are presented in his right hand. Behaviourally tactile recognition thus consists of a series of fast tactile exploratory movements and eventually of some quick raises of the thumb. Formally the task consists of a sampling of sensory information. The sampled information is then compared to the information stored in a tactile memory. Contingent on the result of this comparison and on a decision as to whether the amount of sampled information is sufficient to define the object either new sampling movements are programmed or the motor programme for thumb extension is executed.

This tactile recognition increased the regional cerebral oxygen consumption in prefrontal areas, parietal cortex, sensorimotor areas, limbic structures, basal ganglia and cerebellum. In the prefrontal cortex the superior frontal polar area (FPS) and the superior prefrontal mid-section (SPFM) were activated in the left hemisphere, the whole midfrontal section (MFA, MFM, MFP) was activated in the right hemisphere, and the intermediate posterior prefrontal cortex was activated bilaterally. In the parietal cortex the left supramarginal (SM) area was activated. The hippocampi, the lingual gyri and the anterior insular region was activated bilaterally. The most pronounced increases in regional cerebral oxygen consumption appeared in the left MI and SI (hand area), and bilaterally in the SMA, PM, SS, SII-RI-PO, thalamus and the putamen-globus pallidus (Plate I). In the cerebellum the parasagittal parts of the anterior lobe were activated bilaterally whereas a minor increase in regional oxygen consumption was seen in the lateral parts of the posterior lobe on both sides.

In eight individuals regional cerebral oxygen consumption was also measured during tactile learning. During the tactile learning sessions the objects to be learnt are placed in the right hand at intervals of 10s. The exploratory movements are considerably slower than during tactile recognition, with the individuals using only about half the number of rolls, rotations and dynamic scanning movements per minute. This resulted in a slight but statistically significant decrease in regional cerebral oxygen consumption in the left SMA, PM and SI hand area compared to tactile recognition ($P<0.01$). However, the increases in the lateral part of lobus posterius in both cerebellar hemispheres were greater during learning ($P<0.01$) (Plate I). Otherwise there were no differences between tactile learning and tactile recognition. Therefore, the extra increase in oxygen consumption in the lateral parts of neocerebellum during tactile learning is assumed to be due to energy-demanding metabolic processes involved in the storage of information.

Exactly what kind of information is stored is not possible to state from these experiments. From the cortical regions which raise their oxidative metabolism, one cannot say whether the observed increase in regional cerebral oxygen consumption in the basal ganglia, ventral thalamus and cerebellum is a consequence of the metabolic increases in the prefrontal cortex or those in the sensorimotor fields. The lateral cerebellum receives connections from the prefrontal cortex as well as from sensorimotor areas (Sasaki 1979). The increases in oxygen consumption in the basal ganglia, thalamus and parasagittal cerebellum could be related to the ongoing sensorimotor activities (Roland et al 1982, Fox et al 1985b). The role of the activated superior prefrontal area in the internal organization of brain work in general and the

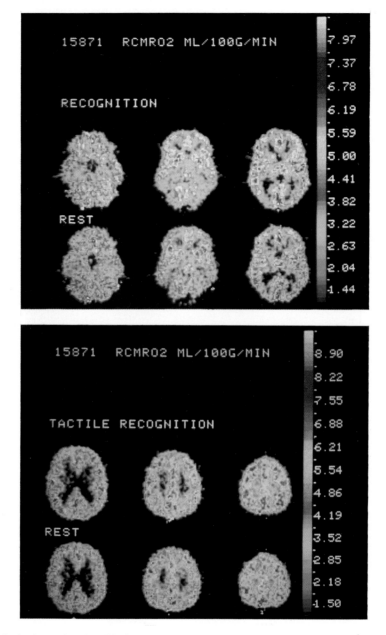

Plate I. 1, 2: regional oxidative metabolism, rCMRO$_2$, at rest and during tactile recognition in a normal young right-handed man. The brain slices are seen from below (right side of slice is left side of brain). The slices were taken 18 and 5 mm below the commissural plane and 8, 20, 32 and 46 mm above it. Hippocampus not shown. Increases in rCMRO$_2$ appear bilaterally in parasagittal cerebellum, basal ganglia, ventral thalamus, anterior insular region, SII, SS, SMA, PM, anterior intraparietal region (IPA) and prefrontal cortex; increases also appear in left MI and SI. *(Plate I continued overleaf.)*

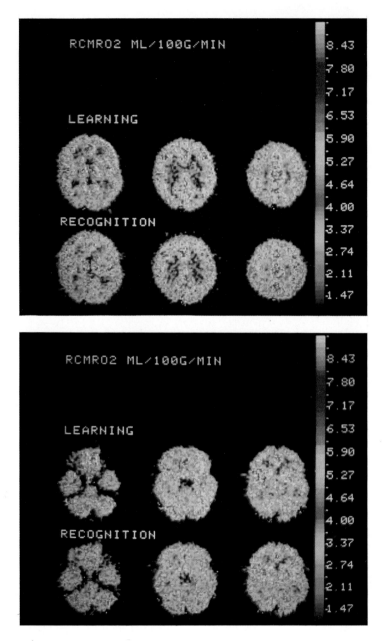

Plate I *(continued)* 3, 4: rCMRO₂ in a volunteer during tactile learning and tactile recognition. Although the frequency of voluntary movements is only 50% of that seen during tactile recognition, the lateral cerebellum (posterior lobe) is more metabolically active during tactile learning. Structures that are metabolically active are identical during learning and recognition. Slices were taken 21 and 7 mm below the commissural plane and 6, 20, 34 and 46 mm above it. (Experiments by P. E. Roland, L. Eriksson, L. Widén and S. Stone-Elander.)

possible roles of the anterior midfrontal and anterior intermediate prefrontal areas have been dealt with in recent reviews (Roland 1984b, 1985b).

Although the PM, SMA, SS and SII frequently work together in sensori-motor tasks this should not lead to the erroneous belief that these soma-tosensory association areas participate whenever a sensorimotor task is undertaken by the brain. So far, no deterministic coactivations between any two areas in the cortex have been demonstrated (Roland 1985b).

References

Cragg BG 1967 The density of synapses and neurons in the motor and visual areas of the cerebral cortex. J Anat 101:639–654

Dauth GW, Gilman S, Frey KA, Penney JB 1985 Basal ganglia glucose utilization after recent precentral ablation in the monkey. Ann Neurol 17:431–438

Fox PT, Fox JM, Raichle ME, Burde RM 1985a The role of cerebral cortex in the generation of voluntary saccades: a positron emission tomographic study. J Neurophysiol 54:348–369

Fox PT, Raichle ME, Thach WT 1985b Functional mapping of the human cerebellum with positron emission tomography. Proc Natl Acad Sci USA 82:7462–7466

Georgopoulos AP 1987 Neural mechanisms of reaching. This volume, p 125–141

Goldman-Rakic PS, Isseroff A, Schwartz ML, Bugbee NM 1983 In: Mussen P (ed) Handbook of child psychology: biology and infancy development, Wiley, New York, p 281–341

Hand P, Greenberg JH, Miselis RR, Weller WL, Reivich M 1978 A normal and altered cortical column. Soc Neurosci Abstr 4:553

Huttenlocher PR 1979 Synaptic density in human frontal cortex—developmental changes and effects of aging. Brain Res 163:195–205

Ingvar DH, Philipson L 1977 Distribution of cerebral blood flow in the dominant hemisphere during motor ideation and motor performance. Ann Neurol 2:230–237

Juliano S, Hand PJ, Whitsel BL 1981 Patterns of increased metabolic activity in somatosensory cortex of macaca fascicularis, subjected to controlled cutaneous stimulation: a 2-deoxyglucose study. J Neurophysiol 46:1260–1284

Juliano SL, Hand PJ, Whitsel BL 1983 Patterns of metabolic activity in cytoarchitectu-ral area SII and surrounding cortical fields of the monkey. J Neurophysiol 50:961–980

Kennedy C, Miyaoka M, Suda S et al 1980 Local metabolic responses in brain accompanying motor activity. Trans Am Neurol Assoc 105:13–17

Larsen B, Skinhöj E, Lassen NA 1978 Variations in regional cortical blood flow in the right and left hemispheres during automatic speech. Brain 101:193–209

Larsen B, Skinhöj E, Lassen NA 1979 Cortical activity of left and right hemisphere provided by reading and visual naming. Acta Neurol Scand Suppl 72:6–7

Mata M, Fink DJ, Gainer H et al 1980 Activity-dependent energy metabolism in rat posterior pituitary primarily reflects sodium pump activity. J Neurochem 34:213–215

Mazziotta JC, Phelps ME 1984 Positron computed tomographic studies of cerebral metabolic responses to complex motor tasks. Neurology 34:116

Melamed E, Larsen B 1979 Cortical activation pattern during saccadic eye movements in human: localization of focal cerebral blood flow increases. Ann Neurol 5:79–88

Olesen J 1971 Contralateral focal increase of cerebral blood flow in man during arm work. Brain 94:635–646

Orgogozo JM, Larsen B 1979 Activation of the supplementary motor area during voluntary movements in man suggests it works as a supramotor area. Science (Wash DC) 206:847–850

Risberg J, Ingvar DH 1973 Patterns of activation in the gray matter of the dominant hemisphere during memorization and reasoning. Brain 96:737–756

Roland PE 1981 Somatotopical tuning of postcentral gyrus during focal attention in man. A regional cerebral blood flow study. J Neurophysiol 46:744–754

Roland PE 1984a Organization of motor control by the normal human brain. Hum Neurobiol 2:205–216

Roland PE 1984b Metabolic measurements of the working frontal cortex in man. Trends Neurosci 7:430–435

Roland PE 1984c Intensity and localizations of cortical activations in man during sensory discrimination, directed attention and thinking. In: Garlick DG, Korner PI (eds) Frontiers in physiological research. Australian Academy of Science, Canberra

Roland PE 1985a Application of imaging of brain blood flow to behavioral neurophysiology: The cortical field activation hypothesis. In: Sokoloff L (ed) Brain imaging and brain function. Raven Press, New York, p 87–104

Roland PE 1985b Cortical organization of voluntary behavior in man. Hum Neurobiol 4:155–167

Roland PE 1985c Somatosensory detection in man. In: Goodwin AW, Darian-Smith I (eds) Hand function and the neocortex. Springer, Berlin. Exp Brain Res Suppl 10:93–110

Roland PE 1987 Somatosensory detection in microgeometry, macrogeometry and kinesthesia after localized lesions of the cerebral hemispheres in man. Brain Res Rev 12:43–94

Roland PE, Friberg L 1983 Are cortical rCBF increases during brain work in man due to synaptic excitation or inhibition? J Cereb Blood Flow Metab (Suppl) 3:S244–S245

Roland PE, Friberg L 1985 Localization of cortical areas activated by thinking. J Neurophysiol 53:1219–1243

Roland PE, Larsen B 1976 Focal increase in cerebral blood flow during stereognostic testing in man. Arch Neurol 33:551–558

Roland PE, Mortensen E 1987 Somatosensory detection of microgeometry, macrogeometry and kinesthesia in man. Brain Res Rev 12:1–42

Roland PE, Skinhoj E, Larsen B, Endo H 1977 Perception and voluntary action: localization of basic input and output functions as revealed by regional cerebral blood flow increases in the human brain. In: Meyer JS et al (eds) Cerebral vascular disease. Excerpta Medica, Amsterdam, p 40–44

Roland PE, Larsen B, Lassen NA, Skinhoj E 1980a Supplementary motor area and other cortical areas in organization of voluntary movements in man. J Neurophysiol 43:118–136

Roland PE, Skinhoj E, Lassen NA, Larsen B 1980b Different cortical areas in man in organization of voluntary movements in extrapersonal space. J Neurophysiol 43:137–150

Roland PE, Skinhoj E, Lassen NA 1981 Focal activations of the human cerebral cortex during auditory discrimination. J Neurophysiol 43:374–386

Roland PE, Meyer E, Shibasaki T, Yamamoto YL, Thompson CJ 1982 Regional cerebral blood flow changes in cortex and basal ganglia during voluntary movements in normal human volunteers. J Neurophysiol 48:467–480

Roland PE, Friberg L, Lassen NA, Olsen TS 1985 Regional cortical blood flow changes during production of fluent speech and during conversation. J Cereb Blood Flow Metab 5 (suppl 1): S205–S206

Roland PE, Eriksson L, Stone-Elander S, Widen L 1987 Does mental activity change

the oxidative metabolism of the brain? J Neurosci 7:
Sasaki K 1979 Cerebro-cerebellar interconnections in cats and monkeys. In: Massion
J, Sasaki K (eds) Cerebro-cerebellar interactions. Elsevier, Amsterdam, p 105–124

DISCUSSION

Calne: Pictures like these are interesting but difficult to interpret. In positron emission tomography scans with fluorodeoxyglucose we tried to find differences between moving a hand and not moving a hand. One problem is how much the images are influenced by stress and attention. All the emphasis of the task is on the motor and sensory activity of the right hand, so I am surprised that there isn't more lateralization between the right and left in your scans.

Roland: We made measurements in 60 s, not during 45 or 60 min as you do with fluorodeoxyglucose. The two techniques and the results obtained are not comparable.

We don't see any lack of lateralization if by this you mean that the presumably active part, the left motor and left sensory hand area, is more metabolically active than the corresponding area on the right.

Calne: The tasks were very difficult and the processes of learning and recognition would generate a great deal of stress.

Roland: That is why we always pace them at the same rate, giving them a new object every 4s, exactly as we have done in all previous studies. We also did cerebral blood flow studies in which we studied the effects of attention. We cannot attribute the changes we see in the lateral part of the cerebellum to differences in attention. All our experience tends the other way. We would expect more metabolic activity during the 'stressful' recognition period than during the relaxed learning period, so we can't attribute the present findings to differences in attention or arousal. We found no statistically significant changes in other areas in the brain, although such changes would have been expected if non-specific factors were present and raised the metabolism more generally. The confidence level we use is 0.01 in eight individuals.

Deecke: How do you compress the long recognition task into 60 s for your measurements?

Roland: We can present 15 objects in the 60s recognition phase. During the tactile learning phase we have 100s for the presentation of 10 objects. When we cut off after 60s only six objects are examined and of course these are not in the same order every time.

Deecke: So the whole thing is a matter of minutes. Was the visual cortex active?

Roland: No; the oxidative metabolism is high in the primary visual cortex but we think this is due to the synaptic density being higher. The metabolic activity in the visual cortex does not change in going from rest to learning, from learning to recognition, or from rest to recognition.

Deecke: At our clinic we do single photon emission computer tomogram (SPECT) experiments (Goldenberg et al, unpublished). Judging from these, I would say that in your experiments the visual cortex may be equally active in both conditions but it is active because the individuals are imagining the objects—that is, they see them in their mind's eye.

Roland: Most of them say that they don't. They have difficulty visualizing these objects because they are too complex.

Marsden: How long do the oxygen metabolic changes last after people stop doing the task?

Roland: I don't know. When we measure the regional metabolic rate for oxygen we assume there is a steady state during the measurement. Transients require other methods.

Marsden: It would be fascinating if one could conclude that the cerebellum is a learning machine on the grounds that it appeared to be more active during the learning phase than during the recognition phase, yet the task during the learning phase was being undertaken with a lower motor load than during the recognition phase.

Roland: We are stuck with a metabolic increase in the lateral part of the cerebellum. It is higher during learning than during recognition. This probably means that a more intense synaptic metabolism is related to synaptic processes. I don't think this proves that the cerebellum is a learning machine; the structures that store information might equally well be distributed. This is just a difference we have found in comparing recognition to learning.

Marsden: An alternative explanation for the increased cerebellar activity is the difference in the nature of the motor acts undertaken during the learning and recognition tasks. Although the motor load is greater because the individuals are working faster while recognizing than during learning, they are probably using a different motor strategy. Those very fast hand movements during recognition are almost ballistic. One would expect a much greater degree of proprioceptive feedback to be guiding the slower movements that occur during the learning phase. That proprioceptive feedback might make the cerebellum work harder. The control for that is to do the recognition task at the same speed as the learning task. Have you done that experiment?

Roland: No. The distinction between ballistic and non-ballistic movement is a matter of definition. When we look at these movements in slow motion on the video we cannot see any change in the strategies. They still use the same dynamic scanning movements with the fingers, although they are faster.

Calne: Why did you change the speed?

Roland: Our intention was to have a paced task with a probability of recognition of between 0.75 and 0.80 for each person, because that is comparable to the other behavioural situations we study.

Calne: So the success rate in the same time is exactly the same for everyone. A standard response like that is quite remarkable.

Roland: There are a few individual variations but the mean differences are very small.

Thach: One might interpret these results as being consistent with cerebellar learning theories. Even though you have slower movements during the learning part, you have increased cerebellar activity. One could suppose that the increased cerebellar cortical activity is due to increased climbing fibre discharge, which would be greater under the 'learning' conditions even though the movement (and the mossy fibre granule cell activity) is less than during the 'recognition' condition. But why should it be bilaterally symmetrical in the cerebellum during learning? The climbing fibre discharge should be lateralized to the hand that is doing the task.

Roland: Some parts of the prefrontal cortex and some parts of the parietal cortex project to the cerebellum. We have bilateral activation in both the parietal and the intermediate part of the prefrontal cortex. This might be one explanation of the bilaterality. I am not sure that the connections in humans and monkeys have been worked out in detail. This would not be the whole explanation because if the information about the shape of the learnt objects was stored there, how would the cerebral cortex get hold of this information? All the connections seem to go to the motor cortices.

Lemon: Is the success rate as good when the same individuals do the recognition task with the other hand?

Roland: These subjects have a catheter in the left arm, leaving the right hand free to explore the objects. We always catheterize the left arm for security reasons.

Calne: I expressed myself poorly in my question about asymmetry. You were thinking about cortex and I was thinking of the whole brain. Areas we didn't get into were the basal ganglia and thalamus. There was not a very striking asymmetry in the thalamic and basal ganglia changes, yet that task was designed to stir up the contralateral basal ganglia and thalamus. Why isn't more change seen there?

Roland: In our experiments with different motor paradigms we have always seen bilateral increases. If the supplementary motor area was engaged it was always engaged bilaterally. If the premotor and supplementary motor area were engaged they were always engaged bilaterally. This holds for the prefrontal cortex, although there is no general rule that says that homologous regions are always activated bilaterally. We and others (Roland et al 1982, Mazziotta & Phelps 1984) have done a few studies on basal ganglia activation during strictly unilateral distal motor tasks with hands and fingers. These studies show that the head of the caudate, the putamen and the pallidum seem to be bilaterally activated during unilateral motor tasks. Also the cerebellum seems to be bilaterally activated during unilateral motor tasks (Fox et al 1985). There might be quantitative differences and we have reported differences between the contralateral and ipsilateral pallidum. There might also be differences in the cerebellum but the general impression is that all these motor structures are bilaterally activated even though the movement is purely unilateral and distal. At present there are only teleological explanations for this.

One approach is to regard the bilateral activation as the activity of neurons involved in transferring motor programmes to the other side. This is purely speculative but there is some support for the idea. If there are lesions of the premotor area it seems that the programmes are still there and individuals can perform extremely well after a very short learning time with the other hand. This is probably not the whole explanation.

Calne: From what we know of the pathways one would expect lateralization in relation to the thalamus and the basal ganglia.

Goldman-Rakic: There are quite extensive bilateral connections from cortex to basal ganglia (Kunzle 1985, Tanaka et al 1980, P.S Goldman-Rakic, unpublished). Bilateral corticothalamic connections also exist (Goldman 1979, (Preuss & Goldman-Rakic 1987). So even one hemisphere might be expected to turn on both sides.

Jones: I don't believe that corticothalamic bilaterality is particularly significant, at least not in the areas we should be concerned with at this level of motor control. It is worth remembering that a lot of activity may have gone round the brain a number of times, even in the 60s required for making metabolic measurements of this sort.

References

Fox PT, Raichle ME, Thach WT 1985 Functional mapping of the human cerebellum with positron emission tomography. Proc Natl Acad Sci USA 82:7462–7466

Goldman PS 1979 Contralateral projections to the dorsal thalamus from frontal association cortex in the rhesus monkey. Brain Res 166:166–171

Kunzle H 1975 Bilateral projections from precentral motor cortex to the putamen and other parts of the basal ganglia. An autoradiographic study in Macaca fascicularis. Brain Res 88:195–210

Mazziotta JC, Phelps ME 1984 Positron computed tomographic studies of cerebral metabolic responses to complex motor tasks. Neurology 34:116

Preuss TM, Goldman-Rakic PS 1987 The crossed cortico-thalamic and thalamo-cortical connections of macaque prefrontal cortex. J Comp Neurol 257:269–281

Roland PE, Meyer E, Shibasaki T, Yamamoto YL, Thompson CJ 1982 Regional cerebral blood flow changes in cortex and basal ganglia during voluntary movements in normal human volunteers. J Neurophysiol 48:467–480

Tanaka DT, Gorska T, Dutkiewicz K 1980 Corticostriate projection patterns and synaptic morphology in the puppy caudate nucleus. Exp Neurol 70:98–108

Differential effects of cortical lesions in humans

Hans-Joachim Freund

Neurologische Klinik, University of Düsseldorf, D-4000 Düsseldorf, Federal Republic of Germany

Abstract. The best-known example of motor deficits after cortical lesions is contralateral paresis and spasticity after damage to the precentral motor strip. After recovery the residual motor functions can be used in a purposive and skilful manner. In patients with lesions of the supplementary motor area (SMA) and cingulate gyrus transient akinesia and mutism have been described. Lesions restricted to more lateral parts of the premotor field interfere with proximal muscle function and interlimb coordination, whereas distal motor activity and bimanual coordination are unimpaired. In contrast, hand function in patients with parietal lesions is severely disturbed. This dysfunction includes deficits such as ataxia, dysmetria and postural instability that are typically observed in deafferented patients. Severe disturbances of the purposive behaviour of the hand during exploratory finger movements and manipulation of objects are seen in patients with posterior parietal lesions.

Observations in human patients are compatible with the hypothesis that lesions of the frontal agranular motor fields interfere with the control of postural and force control whereas parietal lesions are associated with motor programme disorders affecting the use of the hand or the eye as a sense organ or affecting more complex motor behaviour.

1987 Motor areas of the cerebral cortex. Wiley, Chichester (Ciba Foundaiton Symposium 132) p 269–281

The study of the effect of cortical lesions on motor behaviour has entered a new era since the invention of organ-imaging techniques and exact methods of recording unrestricted movements. Since this kind of study has only become possible in the last few years, the bulk of the information about the effects of cortical lesions in humans still stems from clinical observations and their correlation with what was found at subsequent neuropathological examination.

The use of the term 'cortical' lesions in human studies implies concomitant damage of underlying white matter. The combined lesion of grey and white matter raises the pertinent question of the extent to which the resulting deficits are due to the cortical lesions or to fibre disconnections. The interpretation of such disturbances is further hampered by uncertainly about the degree of neuronal dysfunction associated with the lesion, as revealed by

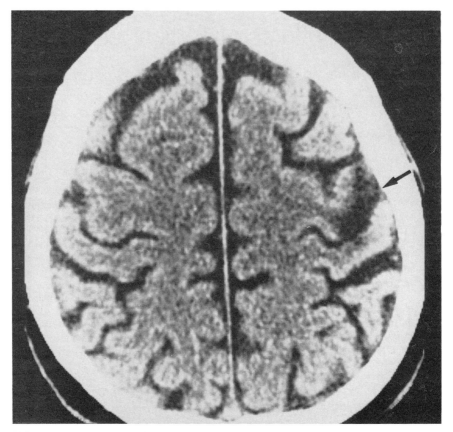

FIG. 1. Computerized tomography scan of right-handed patient with small lesion involving hand area of left precentral gyrus. Left of brain is on the right of the figure. Arrow points to lesion. (From Freund 1987.)

organ-imaging techniques. These obvious limitations of human studies impose considerable constraints on the allocation of functional deficits to the site of a lesion. What remains for the present approach is to collect cases with similar lesions, assess their clinical deficits, measure their sensorimotor performance and evaluate the consistency of certain deficits. The advantage of humans studies is obvious and lies in the accessibility of conceptual, perceptive, associative and executive functions to thorough examination.

Lesions of the precentral gyrus

Examples of well defined small lesions of the primary motor cortex are rare. One patient we saw recently had a small lesion restricted to the hand area of the precentral gyrus (Fig. 1). The only abnormality was the impairment of dexterity and force in the contralateral hand and fingers. Tonus of the arm was normal and reflexes were only slightly increased. Quantitative studies showed that the control of residual force after some recovery was precise. The patient, a skilled dentist, could hold an egg between his fingers without squeezing or dropping it, even without visual control. His residual finger movements were clumsy and slow but purposive and included proper formation of the hand aperture during grasping. These observations are in accordance with previous reports of distally accentuated paresis, disturbance of dexterity and independent finger movements but no major increase in tonus or reflexes. Similar observations have been made since the classical ablation studies in non-human primates of Leyton & Sherrington (1917). The effects of such 'cortical' lesions must be distinguished from those at the level of the internal capsule or the medullary pyramid. Although the effects of such subcortical lesions are commonly referred to as 'pyramidal', they are quite different. Capsular lacunes are usually associated with severe spasticity (Mohr 1982) whereas damage of the medullary pyramid causes hypotonic paresis in humans (Meyer & Herndon 1962) and monkeys (Chapman & Wiesendanger 1982, Gilman & Marco 1971). These major differences are obviously due to the different fibre composition of the pyramidal tract at different cranio-caudal levels. In consequence, the pyramidal syndrome in humans, although frequently regarded as an entity, comprises a range of functional deficits dominated by deficient force control, preferentially in distal muscles.

Lesions of the supplementary motor area and of premotor cortex

Excision of a strip of medial frontal cortex in humans, including the supplementary motor area (SMA) and cingulate cortex, resulted in severe reduction of spontaneous motor activity, more pronounced contralaterally than ipsilaterally (Laplane et al 1977, Talairach & Bancaud 1966). The motor changes in these patients were accompanied by a reduction of speech and an emotional facial palsy. Bimanual coordination and motor copying were also impaired. The nearly complete akinesia predominating in the limbs contralateral to the lesion receded after two weeks. The only persistent deficit was a slowing of alternating serial movements of both hands, called a reciprocal coordination disorder, whereas serial unimanual activities were normal. The results agree with older observations on patients with less well defined lesions, with bilateral medial frontal lobe damage leading to persistent complete akinesia and mutism. Recordings of electrical scalp potentials (Kristeva et al 1979) and investigations of regional cerebral blood flow in humans have corroborated the view that the supplementary motor cortex contributes to motor planning and the initiation of movement (Orgogozo et al 1979, Roland et al 1980). The long controversy about the existence of a premotor syndrome in humans, initiated by the debate between Fulton (1934) and Walshe (1935), has recently been complemented by observations on a group of patients with a disturbance of proximal movements contralateral to the premotor lesions (Freund & Hummelsheim 1985). The most prominent dysfunction was the inability of the patients to coordinate proximal movements between both sides, as disclosed by their grossly disordered movement patterns during the performance of simple windmill movements with both arms or of pedalling movements with both legs. Surprisingly, the patients were unable to improve on this after weeks of training. Electromyographic recordings provided evidence that the sequencing of muscle activation along the limb was altered, so these abnormalities reflect a disturbance in a time domain affecting coordination between muscles rather than a severely deficient force control. We now have evidence that more lateral lesions of the premotor cortex (anterior to the hand area of the precentral gyrus) cause distal dysfunctions similar to those reported for the proximal musculature.

In contrast to the impairment of alternating arm or leg movements, various types of interdependent and independent finger and hand movements could be flawlesly executed by our patients. Bimanual everyday activities such as tieing shoelaces or buttoning clothes were not disturbed. Dexterity, exploration and manipulation of objects were normal. The only distal abnormality was a minor slowing of finger movements in some patients. Reflexes and tonus were normal or slightly increased on the affected site. Eye movements and head and gaze control showed no obvious disturbances. There were no differences between the observed deficits with respect to the side of the lesion.

Parietal lesions

Two types of motor disturbances have been observed after parietal lobe damage. The first category comprises the complex forms of apraxia such as ideational and ideokinetic (or ideomotor) apraxia as defined by Liepmann (1908), and constructional apraxia (Kleist 1907). These disturbances are characterized by an impairment in the generation of complex motor behavioural patterns and by their laterality dependence, such that ideational and ideokinetic apraxia is only seen after damage of the speech-dominant hemisphere, whereas constructional apraxia is usually observed after lesions of the non-dominant hemisphere.

The second category of movement disorders in parietal cases is—in analogy to deafferentation—attributed to the sensory dysfunctions associated with damage to the somatosensory areas. This type of deficit does not depend on the side of the lesion and it comprises motor deficits such as ataxia, postural instability, dystonia and muscle hypotonia. Since the turn of the century neurologists have reported that the ratio of motor to sensory deficits varied considerably. Sometimes the motor signs were too severe to be considered a consequence of the sensory disturbance. Since these observations remained anecdotal, without quantitative studies on deafferented patients (Rothwell et al 1982, Sanes et al 1985), the matter remained unsettled. In a recent study of patients with parietal lesions, however, quantitative evaluation of somatosensory and motor functions of the hand confirmed that the ratio of sensory to motor deficits differed greatly (Pause & Freund 1987).

Analysis of the motor disturbance of the hand

Closer analysis of the impaired motor function of the hand showed that, where the motor deficit was negligible or only moderate, the disturbance closely resembled that seen after deafferentation. All these deficits improve considerably under visual control. In the more severely affected hand movements the situation is different. The characteristic feature of the dysfunction is the loss of purposiveness of the movement. As this is traditionally defined as apraxia. Delay (1935) coined the term tactile apraxia for these deficits. Tactile apraxia appears most clearly in tests on object exploration and manipulation. In all our patients apraxia was associated with astereognosis, whereas cutaneous sensibility was less affected. It was impossible to recognize any meaningful pattern in the hand and finger movements. Not only were the spatial trajectories of the explorative pattern of the finger movements lost but also their typical kinetic profile. Quantitative analysis showed not only derangement of the tactile scan paths but also breakdown of the kinetic profile. Since the motor deficits in the three patients with tactile apraxia were much greater than in patients who were almost completely deafferented we concluded that damage to the parietal cortex may cause a gross motor dysfunction, tactile apraxia, which is not secondary to sensory impairment (Pause & Freund 1987).

The range of disturbances of hand function seen in patients with parietal lobe damage thus extends from severe somatosensory deficits with secondary motor dysfunction to patients with severe motor deficits with minor somatosensory impairment. Evaluation of the patients with the two types of deficit showed that in the first category the lesions lay in the anterior part of the parietal cortex, whereas in those with tactile apraxia the lesions involved mainly the posterior parietal cortex. Since these observations are based on only eight patients further corroboration is needed.

Visuomotor apraxia

Optic ataxia (Balint 1909), visuomotor ataxia (Rondot et al 1977) and visuomotor apraxia (Freund 1987) are some of the terms used for the deficits in patients who can see but who have difficulty in directing their eyes or hands to targets. The resulting movement is ataxic but, like the patients with tactile apraxia, these patients have also lost their purposive pattern, resulting in grossly abnormal, deranged reaching movements. In Rondot's patients and in his survey of the literature the lesions were located near the parieto-occipital border zones. It was concluded that, as in the monkey experiments with lesions severing the occipito-frontal connections (Haaxma & Kuypers 1975), the deficit represents a disconnection syndrome depriving the frontal motor centres of visual information. There are two problems with this straightforward explanation.

(1) Motor behaviour in such patients is much more grossly disturbed than it is in acutely blind people and is quite different from their behaviour. Whereas acutely blind people easily and rapidly acquire strategies for guiding their movements by other cues and can perform them properly, except for missing their targets, patients with visuomotor apraxia have a similar type of motor deficit to that described for patients with tactile apraxia. I have therefore regarded tactile and visuomotor apraxia not as unimodal deafferentation or disconnection syndromes but rather as deficits of sensory-guided motor behaviour due to lesions of the posterior parietal cortex (Freund 1987). This is further supported by the observation that the patients can barely learn to use other sensory cues to improve on their dysfunction.

(2) To my knowledge there is no report from either animal experiments or human observations about visuomotor apraxia occurring after more anteriorly located lesions of the occipito-frontal fibre bundles. On the other hand there is evidence for a powerful projection from the parietal cortex down to the brainstem and cerebellum that conveys visual information to the premotor cortex via the transcerebellar route.

Conclusions

Lesions of the frontal motor cortex interfere with force control and with temporal adjustment of the activity of different muscle groups, including interlimb coordination. There is evidence that damage to the parietal—possibly mainly the posterior parietal cortex—interferes with sensorimotor integration and the elaboration of motor programmes that can generate purposive movements adequate for exploring and manipulating objects with the hand. Gross motor deficits such as tactile or visuomotor apraxia make the hand or arm useless for the patients and cause as much motor impairment as do lesions of the motor cortex. From the clinical evidence the parietal cortex seems of critical importance for the use of the hand as a sense organ, whereas the primary motor cortex provides adequate and precise force control. The premotor cortex contributes to the postural activity of the shoulder and arm muscles as these are necessary for the act of reaching. The close anatomical connections of the SMA and premotor cortex with the basal ganglia and cerebellum are in agreement with a prominent role of the frontal motor fields in postural and force control. Although the predilection type of lesion of the primary motor cortex is a distally pronounced paresis, adequate use of the fingers to explore or manipulate objects reappears as soon as recovery of function provides sufficient strength, in contrast to the deranged, purposeless finger movements seen after damage of the parietal lobe. This is compatible with the hypothesis, derived from experiments on non-human primates, that the parietal cortex processes sensory information from the hand not only for perceptive but also for motor functions (Mountcastle 1975). This brings the issue close to the more complex apraxias such as ideational and ideokinetic apraxia seen after lesions of the temporo-parietal cortex of the speech-dominant hemisphere, representing disturbances in the generation of complex motor behaviour.

References

Balint R 1909 Seelenlähmung des Schauens, optische Ataxie, räumliche Störung der Aufmerksamkeit. Monatsschr Psychiatr Neurol 25:51–81

Chapman CE, Wiesendanger M 1982 Recovery of function following unilateral lesions of the bulbar pyramid in the monkey. Electroencephalogr Clin Neurophysiol 53:374–387

Delay H 1935 Les astereognoises, pathologie du toucher. Masson, Paris

Freund HJ 1987 Abnormalities of motor behavior after cortical lesions in man. In: Plum F (ed) The nervous system. Higher functions of the brain. American Physiological Society, Bethesda, MD (Handb Physiol sect 1: The nervous system, vol 5)

Freund HJ, Hummelsheim H 1985 Lesions of premotor cortex in man. Brain 108:697–733

Fulton JF 1934 Forced grasping in relation to the syndrome of the premotor area. Arch Neurol Psychiatry 31:221–235

Gilman S, Marco LA 1971 Effects of medullary pyramidotomy in the monkey. I. clinical and electromyographic abnormalities. Brain 94:495–514

Haaxma R, Kuypers HGJM 1975 Intrahemispheric cortical connections and visual guidance of hand and finger movements in the rhesus monkey. Brain 98:239–260

Kleist K 1907 Kortikale (innervatorische) Apraxie. Jahrb Psychiatr Neurol 28:46–112

Kristeva R, Keller E, Deecke L, Kornhuber HH 1979 Cerebral potentials preceding unilateral and simultaneous bilateral finger movements. Electroencephalogr Clin Neurophysiol 47:229–238

Laplane D, Talairach J, Meininger V, Bancaud J, Bouchareine A 1977 Motor consequences of motor area ablations in man. J Neurol Sci 31:229–238

Leyton ASF, Sherrington CS 1917 Observations on the excitable cortex of the chimpanzee, orang-outan and gorilla. Q J Exp Physiol 11:135–221

Liepmann H 1908 Drei Aufsätze aus dem Apraxiegebiet. Karger, Berlin

Meyer JC, Herndon RM 1962 Bilateral infarctions of the pyramidal tracts in man. Neurology 12:637–642

Mohr JP 1982 Lacunes. Stroke 13:3–11

Mountcastle VB, Lynch JC, Georgopoulos AP, Sakata H, Acuna C 1975 Posterior parietal association cortex of the monkey: command functions for operations within extrapersonal space. J Neurophysiol 38:871–908

Orgogozo JM, Larsen B, Roland PE, Lassen NA 1979 Activation de l'aire motrice supplémentaire au cours des mouvements volontaires chez l'homme. Rev Neurol (Paris) 135:705–717

Pause M, Freund HJ 1987 The role of parietal cortex for sensory-motor transformation. Evidence from clinical observations. Brain Behav Evol Suppl, in press

Roland PE, Larsen B, Lassen NA, Skinhoj E 1980 Supplementary motor area and other cortical areas in organization of voluntary movements in man. J Neurophysiol 43:118–136

Rondot P, De Recondo J, Ribadeau Dumas JL 1977 Visuomotor ataxia. Brain 100:355–376

Rothwell JC, Traub MM, Day BL, Obeso JA, Thomas PK, Marsden CD 1982 Manual motor performance in a deafferented man. Brain 105:515–542

Sanes JN, Mauritz KH, Dalakas MC, Evarts EV 1985 Motor control in humans with large-fiber sensory neuropathy. Hum Neurobiol 4:101–114

Talairach J, Bancaud J 1966 The supplementary motor area in man. Int J Neurol 5:330–347

Walshe FMR 1935 On the 'syndrome of the premotor cortex' (Fulton) and the definition of the terms 'premotor' and 'motor' with a consideration of Jackson's views on the cortical respresentation of movements. Brain 58:49–80

DISCUSSION

*Rizzolatti:*Were you saying that in humans the lateral premotor area does not use visual information, since the movements it controls are too fast? This may be true for foveal vision but it is not true for peripheral vision, which must be very useful for writing. If I close my eyes my writing changes considerably.

Freund: My point is that precise visual guidance of rapid learnt movements is not possible because the ocular pursuit system can only follow moving objects up to frequencies between 1 and 2 Hz (Mather & Putchat 1983, Von Noorden & Mackensen 1962, Leist et al 1987). Writing is usually performed at alternation rates in the 5–8 Hz range. It is not possible to pursue rapid automated movements (Freund 1986); for this purpose the visuomotor processes have to switch to a different control mode involving the retinal periphery.

*Georgopoulos:*Paillard (1982) has shown conclusively that in some tasks central vision is very important. In others peripheral vision is also very important.

Freund: It would be interesting to investigate whether the two types of visual control, foveal pursuit and peripheral vision, are linked to different types of movement. I have recently proposed (Freund 1986) that pursuit control is linked to the slow sensory controlled hand movements (type I movements, <2Hz), whereas the retinal periphery exerts some sort of 'range control' during rapid automated hand movements as they are employed in a wide range of everyday activities, such as writing, pencil shading, typing, stroking, hammering, etc. (type II movements, > 2 Hz).

Passingham: Where are these posterior parietal lesions on the cytoarchitectonic map?

Freund: Some of them are in the anterior, some in the posterior parietal lobe, and some cover the whole parietal cortex.

Passingham: We don't really know the extent of the supplementary motor area in humans. It may come over the medial surface onto the lateral surface. We have only recently learnt, from the work of Peter Strick and others, where the hand area of the premotor cortex is in the monkey. In a human map of the sort you showed, we still don't know where the various premotor areas are. We need to be cautious in making comparisons with animals.

Roland: I disagree; we know where the supplementary motor area is in humans. It is known exactly where to put electrodes to get responses character-istic of the supplementary motor area (Buser & Bancaud 1967, Chauvel 1976). Larsen et al (1979) have examined regional cerebral bloodflow increases in patients doing motor sequence tasks. When these patients were operated on, exact correlations were found between the stereotaxic stimulation sites from the SMA electrodes. We have nuclear magnetic resonance scans on subjects that match the metabolic changes we see in the same stereotactical frame. The subjects can't move a millimetre in this frame. So I think we have a reasonably good idea about where the supplementary motor area is located. What we don't know are the cytoarchitectonic areas that are territorially defined by these macroscopic means.

Calne: Professor Freund gave us an elegant statement of the limitations and possibilities of clinicopathological correlation, which, as he said, is the oldest tool we have. There is now a potential for acquiring important new knowledge from studies on multiple sclerosis. Patients develop clear demyelinating le-sions, seen on MRI scans, without any symptoms. These lesions come and go in just the sort of regions we are interested in, including the white matter under-lying the cortex. We know that a demyelinating lesion is a functional lesion because such a lesion in the cord is devastating. The lesions underneath the cortex will therefore produce functional impairment, and within-patient stu-dies are possible because the lesions come and go.

As clinicians, we must use the expertise generated from studies in animals to decide to what kinds of tests we can submit symptomless patients, if we are to determine the significance of these transient, demyelinating pathological epi-sodes. These events are so frequent that there will be no shortage of clinical material from which to gather valuable information. Over a decade or so we should have enough information to answer some of the questions that have been posed about fibre linkages under the cortex, as long as we know what questions to ask.

Freund: We have no material from such patients but that may be a very interesting approach because they have small lesions. But they may have lesions in other parts of the sensorimotor pathways that are not seen on the scan.

Marsden: With high and low premotor lesions did you get an identical functional deficit but in a different segment of the arm (proximal for the high lesions and distal for the low lesions)? Or were there differences, other than in the site, in the nature of the deficits produced by high and low lesions?

Freund: We are still collecting patients with low premotor lesions; we have only two so far. One patient has a lesion extending into the precentral strip and I would not dare to interpret his data. He had apractic agraphia and could not do rapid alternating hand or finger movements. The one clear-cut case with a low premotor lesion was really the distal mirror-image of what we had seen in our proximal cases with high premotor lesions. In addition there was impairment of rapid automated hand movements.

Marsden: And that clear-cut case included a failure of bimanual coordination of the hands?

Freund: Yes, that was disturbed.

Marsden: On reconsideration of the site of the lesions high in the premotor cortex (Freund & Hummelsheim 1985), to what extent do you think the lesions were intruding into the supplementary motor area, if at all?

Freund: Some of them clearly did, and some of them intruded into the frontal eye fields. At that time we saw no difference in the clinical signs. Adequate testing involving quantitative measurement of movement initiation and preparation, or of eye movements, may well disclose additional deficits.

Marsden: To what extent did the patients with high premotor lesions and the one with a clear low premotor lesion exhibit the phenomenon that we call neglect, in which people neglect or fail to use the arm in voluntary actions? Is this typical of the higher, more medial lesions which may involve the supplementary motor area?

Freund: Only one patient who had a large lesion had a motor neglect of the arm.

Kuypers: With caudal parietal lesions you saw deficits in both somatosensory and visual guidance of hand and finger movements. Our findings in the monkey were slightly different. After transection of the parietal white matter in monkeys (Haaxma & Kuypers 1975), which produced a limited cortical lesion, the animals still had very fine finger play and no obvious somatosensorimotor deficit. However, they displayed a clear-cut visuomotor deficit. Animals with lesions in the postcentral gyrus had a clear-cut tactile exploratory deficit of hand and fingers, yet several of them displayed no deficit in visuomotor guidance of hand and fingers.

Your data and your emphasis on the parietal lobe suggest that your frontal deficits in the guidance of hand and fingers were less pronounced than the parietal deficits. In experiments with Dr L. Moll, deficits in visually guided movements in the monkey were present after frontal premotor lesions but were less persistent than after parietal lesions. Transection of the tectospinal and rubrospinal decusssations, in addition to the commissurotomy, made the deficit more persistent.

As a control for the frontal premotor lesions, in a separate group of animals Dr Moll and I made extensive electrolytic thalamic lesions involving a major part of the arm-hand slice through the VLo and the VPLo without damaging the internal capsule. From the first day, those animals showed no visuomotor deficit, in marked contrast to the findings in monkeys with lesions of the premotor cortex. Obviously, such thalamic lesions should be repeated using neurotoxins, to make very large thalamic lesions without involving the internal capsule.

Kalaska: We know there is a substantial corticospinal output from the postcentral gyrus but it is not yet established whether these outputs have a strictly sensory function or whether they assist or guide or even initiate movements. In patients with precentral lesions, is there any evidence of an increase in either motility or dexterity of the hand movements when they are manipulating an object and receiving a fairly substantial tactile and proprioceptive input from the hand, compared with the condition where you ask them to make isolated movements of single digits, when presumably there may be a lower degree of somatosensory activity? Such a finding would suggest that the postcentral corticospinal outputs play some role in assisting or even initiating movement and compensating for the precentral lesions.

Freund: The clinical observations we were able to make in one patient with a small precentral lesion showed no such 'somatosensory facilitation'.

Lemon: Some years ago Professor Marsden reported a very interesting case of peripheral neuropathy in a patient who was deafferented from the elbow downwards (Rothwell et al 1982). This patient performed quite well on what we might call laboratory motor tasks but his purposive movements were clearly limited. What sort of message does this have for people who are trying to investigate these structures in experimental animals?

*Marsden:*Peripheral deafferentation does not destroy the concept of the movement that the individual wishes to undertake. That patient had a remarkable range of what one could call programmed movements in the complete absence of peripheral sensory feedback. The most dramatic thing was that he could still drive his old car, though he couldn't drive the new car he had bought just before this illness struck. The mass of motor detail stored in his brain allowed him to execute a whole range of bilateral actions with no sensory feedback at all. It was only when he required feedback for something new that his performance collapsed.

Freund: We are interested in dissociating certain functional demand groups in patients with parietal or premotor lesions. For example, we wanted to check on automatic performances in learnt movements such as writing. Patients with parietal lesions can move their hands but they can't write because the pen falls out of their hand. Now that we have the Selspot system we can fix the LED to the forefinger and test them in that way. This will clarify which category of movement is disturbed by the different lesions.

*Goldman-Rakic:*I was struck by the dissociations you found between parietal and premotor. Most of us who are doing lesion research, whether in animals or humans, are trying to find double dissociations because that convinces us that what we are studying is specifically related to a particular area. However, now that we have found the interconnections between the cortical areas and the networks of conductivity that I showed earlier, we would like to design experiments to show not double dissociation but common cooperativity in a particular functional system. We can see this in Dr Deecke's experiment where he had visual tracking and then added one perturbation, inverted tracking. If we take a class of tasks and then build up the memory component or the sensory component we might be able to show the contribution of, say, frontal and parietal areas, which are interconnected, to a common information-processing domain. Everybody is using slightly different tests in animals and humans. If we could use tests with common elements we might progress further.

Freund: I agree. There is much evidence for cooperative action. But at present the test repertoire does not include tests for complex interactions that could disclose how patients who have parietal or premotor lesions, possibly including the frontal eye-fields, explore complex visual scenes or how they direct their eyes and organize their scanning paths. This should be measured.

Deecke: Everything behind the rolandic fissure is sensory and can be discussed in terms of attention. Everything anterior to the rolandic fissure is motor or motivation. In our experiments we measured the negativity after the stimulus in order to analyse this point. We call this negativity 'directed attention potential' just to give it a name. Everything retrorolandic has this sensory aspect of attention to a stimulus from the outer world. Everything anterior to the central sulcus relates the input from the outer world to the inner needs of the body. The result is a compromise that takes into account both aspects. Now we need a brain area that determines *when* to start the movement, in our opinion a key function of the SMA, which, thus, is a prerequisite to self-pacing a movement. In short, there is an attentional brain at the back and a motivational brain or motor brain in the front of each hemisphere.

References

Buser P, Bancaud J 1967 Bases techniques et méthodologiques de l'exploration fonctionelle stéréotaxique du télencéphale. In: Talairach J et al (eds) Atlas d'anatomie stéréotaxique du télencéphale. Masson, Paris, p 251–322
Chauvel 1979 Les stimulations de l'aire motrice supplémentaire chez l'homme. Thesis, Université de Rennes
Freund HJ 1986 Time control of hand movements. Prog Brain Res 64:287–294
Freund HJ, Hummelsheim H 1985 Lesions of premotor cortex in man. Brain 108: 697–733
Haaxma R, Kuypers HGJM 1975 Intrahemispheric cortical connections and visual guidance of hand and finger movements in the rhesus monkey. Brain 98:239–260

Larsen B, Orgogozo JM, Rougier A, Sageaux JC, Cohadon F 1979 Regional cortical blood flow with the 254 channels gamma-camera. A stereotactic study. Acta Neurol Scand 72 (suppl):234–235

Leist A, Freund H-J, Cohen B 1987 Comparative characteristics of eye and hand tracking in humans. Hum Neurobiol 6:

Mather JA, Putchat C 1983 Parallel ocular and manual tracking responses to a continuously moving visual target. J Motor Behav 15:29–38

Paillard J 1982 The contribution of peripheral and central vision to visually guided reaching. In: Ingle DJ et al (eds) Analysis of visual behavior. MIT Press, Cambridge, Massachusetts, p 367–385

Rothwell DC, Traub MM, Day BL, Obeso JA, Thomas PK, Marsden CD 1982 Manual motor performance in a deafferented man. Brain 105:515–542

Von Noorden GK, Mackensen G 1962 Pursuit movements of normal and amblyopic eyes. I. Physiology of pursuit movements. Am J Ophthalmol 53:325–336

What do the basal ganglia tell premotor cortical areas?

C.D. Marsden

MRC Movement Disorders Research Group, University Department of Neurology and Parkinson's Disease Society Research Centre, Institute of Psychiatry & King's College Hospital Medical School, Denmark Hill, London, SE5 8AF, UK

Abstract. The defects in execution of simple single arm movements at one joint, and of complex arm movements simultaneously or sequentially at two joints, in Parkinson's disease are analysed as a clue to the formal functions of the basal ganglia in human motor control. Slowness in execution of single movements, due to failure to scale the size of the initial electromyographic burst of activity in the agonist, is one characteristic abnormality. However, patients with Parkinson's disease are also shown to have added difficulty with complex motor tasks. When they attempt to undertake a hand 'squeeze' at the same time as an elbow 'flex', both movements are even slower. When they try to perform an elbow flex as quickly as possible after a hand squeeze with the same or opposite arms, the second movement is slowed and the interval between movements is prolonged. Similar movement abnormalities have been found in patients with Huntington's disease—even in those with chorea alone, and irrespective of drug therapy—and in a patient with an infarct involving the right supplementary motor area.

These observations suggest that the basal ganglia in humans are required to set up the correct motor programmes to execute complex simultaneous and sequential movements. It is suggested that the basal ganglia, acting on a read-out of existing sensorimotor cortical activity, direct the premotor cortical areas to select the correct parameters of the motor programmes required for subsequent motor action.

1987 Motor areas of the cerebral cortex. Wiley, Chichester (Ciba Foundation Symposium 132) p 282–300

The motor areas of the cerebral cortex receive major subcortical inputs from the peripheral sensory apparatus, the cerebellum and the basal ganglia. Here I will discuss those from the basal ganglia, concentrating on the question 'What is the nature of the instructions that the basal ganglia deliver to the motor cortical areas?'

The basal ganglia do not project directly to the primary motor cortex. A major portion of their output from the globus pallidus and substantia nigra zona reticulata is directed, via the thalamus, to the supplementary motor area

---

* *Present address*: Department of Neurology, Institute of Neurology, National Hospital for Nervous Diseases, Queen Square, London, WC1N 3BG, UK.

and (probably) the lateral premotor cortical regions (see Jones, this volume). Supplementary motor area and lateral premotor cortex influence the motor system via direct corticospinal projections (especially to proximal limb and axial structures: see Wiesendanger et al, this volume), as well as by projections to motor cortex itself. This basal ganglia output is thus likely to control the organization of movement. Other parallel basal ganglia pathways are directed, via other thalamic relay nuclei, to prefrontal cortex. The extent to which these basal ganglia outputs are concerned with thought rather than movement is not certain. However, basal ganglia projections to area 46 may also be involved with higher order control of movement (see Goldman-Rakic, this volume).

The basal ganglia must thus provide an important influence on supramotor areas of the cerebral cortex. However, the motor instructions they deliver to these regions are not known. Evidence on this has been obtained from lesion experiments and single unit recordings in animals, especially non-human primates (see Ciba Foundation 1984).

Our work has been in humans. In particular, we have concentrated on the nature of the motor defects of Parkinson's disease, for this illness provides one of the best human models of disordered basal ganglia function (Marsden 1982). Elsewhere (Marsden 1984), it has been argued that the tremor and rigidity of Parkinson's disease are not valuable indicators of the normal functions of the basal ganglia. They are, in Hughlings Jackson's terms, positive symptoms resulting from abnormal activities of distant brain mechanisms, released by basal ganglia damage. It is the negative symptoms, functions that are lost, that provide the crucial clues. In Parkinson's disease, these are akinesia/hypokinesia (inability or slowness to initiate movement) and bradykinesia (slowness of the movement itself). (Difficulties in locomotion, postural instability and loss of postural reflexes are other classes of negative symptoms in Parkinson's disease. However, these may represent, in part at least, loss of basal ganglia output to lower brainstem centres concerned with postural and locomotor control. They are not considered further here.)

We have investigated the breakdown of upper limb movements in patients with Parkinson's disease at a relatively early stage of their illness, when general cognition is preserved and more diffuse brain damage is unlikely. Most patients were studied after withdrawal of their regular levodopa or other dopamine agonist therapy on the day of investigation. The studies to be described were undertaken with Drs R. Benecke, J.C. Rothwell, B.L. Day, A. Berardelli, J.P.R. Dick and P.D. Thompson.

Simple arm movements in Parkinson's disease

When a patient with Parkinson's disease attempts a self-paced simple fast movement of one joint of the upper limb, the movement is executed slowly.

In reaction paradigms it is the movement time, rather than response time, that is most compromised in Parkinson's disease (Evarts et al 1981).

A normal person who executes a simple fast or ballistic movement shows a stereotyped pattern of EMG activity in agonist and antagonist muscles (accompanied as necessary by similarly stereotyped activity in synergists and postural fixators). The agonist fires first to provide the impulsive force, then is silent while the antagonist fires to provide any required braking force; the agonist may then fire again to provide any required final correction. Movements of increasing amplitude and velocity are achieved by increasing the size and, to a lesser extent, the duration of the first agonist burst of EMG activity.

The parkinsonian patient activates agonist and antagonist muscles in the correct sequence and brings in appropriate anticipatory activity in postural muscles (Dick et al 1986a). In other words, the selection of muscles and the relative timing of their activation is correct, so the basic form of the motor programme is preserved.

The reason why a fast ballistic movement in Parkinson's disease is slow is that the force of the initial impulsive activity in the agonist is inadequate. This is because the size of the initial EMG burst in the agonist is reduced (Hallett & Khoshbin 1980) (Fig.1). This is true even for distal limb movements involving no postural support (Berardelli et al 1984). The size of the first agonist burst can be graded to make larger movements (Berardelli et al 1986) but it is consistently underscaled for the amplitude of movement intended. As a result, the velocity of the resulting movement is too slow and the displacement achieved undershoots the point of aim. The latter is finally reached by a subsequent series of additional small bursts of EMG activity, which adds to the overall delay in achieving the required movement.

This failure to scale the initial agonist activity appropriate to the intended amplitude and velocity of movement is undoubtedly a fundamental abnormality of limb motor control in Parkinson's disease. But is it sufficient to explain all of the akinesia and bradykinesia so characteristic of that illness? There are good reasons to think not. For example, there is no close correlation between the extent of slowness of such simple ballistic movements of a single joint and the degree of clinical disability. Patients who were remarkably mobile when taking dopaminergic therapy showed only modest improvement in their capacity to execute such simple movements, compared to their performance when drugs were withdrawn and they were dramatically immobile (Berardelli et al 1986); the degree of slowing was not closely related to the degree of clinical bradykinesia.

Motor behaviour in daily life demands much more complex control than that required for the regulation of simple single movements of one joint. Many goal-directed motor acts require the performance of a series of movements, sequentially and/or simultaneously, at different joints and of different limbs. For instance, to drink we need to advance one or both arms to the cup, grasp it, then lift it to the lips, before engaging the sucking and swallowing

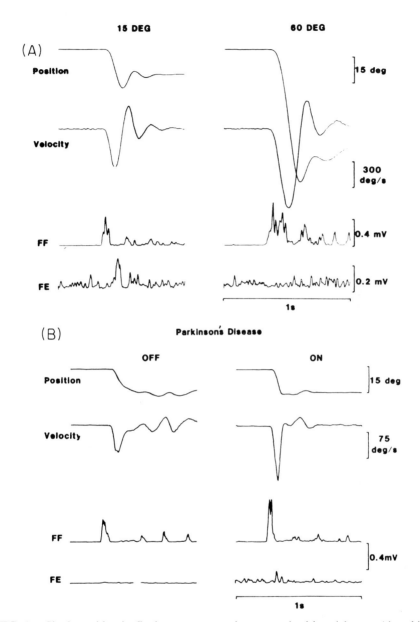

FIG. 1. Single rapid wrist flexion movements in a normal subject (above , A) and in a patient with Parkinson's disease when OFF and ON drug therapy (below, B). In A, a movement of 15° (left) is contrasted with a movement of 60° (right). In B, a 15° movement made when OFF drugs (left) is contrasted with the same movement made when ON drugs. Records are, from top to bottom, wrist position, velocity and rectified surface EMG activity from the flexor (FF) and extensor (FE) muscles in the forearm. The EMG activities were filtered digitally with a three-point moving-average filter. Background activity can be seen in the extensor muscles before the onset of movement. This is because the individuals tested began to move from an initial angle of 30° extension. (From Berardelli et al 1986, with permission.)

mechanisms. Each of these actions involves an individual motor programme, but the whole act requires appropriate sequencing and superimpostion of the individual motor programmes to achieve a smooth and accurate overall performance.

Patients with Parkinson's disease exhibit may problems in executing complex motor actions such as repetitive, simultaneous or sequential motor acts. Commonplace clinical observation reveals that parkinsonian patients have particular difficulty in repeatedly tapping the finger on the thumb or the ball of the foot on the floor. The initial movement is slow and undershoots, but subsequent repetitions progressively decrease in amplitude and velocity until the movement may cease. There is also a progressive decrease in the size of letters in micrographia. More complex motor acts, involving switching from one to another motor programme in a sequence or the execution of two different motor acts with opposite limbs, are obviously compromised (see Marsden 1984).

The clinical observations suggest that there is something more to the motor deficits of Parkinson's disease than just the underscaling of the initial agonist burst. For this reason, we have turned to the analysis of simultaneous and sequential movements. The Bereitschaftspotential, believed to arise at least in part from activity in supplementary motor areas, preceding such simultaneous and sequential movements is larger and longer than that before similar simple movements (Benecke et al 1985), suggesting greater activation of premotor cortical areas with complex movements.

Simultaneous motor actions in Parkinson's disease (Benecke et al 1986a)

The basic paradigm for testing the execution of simultaneous voluntary movements is shown in Fig. 2. Patients and controls were asked to perform a 15° fast isotonic elbow flexion ('flex') and an isometric opposition of the thumb to the fingers against a strain gauge to exert a force of 30 N ('squeeze'), separately or simultaneously. All movements were self-paced and performed with maximal speed. Duration of the elbow flex movement time (MTfl) was measured from the velocity signal; duration of the finger/thumb squeeze (Tsq) was measured from the force signal. Starting and target positions, as well as the elbow position and hand force, were displayed to the individual on an oscilloscope screen. The individuals undertook (a) elbow flex by itself, (b) hand squeeze by itself, or (c) both movements simultaneously ('squeeze and flex'). After five practice trials, 10 single trials of each type were recorded in cyclical order. Ten patients with Parkinson's disease were compared while they were off treatment with an age-matched group of normal individuals.

The results may be summarized as follows.

(1) The movement times of flex and squeeze varied from trial to trial in each individual, but there was no correlation between them in the simultaneous flex-and-squeeze task, in either normal people or parkinsonian pa-

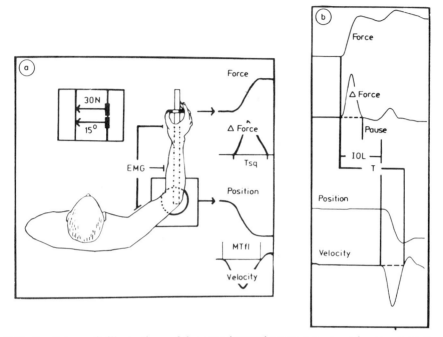

FIG. 2. Schematic illustrations of the experimental arrangements and measurements of movement performance. (a) shows the arrangement for the 'squeeze' and 'flex' tasks. Fixed starting and target positions (1 cm apart), as well as the movement response, were displayed as vertical bars on an oscilloscope screen 60 cm in front of the subject. Movement times (Tsq, MTfl) were measured by means of Δ- force (first derivative of the force signal) and velocity of flex (onset to zero crossing). (b) shows the measurement of mutual timing in the sequential squeeze-then-flex task. Total movement time (T) was measured from onset of squeeze to the termination of flex. The inter-onset latency (IOL) is the time between the onsets of both movements. The pause was measured between termination of the first (squeeze) and onset of the second movement (flex). (From Benecke et al 1987b, with permission.)

tients. This indicates that the complex task was executed by superimposition of two separate motor programmes rather than by the use of a new single generalized motor programme (see Schmidt 1975, Carter & Shapiro 1984).

(2) The separate individual movements of flex or squeeze with the same arm were performed more slowly by the parkinsonian patients than by the normal individuals (mean MTfl 349 ms versus 229 ms for flex; Tsq 221 ms versus 156 ms for squeeze).

(3) When the two movements were performed simultaneously with the same arm (flex and squeeze), there was no change in the duration of either movement in normal individuals compared with their performance of each movement by itself (mean MTfl alone compared to MTfl when combined with squeeze: 229 versus 216 ms; Tsq alone compared to Tsq when combined with flex: 156 versus 156 ms).

(4) However, in the parkinsonian patients there was an additional slowness of both movements when performed together with the same arm, compared with that seen for the separate movements alone (mean MTfl alone compared to MTfl combined with squeeze: 349 versus 557 ms, extra time in combined task 208 ms; Tsq compared with Tsq combined with flex: 221 versus 309, extra time in combined task 88 ms).

(5) Similar results were obtained when patients and controls squeezed with one arm but flexed with the opposite limb, although the extra slowness of the movements when done together by the parkinsonian patients was less marked than when the same arm was used for both tasks.

The conclusion from this study was that patients with Parkinson's disease have added difficulty (expressed as extra slowness) when they try to execute two motor programmes simultaneously, especially with the same arm. In other words, they have added difficulty superimposing two motor programmes simultaneously for separate joint movements, over and above the difficulty that is evident when they execute either movement by itself.

Sequential motor actions in Parkinson's disease (Benecke et al 1987a, b)

The same paradigm as above was used to test sequential motor actions (Fig. 2). Patients and controls were instructed to (a) squeeze to 30 N with the right hand, then flex the right elbow through 15°, and (b) squeeze with the left hand then flex with the right elbow. They were given two instructions: (i) move as rapidly as possible, and (ii) start the second movement immediately after the end of the first. Their performance on these ipsilateral and contralateral sequential tasks was compared with their performance when they undertook the individual movements by themselves. In addition, the interval between the onset of the first movement and that of the second (the inter-onset latency, IOL) and the interval between the termination of the first movement and the onset of the second (the pause) were also measured, as was the total time taken to complete both movements.

The results may be summarized as follows.

(1) As with simultaneous movements, there was no correlation between the times for squeeze and flex in sequential movements, or between movement times and the pause between movements, in either normal individuals or parkinsonian patients. Again this indicates that the complete movements of squeeze-then-flex were executed by two separate motor programmes.

(2) The separate single movements were slower in the parkinsonian patients than in the control individuals and there was a further decrease in speed in the parkinsonian patients, when the two movements were executed sequentially. The findings for the unilateral test of squeeze-then-flex with the same arm are summarized in Table 1. Similar results were observed for the bilateral squeeze with the left hand, then flex with the right.

TABLE 1.   Sequential movements in patients with Parkinson's disease and age-matched normal controls (Benecke et al 1987a)

	Controls (n = 9)	Parkinson's disease (n = 10)
Single movements		
Tsq	156 (23)	221 (29)*
MTfl	229 (41)	349 (77)*
Sequential movements		
Tsq	150 (25)	254 (38)*†
MTfl	244 (35)	445 (110)*†
IOL	244 (33)	425 (46)*
Pause	94	171 *
Total time	488 (42)	870 (147)*

The subjects squeezed then flexed with the right arm.
Means (SD) are shown in milliseconds.
Tsq: hand squeeze;
MTfl: elbow flex;
IOL: inter-onset latency between the two movements;
Pause: interval between the end of the first and the beginning of the second movement;
Total time: time required to complete the sequence of two movements.
*: Parkinson's disease slower than normal, p <0.01 or less.
†: Sequential movement times slower than single movements, p <0.01 or less.

(3) The IOL between the beginning of the first squeeze and the second flex movements was automatically chosen at about 244 ms by normal individuals. The first movement was completed in about 150 ms, so there was a pause of some 70—100 ms before the second movement was started. This pause occurred despite the instruction to execute the second movement as soon as possible after the first. When normal subjects were asked to vary the interval between the two movements, by making it shorter or longer at will, it transpired that at IOLs of less than about 200 ms the speed of the second elbow flex decreased; the shorter the IOL below 200 ms, the slower the second movement (Fig. 3A). This is interpreted to indicate that normal individuals automatically switch from one motor programme to another with an optimal minimal delay of a little longer than about 200 ms, in order to execute the second movement with maximum speed (Benecke et al 1986b). This optimal interval between movements corresponds to the known maximum rate of tapping movements of the hand at around 5 Hz.

(4) Patients with Parkinson's disease found it difficult to learn the sequential task of squeeze-then-flex. When they had done so, the IOL was longer than normal (about 425 ms), as was the pause between the two movements (around 171 ms). If they tried to execute the two movements with IOLs of less than 400 ms they found it extremely difficult; when they succeeded the speed of the second movement declined progressively (Fig. 3B). In other words the

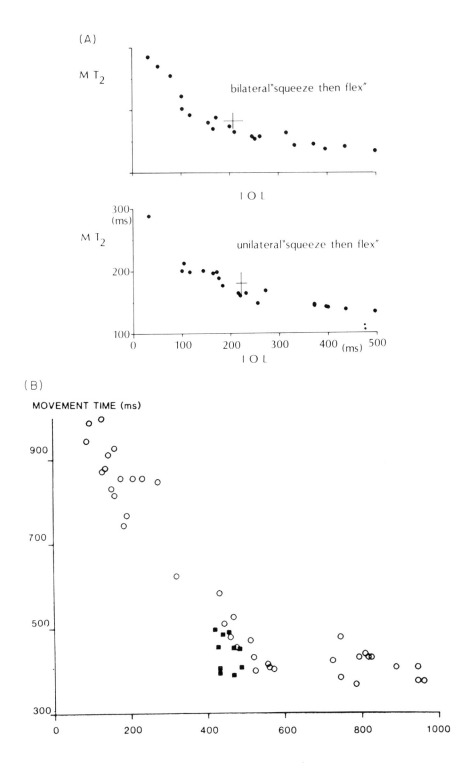

optimum interval between movements so as to maintain the speed of the second movement was considerably longer in the parkinsonian patients than in the controls.

The conclusion is that patients with Parkinson's disease have added difficulty when attempting to execute two motor programmes sequentially with the same or opposite arms. They perform the individual movements in the sequence more slowly than when each is carried out alone, and the interval between the two movements is prolonged. It turned out that the extra slowness in executing such a complex motor sequence was more closely related to the degree of clinical bradykinesia than to the slowness of single movements.

Complex motor actions in other diseases

So far, results for patients with Parkinson's disease have been presented, but similar deficits have been shown in patients with Huntington's disease (Thompson et al 1987) and in a patient with an infarct involving the right supplementary area (Dick et al 1986b).

Simple wrist flexion movements were slower than normal in 15 patients with Huntington's disease, even in those who exhibited only chorea, and irrespective of drug therapy. In four of six patients studied on the simultaneous squeeze-and-flex task, the speed of the elbow flex fell when the two movements were performed together. Only three of five patients studied doing the sequential squeeze-then-flex test with the same arm could complete the task. Those who could complete it had extra slowness of the second movement and longer IOLs and pauses between the two movements than normal. These findings show that patients with Huntington's disease have deficits in simple and complex simultaneous and sequential arm movements

---

FIG. 3.   (A) Uniform relationship between inter-onset latency (IOL) and duration of the second movement (MT_2) in the performance of two different types of sequential movements in one representative normal person. The cross in each diagram indicates the mean IOL and $MT_2\pm$ SD measured in trials when the individual was asked to squeeze then flex as fast as possible. The individual was then asked to modify voluntarily the IOL between the two movements. In each diagram the values of 20 sequential movements are plotted. Calibrations of the lower diagram in A apply to both diagrams. Note the prolonged movement times (MT_2) in both tasks at IOLs less than 200 ms ('refractory period' of movement speed production). (From Benecke et al 1986b, with permission.)

(B) relationship between inter-onset latency (IOL) and duration of the second movement (MTfl) in a patient with Parkinson's disease. Unilateral squeeze-then-flex task. First, the patient performed the task with the normal instruction (solid squares). Then he was asked to modify voluntarily the IOL between the two movements (open circles). Note the prolonged movement times at IOLs of less than 400 ms ('refractory period' of movement speed production). When the patient followed the normal instruction, he automatically chose an IOL which enabled him to perform relatively rapid second movements. (From Benecke et al 1987a, with permission.)

very similar to those in patients with Parkinson's disease, even if the former exhibit only chorea clinically, and irrespective of drug therapy. Patients with Huntington's disease, like those with Parkinson's disease, have difficulty superimposing or sequencing two separate motor programmes, which must contribute to a basic bradykinesia in both conditions.

Similarly, the patient with an infarct involving the right supplementary motor area exhibited slowness of elbow flex when this movement was combined simultaneously with a hand squeeze with either the right or left arm; inability to squeeze-then-flex sequentially with the left arm; slowness of elbow flex after hand squeeze with the right arm; and a prolonged IOL and pause when a right-hand squeeze was followed sequentially by a left-arm flex. Thus, this patient had evidence of bilateral difficulty in executing simultaneous movements, profound inability of the left arm to execute sequential movements (with lesser difficulties in the right arm), and considerable delay in sequencing bilateral movements started by the right arm and finished by the left (with lesser difficulty for movements started with the left arm and finished by the right). A right supplementary motor area lesion thus appears to disrupt the superimposition of two motor programmes in the same limb, on both sides, and also disrupts the sequencing of two programmes with the left more than the right arm, or with both arms each performing one of the two movements.

Discussion

The studies reviewed here have shown that damage to the basal ganglia in humans (as seen in patients with both Parkinson's and Huntington's disease) causes (1) slowness of single simple arm movements with one joint and (2) extra difficulties in the execution of simultaneous or sequential complex arm movements with two joints.

Can the first abnormality explain the second? Wing (1984) wondered whether the difficulty that patients with Parkinson's disease have in single movements might be sufficient to explain their problems with movement sequences: 'the question is whether their difficulty with sequences exceeds what one would expect, given that there are deficiencies in activating even a single preplanned movement? . . . If none of the components in a sequence are activated normally I would suggest that they may all be related to the first element of the sequence.'

The more recent findings presented here suggest that the slowness of simple single movements (due to underscaling of the size of the first agonist EMG burst) is not in itself sufficient to explain the added problems encountered in complex simultaneous and sequential motor acts. Not only does the performance of two movements expose the extra slowness of each component, but in the sequential task there is also extra delay between the two movements in parkinsonian patients compared to normal individuals.

This analysis suggests that the basal ganglia in humans are concerned with the accurate execution of complex movements requiring simultaneous or sequential operation of separate motor programmes. In the experiments described here we studied tasks requiring simultaneous or sequential delivery of two motor programmes. It might be predicted that the extra problems encountered with two motor programmes would become even more evident if even longer sequences involving three or more motor programmes were examined. Indeed, the extra slowness and delay of the next movement in a long sequence might get more evident as the sequence progresses, to produce the progressive fade and collapse of complex repetitive or sequential motor actions so characteristic of Parkinson's disease. As suggested earlier (Marsden 1982, 1984): 'Each motor programme in itself is imprecise, so it is not altogether surprising that, when repeated, the whole sequence is in error. However, the details of the impairment of repetitive action suggests that there is more than this. The critical feature is that, as the sequence is continued, the individual movement or motor programme progressively degrades. The time to initiation gets slower and the size of the movement progressively fades. Thus the final movement in a sequence is far worse than when that individual movement is performed by itself. Repetition of the movement unearths a greater deficit than is apparent in single movements. Likewise, when two movements are made together, they are each performed much worse than if they are undertaken alone. This suggests that there is a fundamental breakdown in the capacity to run the sequence of movements that comprises a motor plan. In particular, there appears to be a major problem in switching from one motor programme to another. In other words, the sequence of the motor plan does not run smoothly in Parkinson's disease.'

On the basis of the human evidence, one would suggest that the output of those parts of the basal ganglia involved in the control of arm movement is concerned with the organization of simultaneous processing or sequencing of the many motor programmes required to execute complex motor acts. This basal ganglia output is likely to be directed to the supplementary motor area (and perhaps also the lateral premotor area). The observation that a lesion of the supplementary motor area produces deficits in complex movements similar to those seen in Parkinson's disease supports this suggestion (although these observations in a single patient require replication in others).

The deficit in sequencing the arm movements seen in patients with Parkinson's and Huntington's disease, and in the patient with a supplementary motor area lesion, leads to another proposition. Perhaps the motor basal ganglia are more concerned with directing what happens to the next movement in a sequence than with the initial movement. It has been difficult to correlate the pattern of single-unit discharges in the basal ganglia of subhuman primates with a single motor act (see DeLong et al 1984). Single units in the output zones of globus pallidus interna and substantia nigra pars reticulata show somatotopic organization, with correlation between cell discharge in localized regions and active movements of specific body parts. However, such neuronal discharges do not clearly or consistently precede the first EMG changes in muscles; overall, changes in neuronal discharge seem to occur later in the basal ganglia than in the motor cortex. This is not surprising, for the basal ganglia receive a 'read-out' of the motor cortex output that drives the movement itself, via corticostriatal pathways from sensorimotor cortex to putamen. Putamen units (and probably those of the globus pallidus) fire in relation to the direction and amplitude of the movement (rather than to the activity in the individual muscles involved), suggesting that these basal ganglia areas monitor parameters of the movement. The suggestion is that this information is used to set up the premotor areas to select the correct parameters for the next movement. To test this hypothesis those who record the activity of basal ganglia units in awake performing primates would need to correlate such neuronal discharge with the next movement the animal performs, not with the immediate obvious motor action as has been done so far.

How would such a theory explain the slowness of a simple single one-joint movement? Why do parkinsonian patients (and those with Huntington's disease) underscale the size of the first agonist EMG burst in relation to the amplitude and velocity required to execute the desired movement? One suggestion is that such simple movements are defective because they must be based on what has gone before. In other words, the correct setting of the parameters of the motor programme required to execute even a single movement must depend on information about the motor state before its execution. If the read-out of existing motor activity from sensorimotor cortex delivered to the basal ganglia is mishandled, the output of the basal ganglia to premotor areas might misdirect the selection of parameters for even a simple single movement. Such a hypothesis has the attraction of encompassing all the defects of arm movement demonstrated in Parkinson's disease within one basic abnormality, namely a failure of basal ganglia direction of premotor areas to select the correct parameters for subsequent motor programmes.

Thus, in conclusion, these studies in humans suggest the hypothesis that the motor regions of the basal ganglia deliver instructions, based on a read-out of ongoing activity in sensorimotor cortex, to premotor areas in such a way as to set up the correct motor programmes required for the next motor actions.

References

Benecke R, Dick JPR, Rothwell JC, Day BL, Marsden CD 1985 Increase of the Bereitschaftspotential in simultaneous and sequential movements. Neurosci Lett 62:347–352

Benecke R, Rothwell JC, Dick JPR, Day BL, Marsden CD 1986a Performance of simultaneous movements in patients with Parkinson's disease. Brain 109:739–757

Benecke R, Rothwell JC, Day BL, Dick JPR, Marsden CD 1986b Motor strategies involved in the performance of sequential movements. Exp Brain Res 63:585–595

Benecke R, Rothwell JC, Dick JPR, Day BL, Marsden CD 1987a Disturbances of sequential movements in patients with Parkinson's disease. Brain 110:361–379

Benecke R, Rothwell JC, Dick JPR, Day BL, Marsden CD 1987b Simple and complex movements off and on treatment in patients with Parkinson's disease. J Neurol Neurosurg Psychiatry 50:296–303

Berardelli A, Rothwell JC, Day BL, Marsden CD 1984 Movements not involved in posture are abnormal in Parkinson's disease. Neurosci Lett 47:47–50

Berardelli A, Dick JPR, Rothwell JC, Day BL, Marsden CD 1986 Scaling of the size of the first agonist EMG burst during rapid wrist movements in patients with Parkinson's disease. J Neurol Neurosurg Psychiatry 49:1273–1279

Carter MC, Shapiro DC 1984 Control of sequential movements: evidence for generalised motor programmems. J Neurophysiol 52: 787–796

Ciba Foundation 1984 Functions of the basal ganglia. Pitman, London (Ciba Found Symp 107)

DeLong MR, Georgopoulos AT, Crutcher MD, Mitchell SJ, Richardson RT, Alexander GE 1984 Functional organization of the basal ganglia: contributions of single-cell recording studies: In: Functions of the basal ganglia. Pitman, London (Ciba Found Symp 107) p 64–78

Dick JPR, Rothwell JC, Berardelli A et al 1986a Associated postural adjustments in Parkinson's disease. J Neurol Neurosurg Psychiatry 49:1378–1385

Dick JPR, Benecke R, Rothwell JC, Day BL, Marsden CD 1986b Simple and complex movements in a patient with infarction of the right supplementary motor area. Movement Disord 1:255–266

Evarts EV, Teräväinen H, Calne DB 1981 Reaction time in Parkinson's disease. Brain 104:167–186

Goldman-Rakic PS 1987 Motor control function of the prefrontal cortex. This volume, p 187–200

Hallett M, Khoshbin S 1980 A physiological mechanism of bradykinesia. Brain 103:301–304

Jones EG 1987 Ascending inputs to, and internal organization of, cortical motor areas. This volume, p 21–39

Marsden CD 1982 The mysterious motor function of the basal ganglia. Neurology 32:514–539

Marsden CD 1984 Which motor disorder in Parkinson's disease indicates the true motor function of the basal ganglia? In: Functions of the basal ganglia. Pitman, London (Ciba Found Symp 107) p 225–237

Schmidt RA 1975 A schema theory of discrete motor skill learning. Psychol Rev 82:225–260

Thompson PD, Berardelli A, Rothwell JC et al 1987 On the Parkinsonism of Huntington's disease and its implications for theories of basal ganglia control of movement. Brain, in press

Wiesendanger M, Hummelsheim H, Bianchetti M et al 1987 Input and output organization of the supplementary motor area. This volume, p 40–62

Wing AM, Miller E 1984 Basal ganglia lesions and psychological analysis of the control of voluntary movement. In: Functions of the basal ganglia. Pitman, London (Ciba Found Symp 107) p 242–253 (and Wing AM, p 254–255)

DISCUSSION

Thach: One can ask patients with Parkinson's disease, in whom it is difficult to feel rigidity or cogwheel tremor in the limbs, to perform manoeuvres with the contralateral limb and then test the passive limb again. That limb is not part of any planned activity but during these activation procedures one can often detect an increase in tone.

Marsden: The story of rigidity in Parkinson's disease rests on the significance of enhanced long latency stretch reflexes. There is a general correlation between the size of long latency stretch reflexes and the degree of clinical rigidity. I would interpret the reinforcement procedure as setting the gain for the long latency stretch reflexes in the cortex, rather than involving the basal ganglia.

Kuypers: The last patient you described could have had a certain amount of spasticity and some forced grasping, which would have interfered with his performance, wouldn't it?

Marsden: No. Immediately after the lesion, which occurred acutely, he had the typical neglect seen in humans after medial frontal lesions: he did not use the arm. However, there was no grasp reflex, there was a slight increase in muscle tone, and one could elicit a Hoffman reflex on that side. There was no weakness: in response to verbal command he could execute a full range of movements with normal power. He did not want to speak, but if you spoke to him he spoke. That neglect receded over the first week to 10 days, and even the Hoffman reflex disappeared. Most studies were done at a stage where there were no crude neurological signs.

Deecke: The Bereitschaftspotential recordings, comparing complex movements with a single sequence, were in normal subjects, weren't they? This can also be interpreted in terms of effort. They need more cortical engagements to execute the complex task. The other recordings show that in patients with Parkinson's disease the Bereitschaftspotential occurs later. Thus, part of the synaptic drive which forms the Bereitschaftspotential must come from the basal ganglia, which is available in healthy individuals but less available in the parkinsonian patient.

Tanji: What were the simultaneous motor task and the readiness potential like in the SMA patients?

Marsden: We did not study either of those. There are so many problems in undertaking such clinical studies that we can only look at certain things in each patient.

Tanji: Our patients with damage to the midline cortex cannot do rhythm tests; the reaching test is not such a problem. Patients given a certain rhythm with a tone-signal could beat in time while they were listening to the signal, but if the signal was turned off tapping out the rhythm became a problem.

Marsden: This was the same for this gentleman; he could not perform that sort of tapping task with the more affected left arm.

Thach: We can now use single-unit recordings to find the command for these kinds of operations. Presumably one might look for a discharge which occurs more readily within the basal ganglia in relation to combinations of movements, rather than in relation to each of those movements independently.

Marsden: There could be a better correlation of the discharge pattern of single units in basal ganglia, not with the parameters of that first movement, but with those of the following movement in a sequence. The single-unit discharge may not be related to the movement being studied but to the next movement in the sequence.

Calne: Clinically, akinesia is the most problematic issue, but the extrapyramidal diseases were initially defined in terms of involuntary, additional and unwanted movements, such as tremor and chorea. How do you think input to the motor cortex might be disturbed to produce these abnormalities?

Marsden: The ability of visual and auditory cues to overcome the akinesia in Parkinson's disease is a striking clinical phenomenon. One interpretation is that there are two methods of accessing motor pathways: one through the basal ganglia, the other via a direct corticocortical loop, which may have only small projections albeit very important and very fast. Everyday, automatic movements that rely on the basal ganglia to set up sequences of movement may be impaired in akinesia. But if you use a corticocortical direct pathway for sudden non-automatic movements you might bypass everything.

Akinesia is a fundamental abnormality of all basal ganglia disease. Professor Freund has shown slowness of finger movements in Huntington's chorea, and we too have found abnormalities of sequential movements in this illness. So although Huntington's chorea is classified as a hyperkinetic disorder, I think that it has the same fundamental akinesia that is evident in Parkinson's disease, on top of which is grafted chorea. The chorea may depend on the role of the subthalamic nucleus, which gates the output of the putamen–globus pallidus motor loop. This might explain how you can get excessive movement (chorea) and bradykinesia at the same time.

Deecke: One should consider which movement best discriminates between normal humans and those with Parkinson's disease. In one experiment, normal subjects had to grasp a weight from the floor, make a few steps and put the weight on a high shelf. Optimally the movement produces a bell-shaped velocity curve (Bizzi & Abend 1983). Although there are many components of the movement—bending, reaching down, grasping, getting up, reaching up, etc.— these components are normally so well arranged that the object makes an ideal flying curve. I think movements like this may be suitable ones for investigation in Parkinson's disease or other basal ganglia diseases.

Marsden: Although the final output is a relatively smooth trajectory in which the weight is lifted onto the shelf, it involves at least four separate motor programmes which have to be welded together. In Parkinson's disease, instead of a smooth continuum it becomes fragmented into separate motor programmes.

As well as the ways of stimulating patients with Parkinson's disease to move, the other fascination for clinicians is how patients freeze in the course of movement. I think that is because they cannot run their motor programmes.

Freund: What disturbs many patients is that simple automatic movements related to the trunk are difficult; for example, they cannot turn over in bed. However, a few of my patients are artists and they can still perform their skilful activity. Could you comment on the notion that automatic movements are more affected than more sophisticated or voluntary motor acts?

Marsden: That varies tremendously between patients and with the stage of illness at which you meet them. Some patients can still paint and type but feel unstable and have difficulty turning over in bed: others cannot write clearly. The question is, why do some patients have axial problems and others distal limb problems? One hypothesis is that selective nigral damage is focused on different parts of the putamen–globus pallidus motor loop. There is a somato-topy of single-unit recordings in the globus pallidus. I like the idea of subdi-vided parallel loops in the basal ganglia, provided that they talk to each other at some point.

Rizzolatti: It may be that supplementary motor area and various premotor areas issue sequential commands to basal ganglia but, since the basal ganglia are slow in computing the movement parameters in Parkinson's disease, the second command in a sequence is not processed because the basal ganglia machinery is still computing the motor act related to the first command.

Marsden: That is a conceivable hypothesis. I favour the notion that the basal ganglia calculate the 'matrix' or requirements for the second movement based on the first. If you looked at basal ganglia unit discharges in a two-movement task and correlated the discharge frequency with the parameters of the second movement, not with those of the first, you might get the right answer.

Passingham: It might not be just the intensity. With our sequence task the monkeys were not doing the movements with the wrong force intensity—they were making the wrong movement.

Marsden: That is not so for patients with Parkinson's disease, nor in our patient with a lesion in the supplementary motor area.

Strick: Are any of the other disorders of movement, like the rigidity and tremor, partially mediated by an intact SMA in patients with Parkinson's disease?

Marsden: Possibly the rigidity in Parkinson's disease is related to exagger-ated long latency stretch reflexes. The gain of the long latency reflex passing through the cortex, irrespective of the route whereby it reaches the cortex, may be modulated by supplementary motor area. Professor Wiesendanger some years ago stimulated the SMA and looked at long latency stretch reflexes. He demonstrated an effect of the SMA on the gain of this stretch reflex.

Thach: Before L-dopa was available the treatment for Parkinson's disease was thalamic surgery, which was said to improve the tremor and the rigidity but sometimes make the akinesia worse. Would you agree that that kind of surgery should make the akinesia very much worse?

Marsden: No, because the optimum site of the lesion for stereotactic operations to eliminate tremor is not in the outflow pathway of the globus pallidus, but in ventralis intermedius. This is the proprioreceptive thalamic relay. Tremor seems to be related to spontaneous bursts of cells in ventralis intermedius, perhaps as a result of deafferentation. It might eliminate rigidity by interfering with a putative proprioreceptive reflex pathway of long latency passing to the cortex via the thalamus.

Jones: I have looked at a number of lesions in this general territory and I think the area damaged is usually much larger than the surgeons claim. The most effective lesions seem to be those that are more ventrally placed. The critical point for damage may not be the ventralis intermedius but the fibres entering it from below, probably with a substantial cerebellar deafferentation of the thalamus.

Marsden: For some stereotactic surgeons, for instance A. Struppler in Munich, the preferred target site is in this subthalamic zone.

Deecke: We should also consider differential access to the motor system. Patients with Parkinson's disease have problems with voluntary access. This is obvious when they try to stand up or turn around. However, when patients are stimulated by visual targets they move more easily. The initial experiments on parkinsonian patients were always of the second type (reaction time experiments), so your experiments using self-initiation of movement are very relevant. Patients with Parkinson's disease, who are unable to get up from a chair, can still catch a ball thrown to them and, if they miss, they can reach after the ball in an appropriate manner quite easily. There are several examples of parkinsonian patients who play football, or ski or drive a car where they have access to the motor system via external stimuli—that is, they react better than they act (cf. Deecke 1985).

Marsden: It all comes back to this same issue of self-initiated rather than externally stimulated movement.

Calne: There is some difficulty in defining externally initiated movement. A stripe on the floor is a visual stimulus that may be used as a cue for stepping, but in itself it is not necessarily associated with movement. There must be some linkage between the cueing stimulus and the motivation for movement. There is no automatic programme such that whenever a ball passes, you try to catch it. There must be the same motivational component to execute the movement for a stripe on floor, or a passing ball.

Deecke: But lines can have an opposite effect. They can act as thresholds, and patients with Parkinson's disease have trouble passing thresholds. One patient was trying to cross the tram lines in Vienna and he froze in the middle of the street. A policeman reproved him but this did not help. Then the tram came and the emotional stimulus of this danger overcame the barrier and he was able to run across the street. He was nearly fined, because the policeman thought he was malingering.

Marsden: How long was Parkinson's disease thought to be a psychiatric illness before the pathology was discovered?

Deecke: Since the time of Dr James Parkinson!

Kuypers: I wonder whether the diffuse descending noradrenergic and serotonergic systems, which increase the responsiveness of the spinal motor neuronal assembly, play an important role in the diseases you described? These systems seem to be very much under limbic control. We have heard several times that a strong emotional stimulus is sufficient to initiate movements. These diffuse systems may therefore play a role in defects that are regarded as being related to higher brain areas but may actually reflect trouble in the spinal cord.

Marsden: The emotional/limbic effects may be an important component but they do not entirely explain the phenomenology of the visual requirement in Parkinson's disease. Experiments in both humans and animals have shown that, given visual information in tracking tasks or handwriting, patients with Parkinson's disease can perform reasonably well. If parts of the visual information are removed, the performance collapses. Patients asked to track patterns drawn on the back of a plexiglass screen can track a very complicated pattern. They can learn that pattern and repeat it perfectly well. If you remove little bits of the pattern, patients can no longer repeat the test, even though they know what the pattern is. In a visually controlled tracking task in monkeys there was virtually no difference from normal behaviour after cooling the globus pallidus, but when elements of the visual control of the tracking task were removed the monkeys were unable to move at all.

Passingham: Doesn't this suggest that your account of what the SMA does might be correct—that is, it is involved in one movement instructing another? Then the reason why these patients can do visually guided tasks is because the SMA is not concerned with these tasks. Other mechanisms could be relatively intact in those patients, such as cerebellar mechanisms influencing the motor cortex, or basal ganglia mechanisms influencing premotor cortex.

Marsden: The crucial question becomes the extent to which the basal ganglia project to the part of premotor cortex that receives a visual input.

References

Bizzi E, Abend W 1983 Posture control and trajectory formation in single- and multi-joint arm movements. In: Desmedt RE (ed) Motor control mechanism in health and disease. Raven Press, New York (Adv Neurol vol 39) p 31–45

Deecke L 1985 Cerebral potentials related to voluntary actions: Parkinsonian and normal subjects. In: Delwaide PJ, Agnoli A (eds) Clinical neurophysiology in Parkinsonism. Amsterdam, Elsevier (Restorative Neurol vol 2) p 91–105

Final general discussion

Wiesendanger: Could we clarify our ideas on the extent to which the basal ganglia are connected to the cortex outside the supplementary motor area, particularly to other areas of the frontal cortex? The SMA is quite small and it seems evident from anatomical work (cf. Alexander et al 1986) that the SMA is not the sole recipient of basal ganglia outflow.

Strick: In that review we emphasized that the basal ganglia participate in multiple loops with the cerebral cortex. Only one of these loops, a skeletomotor loop, is focused on the SMA. Others appear to feed back on the frontal eye fields and several additional regions of cortex in the frontal lobe. I find it very interesting that Professor Marsden has found significant similarities between the movement disorders in Parkinson's disease and those observed after damage to the SMA.

Goldman-Rakic: I agree, but we find that substantia nigra, at least, projects very densely on the paralamellar portion of mediodorsal nucleus (MD) (Ilinsky et al 1985). An injection that shows a dense projection to this portion of MD also gives a patchy and less dense projection to the parvocellular and magnocellular portions. The substantia nigra must therefore be added to the areas that have access to the prefrontal cortex.

The parallelism in the descending projections is impressive. Almost the entire cerebral cortex seems to project on the basal ganglia and the prefrontal cortex projects on at least a third of it, from the head of the nucleus in the frontal lobe all the way to the tail in the temporal lobe. The question of whether the descending projections are organized strictly in parallel or whether there is some divergence has not been settled. I feel that there is some divergence and some parallelism, not one or the other.

Professor Marsden, your behavioural results were very elegant. Is the nature of the prefrontal contribution to basal ganglia function known?

Marsden: I don't think we can begin to answer that from human experience. There is some evidence from humans with frontal lobe lesions, but to what extent their deficits are due to failure of frontal lobe input into basal ganglia is unknown. Planning seems to be impossible for patients with frontal lobe damage. They can carry out many everyday activities but if they have to lay the dinner table for a party, for example, they can't manage it.

Calne: Is that because they can't plan or because they can't be bothered?

Goldman-Rakic: The patients with Parkinson's disease, at least in the early stages, showed no delays in initiating movements. In those patients only the more SMA-related part of the basal ganglia may be involved. As the disease advances, perhaps damage of the portions that affect the prefrontal and other afferents causes bradyphrenia and bradykinesia.

Marsden: The neuronal system responsible for starting the sequence of motor programmes that one might call a motor plan is not necessarily the system required to execute that plan. The starting button may be something totally different from what is required for driving a car, for example.

Thach: Hikosaka & Wurtz (1983) in their work on eye movements provide a model different from yours. Their observation was that the sustained discharge of activity in substantia nigra pars reticulata seen in single-unit studies in monkeys diminished at the time, or shortly after, the eye movement was initiated. Inhibitory GABAergic neurons projected to the superior colliculus. The interpretation was that this was a tonic braking action which was turned off in order to permit the eye movement to be initiated, perhaps from colliculus. In their view, an impulse—say from frontal eye fields—could activate colliculus and turn off the basal ganglion brake on it at the same time.

Marsden: That is not necessarily different from our interpretation. The breakdown of sequential movements and the failure to link them together could well be due to incorrect formulation of the signal that allows the second movement to proceed. The burst of pallidal neurons that you might see in relation to the first movement may be the beginning of the signal which allows the final timing of the second movement.

Jones: We know that the pallidal outflow reaches the SMA and that this hard-wiring is independent of the cerebellar terminus in the cortex. I feel sure that the pallidal outflow nucleus in the thalamus also gains access to other areas of premotor cortex—areas that we generally call the rest of area 6. It is remarkable that so much anatomical work has been done on these systems, yet a gap as large as that remains.

Calne: In patients with Parkinson's disease who undergo fluctuations in response to L-dopa the most marked manifestation of the change is akinesia. As they are coming out of 'off reactions' the patients know they will be able to move before they try to move. Are there any analogies of transient changes in pyramidal function that one can compare with this, or any other clues that can be drawn from this observation?

Deecke: Maybe they make small test movements that tell them they can move.

Calne: I don't think so. The patients say it is almost a sensory experience in the limbs.

Deecke: One of our patients knew that if he took his morning tablet of L-dopa at 7.00 a.m. he would be able to move at 7.32 sharp.

Passingham: When we made anterior thalamic lesions in monkeys the animals were temporarily akinetic, which surprised us. We were even more surprised that SMA lesions do not produce akinesia; nor does a cingulate lesion that includes the lower bank of the cingulate sulcus. That made us wonder whether akinesia is the state when no premotor cortex can work. You won't see it if you only remove a single premotor area. It may simply be the state in which no instructions are getting through to the motor cortex. It is as if the whole of the premotor cortex were removed.

Wiesendanger: An alternative interpretation is that these monkeys with subcortical lesions or the patients with Parkinson's disease also suffer from a dysfunction of the direct ascending dopaminergic fibres from the ventral tegmental area, with their widespread innervation of the prefrontal cortex.

Porter: Dr Tanji, would you comment on bilateral cooling of the SMA? Your work (Tanji et al 1985) indicated that, at least in early trials, animals failed to perform a learnt movement, although they could recover from that disability.

Tanji: The animals were unable to perform a variant of the task which required them to respond properly to the upcoming sensory signal. Oddly, if we removed the restraining casts the animals still made freely initiated movements. I did not specifically try the reaction-time task in restrained or unrestrained animals.

Passingham: Both SMA and the cingulate cortex seemed to be involved in all the patients who showed akinesia and an infarct of the medial wall.

Thach: Going back to loops again, what are thought to be the brainstem targets of pallidal output of substantia nigra pars reticulata? How significant are these in relation to other thalamic targets?

Kuypers: In the rat the fibres from the pars reticulata of the substantia nigra to the superior colliculus give rise to numerous collaterals to the thalamus. We assumed that this thalamic projection was related to eye movements (Bentivoglio et al 1979). From what Patricia Goldman-Rakic said, I conclude that the collaterals from the reticulata to the thalamus in monkey are actually distributed to those thalamic areas which lead to the area of the frontal eye field that in turn projects back to the superior colliculus. Thus, the thalamic collaterals of the nigrocollicular fibres close a cortical circuit leading back to the superior colliculus.

Armstrong: Although the connections from the basal ganglia to the pedunculopontine nucleus may not be enormous, that area is more or less co-extensive with the mesencephalic locomotor region, where microstimulation can trigger locomotor sequences very easily in decerebrate animals (see Armstrong 1986, Garcia-Rill 1986). As Garcia-Rill has suggested, there may be some tie-up between that descending system and the inability of patients with basal ganglia disorders to initiate locomotion properly.

Goldman-Rakic: There might be another mechanism in addition to those mentioned for some sort of integration in the neostriatum. In double-labelling experiments we injected the temporal cortex with one tracer and the prefrontal with another, injecting areas that are cortically interconnected (Solomon & Goldman-Rakic 1985). These two areas project to the same general area of the basal ganglia but they interdigitate their terminal distributions. Small 500 µm wide clusters of cells in the parietal cortex are interlaced in a mosaic fashion with similar sized territories of the prefrontal projections. It is even possible that prefrontal and parietal afferents might terminate on the same dendrites. That is something neuroanatomists could look at in the future. It would be a different kind of convergence.

Marsden: We have heard almost no discussion of the microanatomy of the premotor cortex, the supplementary motor cortex or the motor cortex itself. Do we know how the supplementary motor area addresses the motor cortex in terms of the microanatomy?

Jones: The same principles of connectivity and cellular organization are probably operating but we don't know the fine details. The outflow layers of the SMA and the other premotor areas are probably primarily the upper layers, II and III, but we cannot rule out contributions from deeper layers as well. There is clear evidence in a number of cortical areas of substantial contributions to these pathways, particularly from layer VI. In other interconnected cortical areas the connection between two areas in one direction may well emanate from one layer and the return connection from another layer. I don't think this has been firmly established in the area we are discussing.

The possibilities for connection between the input pathway and the recipient cells in, say, area 4 have not been well looked at. There is evidence that in rodents there are inputs not simply to the interneurons of the motor cortex but also to particular pyramidal tract neurons. The population of non-pyramidal neurons and the populations of pyramidal neurons are the same in general as those described in visual and somatosensory cortex, but this aspect has not been much studied in the motor cortex.

Porter: Yet the influence of a given incoming fibre from another area of cortex on that receiving zone could be quite different, depending on whether predominantly inhibitory neurons or predominantly output cells were activated by that input.

Jones: We would like to know this. The only quantitative data come from the work of E.L. White on the somatosensory cortex of mice. This is primarily in relation to thalamic inputs but he has data on corticocortical inputs. A particular population of output neurons may receive radically different percentages of thalamic synapses, ranging from about 27% for corticothalamic neurons to close to 3% for corticostriatal neurons. These observations are fundamentally important, but despite much work of this kind, and the work on single cells that has been done on the visual cortex, there are no comparable data in other areas.

Deecke: One SMA sends output fibres to the motor cortices on either side. Is this projection as strong on the ipsilateral side as it is on the contralateral side? If so, one must be careful in evaluating lesions, because if the lesion also damages the corpus callosum, this is a different story.

Strick: The ipsilateral projection is more substantial than the contralateral one. The SMA also projects bilaterally to the spinal cord and contributes to the contralateral and ipsilateral corticospinal tracts in the dorsolateral funiculus.

Wiesendanger: Is that via the corpus callosum?

Strick: No, the cortical connections are via the corpus callosum; the spinal connections are not.

Fetz: The prevailing assumption seems to be that different motor functions can be ascribed to different cortical regions. While cortical areas are undoubtedly specialized, the evidence from single-unit recordings suggests that sets of cells with the same response properties are distributed over many regions. For example, cells related to motor 'set', and cells responsive to active and passive limb movements, even to the sight of approaching objects, are encountered in quite different cortical fields. This suggests that cells with common response properties may be involved in similar functions, and consequently each cortical region is involved in multiple functions.

The most extreme example of a functional dichotomy is the notion that precentral and postcentral cortex subserve exclusively motor and somatosensory function. If this dichotomy is considered to be absolute, rather than relative, identical response properties of single units must be interpreted in totally different functional terms. While the passive responses of postcentral cells are interpreted as subserving somatic sensation, the equally clear passive responses of precentral cells are considered to subserve unconscious reflex functions. Similarly, the early responses of precentral cells preceding active limb movement are thought to be involved in generating the movement, while identical early responses in postcentral cells are thought to subserve some sensory 'corollary discharge'. The rationale for these diverse interpretations rests largely on the different effects of cortical stimulation. Yet here the same double standard is applied to the experimental evidence. The somatic sensations evoked by stimulating precentral cortex in conscious humans are ascribed to spread of activity to postcentral sites. The movements evoked by stimulating postcentral cortex are similarly ascribed to precentral mediation, and reports that such movements can be evoked after ablation of precentral cortex are taken as evidence that the lesions were incomplete.

Thus, the notion that cortical functions are segregated into different cortical areas can be preserved only by imposing different interpretations on identical experimental evidence! A plausible alternative is to consider the similar response properties of cells in different cortical regions as evidence that they are performing similar functions; the substrate for these functions is then correspondingly distributed. To the extent that a given cortical region contains diverse cell types, it would be involved in correspondingly diverse functions. This view provides a basis for distributed interactions between these functional sets of cells and helps to explain the recovery of function after lesions.

Jones: What is the role of the postcentral gyrus in motor control, and what is the role of the corticospinal pathways emanating from this area or from any other areas posterior to the central sulcus? There is a general assumption, which I do not believe is valid, that corticospinal outflows from different areas are equivalent to each other. One has only to consider that the corticospinal neurons of the postcentral gyrus terminate high in the dorsal horn, including the substantia gelatinosa, to see that they are very unlikely to play a direct role in movement control other than in sensory tracking or feedback of some kind. One does not often hear this expressed: is that because we have no good ideas about it?

Kuypers: That pattern is familiar to neuroanatomists: postcentral gyrus projects to dorsal horn, motor cortex projects to motor neurons and to propriospinal neurons (Coulter & Jones 1977, Kuypers 1960).

Cheney: Our recent stimulation experiments in awake monkeys support the conclusion suggested by the anatomy that postcentral cortical areas are unlikely to exert any direct control over motor neurons. We applied microstimuli to precentral and postcentral areas during movement and computed averages of muscle activity from those stimuli. Effects elicited from postcentral areas differ dramatically from those elicited from precentral cortex. Averages of rectified EMG activity triggered from individual stimuli rarely showed any effect for sites in postcentral cortex. Trains of stimuli elicited some effects from postcentral cortex but the majority of these consisted of weak suppression. So again there is a sharp contrast between the motor effects that can be elicited from precentral and postcentral sites. Our results suggest that the linkages available to postcentral cortical areas for influencing muscle activity are relatively indirect and weak.

Tanji: Are those data from area 3b, 1 or 2? What about area 3a, which may be a specialized area?

Cheney: We have stimulated sites in all cytoarchitectonic areas of the first somatic sensory area, including area 3a, with similar results. In addition to area 3a, area 2 is of particular interest since it projects heavily to area 4 and, hence, might be linked tightly with primary motor cortex corticospinal output to motor neurons. Surprisingly, we found no clear excitatory effects on average muscle activity from area 2, even at sites where cells had properties similar to those of motor cortex cells and using trains of 10 stimuli at intensities up to 40 and 60 μA. Therefore, it seems quite unlikely that these postcentral sites relay directly with corticospinal neurons in the primary motor cortex; neither are they likely to be the origin of corticomotoneuronal cells.

Kalaska: That is an important observation; these corticospinal axons arising from motor, premotor and postcentral cortex may be parallel in the most macroscopic anatomical sense but there is no reason to assume that they are functionally equivalent. What sorts of signals these various corticospinal axons transmit to the cord and what role these signals play in cord function are questions that await further investigation.

Kuypers: During sleep is there still cellular activity similar to that seen in alert monkeys?

Porter: Ed Evarts (1964) demonstrated that pyramidal tract neurons in area 4 of the cerebral cortex of the monkey showed an increase in activity during sleep. The rates of discharge were higher during sleeping than during wakefulness. The only thing that had to be excluded was the phasic activity of those cells which accompanied movement of the animal.

Thach: It was not slow wave sleep but rapid eye movement (REM) sleep in which the discharge of motor cortex neurons was more intense than during waking, yet with the conspicuous absence of movements other than eye movements.

Kuypers: This point is worth emphasizing because we are probably dealing with separate systems which we have not discussed at all, but which determine whether movements will occur.

Marsden: Hess et al (1987) have shown that the human motor cortex is inexcitable to magnetic stimulation during rapid eye movement sleep at a time when patients with involuntary movement disorders could exhibit tics, chorea and a variety of other phenomena, suggesting that there are indeed alternative motor pathways for some of these dyskinesias.

Kalaska: Although it is true that any individual neuron may show phasic discharge during REM sleep, it is not known whether there is synchronicity in this discharge across populations any larger than the cell's nearest neighbours. What you may see is a strong discharge in single neurons but desynchronization of the activity of the total population. For any meaningful movement to occur, there must be both activation of single neurons and a meaningful pattern of activity changes across the relevant neuronal population. This latter requirement may not be met during REM sleep. Of course, this cannot be the sole factor involved, since the activation of a small local population of motor cortex cells by intracortical microstimulation will evoke twitch-like movements. This suggests that there is another system somewhere that can modify or even block the access of this enhanced cortical output to the spinal motor apparatus during REM sleep.

This dissociation is also seen in the instructed-delay task used by Drs Tanji, Evarts, Wise and others. During the delay period in these tasks, when the monkey knows what movement to make but must wait for a second signal before he can perform it, there is considerable activity in premotor and supplementary motor cortex, and even some in the motor cortex, if I am not mistaken. Yet there is no measurable change in muscle activity despite this increase in cortical activity. Once again, this suggests that, provided some of this cortical activity is being relayed down the corticospinal tract and would under normal conditions result in a movement, some other system must be preventing movement during the delay period.

Kuypers: The descending systems are derived from the noradrenergic coeruleus and subcoeruleus nuclei and from the serotonergic medullary (mid-line) raphe nuclei. Neurons in these areas distribute fibres throughout the length of the spinal cord, and these fibres distribute collaterals to the spinal grey matter along their trajectory. Some of the fibres which descend mainly through the dorsolateral funiculus are distributed to the dorsal horn, while the others which descend through the ventral and ventrolateral funiculi distribute collaterals to the intermediate zone and the motor neuronal cell groups. The cells of origin of these pathways receive fibres especially from limbic areas, such as amygdala and hypothalamus. The activity of some of these neurons is strongly increased when novel stimuli are presented, and their activity seems to go up and down with wakefulness and sleep. Further, the transmitters involved apparently increase the responsiveness of motor neurons to other stimuli. In view of these findings, I expect these diffuse systems to determine whether other descending pathways are able to elicit movements. It is an aspect of motor control which is worth considering (see Kuypers 1985).

Lemon: When a monkey is becoming drowsy the discharges from a pyramid-al tract neuron are preceded and succeeded by long interspike intervals. Recently (Lemon & Mantel 1985) we looked at the structure of the spike change during voluntary movement. If we look simply at the individual spikes which are preceded and succeeded by long periods of silence in that particular neuron the individual events produce quite powerful effects on the muscle. Looking at the spike train alone doesn't tell you whether the movement will occur. This suggests that other influences must exist to allow impulses from the corticospinal neuron to be expressed in movement.

Porter: The challenge there is for the physiologists to discover what the other influences are, where they are and how they are activated by the outflow from the cerebral cortex.

References

Alexander GE, DeLong MR, Strick PL 1986 Parallel organization of functionally segregated circuits linking basal ganglia and cortex. Annu Rev Neurosci 9:357–381

Armstrong DM 1986 Supraspinal contributions to the initiation and control of locomotion in the cat. Prog Neurobiol 26:273–361

Bentivoglio M, van der Kooy K, Kuypers HG 1979 The organization of the efferent projections of the substantia nigra in the rat. A retrograde fluorescent double labeling study. Brain Res 174:1–17

Coulter JD, Jones EG 1977 Differential distribution of corticospinal projections from individual cytoarchitectonic fields in the monkey. Brain Res 129:335–340

Evarts EV 1964 Temporal patterns of discharge of pyramidal tract neurons during sleep and waking in the monkey. J Neurophysiol 27:152–171

Garcia-Rill E 1986 The basal ganglia and the locomotor regions. Brain Res Rev 11:47–63

Hess CW, Mills KR, Murray NMF, Schriefer T 1987 Magnetic stimulation of the human brain during natural sleep. J Physiol (Lond), in press

Hikosaka O, Wurtz RH 1983 Visual and oculomotor functions of monkey substantia nigra pars reticulata. I. Relation of visual and auditory responses to saccades. J Neurophysiol 49:1230–1253

Ilinsky IA, Jouandet ML, Goldman-Rakic PS 1985 Organization of the nigrothalamo-cortical system in the rhesus monkey. J Comp Neurol 236:315–330

Kuypers HGJM 1960 Central cortical projections to motor and somato-sensory cell groups. An experimental study in the Rhesus monkey. Brain 83:161–184

Kuypers HGJM 1985 In: Swash M, Kennard C (eds) Scientific basis of clinical neurology. Churchill Livingstone, Edinburgh, p 3–18

Lemon RN, Mantel GWH 1985 The impact of differences in cortico-motor (CM) neurone firing frequency upon hand muscles in the conscious monkey. J Physiol (Lond) 372:15P

Selemon LD, Goldman-Rakic PS 1985 Longitudinal topography and interdigitation of corticostriatal projections in the rhesus monkey. J Neurosci 5:776–794

Tanji J, Kurata K, Okano K 1985 The effect of cooling of the supplementary motor cortex and adjacent cortical areas. Exp Brain Res 60:423–426

Chairman's closing remarks

R. Porter

The John Curtin School of Medical Research, The Australian National University, GPO Box 334, Canberra City, ACT 2601, Australia

1987 Motor areas of the cerebral cortex. Wiley, Chichester (Ciba Foundation Symposium 132) p 310–312

We have all benefited from the opportunity to hear and comment on what our colleagues have had to say at this symposium. It is difficult to summarize the territory we have covered in the last few days, but some issues have been raised that are worth recording for the future.

Charles Phillips started us off where we have now finished, on the electrical stimulation of the cerebral cortex and the observation of motor responses. As Hans Kuypers has pointed out, we may still have a lot to learn about the relationship between the two and about the multiplicity of the pathways and systems that may be activated by such a complex event as an electrical stimulus to the cerebral cortex. That comment achieves greater meaning now that these methods are being used in studies of motor responses and motor pathways in humans, either in the cruder form of electrical shocks through the head or in what appears to be a modified form, perhaps activating different systems or the same system in different ways, using a magnetic pulse to activate those structures within the head.

Another major element of our discussions has concerned deficits of movement performance produced as a result of brain lesions, either those purposely inflicted by the experimentalists or those resulting from disease or damage to the brain. These deficits can provide important information about the essential elements of movement which require those parts of the central nervous system to be intact. Most people would agree that the precentral motor cortex has within it a structural component which is essential for the fine control of distally acting muscles, and that, in the absence of function in precentral motor cortex, an inability to fractionate the use of muscles acting about the digits is a common phenomenon.

Although our attention has recently been drawn to the role of the postcentral cortex in relation to the performance of movement, it seems to be clear—and I think it was clear to Sherrington at the turn of the century—that purposeful lesions in the postcentral cortex might appear to give an animal a useless limb. That uselessness, however, followed from the fact that the animal had no knowledge of the existence of its limb and therefore neglected it, yet movement functions in that limb could be shown to be intact. As one goes further back into the parietal cortex it seems that disorganization of movement performance may be demonstrated after lesions in the parietal lobe, and the term 'apraxia' has been used in a number of our discussions.

As a result of these sorts of studies our attention has been focused on the separate global functions that may be associated with a number of other regions of cortex, such as the premotor, supplementary motor and prefrontal cortex. In studies on monkeys it appears that intactness of the arcuate premotor cortex is important if animals are to re-learn the performance of actions based on visual cues about their external environment. In contrast, the supplementary motor area needs to be intact if monkeys are to re-learn movements requiring the use of information about proprioceptive aspects of the movement that have been internalized. Our attention has been drawn to the extensive literature relating lesions in the prefrontal areas of monkeys to a deficit in delayed responding, whether that responding is carried out with the hand or with the eyes.

Some of these observations may have their counterparts in humans, but the discussions have made it clear that there are areas of overlap in these observations and also that areas of disagreement exist. Perhaps we need to give more thought to the reasons for these possible discrepancies. Disease processes may not always respect cytoarchitectonic boundaries, and may even fail to respect the boundary between grey and white matter, so that disconnections may occur for areas of cortex remote from those which appear to be the site of the lesion involving the cerebral cortex. Further, although newer methods of studying the metabolism, blood flow, and electrical and magnetic field potentials of the human brain have allowed dramatic improvements in both temporal and spatial resolution, the capacity of these methods in human studies is limited by the requirement, in some cases, to study averages over a number of repeated performances which smooth out some of the most interesting aspects related to motor performance. Their capability is also limited even when the time-scale for metabolic studies is reduced to 60s or thereabouts. In that time, repetitive events in many parallel pathways could have circulated in the brain structures and gone around some loops several times.

Lesion studies have in the past allowed anatomical connections to be explored. Several participants referred to the way in which refinements in our understanding of those anatomical connections have been generated by newer tracing methods. To some degree that anatomical information provides a substrate which helps to explain the behaviour with which brain regions are associated. But I submit that a too simplistic view of the relationship between such regional anatomy and brain regional function could get us into a great deal of trouble, in that we would fail to understand the subtleties of the activities which may be generated within those brain regions.

Further, the tracer studies give us essentially regional information. Much more detailed descriptions of cell-to-cell connectivity are required if we are to understand the functions subserved by the connections between one part of the brain and another. We need to understand what impact the incoming fibres have on which particular cells within those regions. I imagine that the anatomists will have a job to do for long into the future in helping to unravel those problems.

We have not talked much about the detail of the transmitter activity that enables a cell in one part of the brain to communicate with another. Ted Jones referred to the transmitters that may operate in some of the cells within a region of the cerebral cortex, but as yet we know little about the interactions. Hans Kuypers reminded us that sometimes the soup in the spinal cord can be as important as the impulses that travel down corticospinal fibres into the spinal cord. That reminded me of the observation that in a spinal preparation the injection into the cord itself, or into the blood supply of the cord, of a substance like serotonin can produce locomotor activity in the spinal cord which otherwise cannot be revealed.

The recording of single neurons also has a number of limitations that have been referred to frequently in these discussions. Those limitations could be partially overcome if the connections of the cell from which the recordings have been made could be established with some degree of certainty.

In spite of all of those problems, this symposium has shown that relevant questions can be asked about the behaviour of cells in different parts of the brain, but those questions achieve their relevance because of knowledge that has been obtained about anatomical connectivity or about behavioural associations from lesion or blood-flow studies, or from metabolic studies or global electroencephalography. My view is that we can have some optimism in continuing our investigations. Some areas may be more fraught with difficulties than others in terms of their interpretations. But I identify enough security in the observations presented to feel that the pursuit of all these methods, and future symposia which attempt to bring them together, are likely to lead us to a much better understanding of how the separable motor areas of the cerebral cortex interact and cooperate in controlling movement in primates.

Index of contributors

Thach, W.T., 18, 56, 80, 112, 114, 123,
    132, 135, 170, 183, 198, **201**, 215, 216,
    217, 218, 219, 227, 249, 267, 296, 297,
    298, 302, 303, 307

Wiesendanger, M., **40**, 53, 54, 55, 56,

57, 94, 149, 168, 169, 245, 301, 303,
    305
*Wiesendanger, R., **40**
Wu Chien-Ping, 76, 133, 247

Xi Ming-Chu, 37, 228, 229

Subject index